D1757302

BISHOP BURTON LRC
WITHDRAWN

ACCESSION No. T049421

CLASS No. 636·089 Ref

Alternative Health Practices for Livestock

Edited by

Thomas F. Morris and Michael T. Keilty

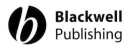

Tom Morris is an associate professor and extension agronomist, Department of Plant Science, University of Connecticut, Storrs, CT. He is currently the coordinator for the Professional Development Program, Northeast Sustainable Agriculture Research and Education (SARE) program.

Michael T. Keilty has been the owner of Maple Spring Farms located in Morris, CT, since 1974, specializing in diversified livestock and plant production. He is currently a sustainable agriculture research associate, Department of Plant Science, University of Connecticut, Storrs, CT.

© 2006 Blackwell Publishing
All rights reserved

Blackwell Publishing Professional
2121 State Avenue, Ames, Iowa 50014, USA
   Orders: 1-800-862-6657
   Office: 1-515-292-0140
   Fax: 1-515-292-3348
   Web site: www.blackwellprofessional.com
Blackwell Publishing Ltd
9600 Garsington Road, Oxford OX4 2DQ, UK
   Tel.: +44 (0)1865 776868
Blackwell Publishing Asia
550 Swanston Street, Carlton, Victoria 3053, Australia
   Tel.: +61 (0)3 8359 1011

Authorization to photocopy items for internal or personal use, or the internal or personal use of specific clients, is granted by Blackwell Publishing, provided that the base fee of $.10 per copy is paid directly to the Copyright Clearance Center, 222 Rosewood Drive, Danvers, MA 01923. For those organizations that have been granted a photocopy license by CCC, a separate system of payments has been arranged. The fee codes for users of the Transactional Reporting Service are ISBN-13: 978-0-8138-1764-4; ISBN-10: 0-8138-1764-1/2005 $.10.

This book is the result of a conference funded by the USDA Northeast Sustainable Agriculture Research and Education (SARE) program.

First edition, 2006

   Library of Congress Cataloging-in-Publication Data

Morris, Thomas F.
  Alternative health practices for livestock / Thomas F.
Morris and Michael T. Keilty.—1st ed.
    p. cm.
  ISBN-13: 978-0-8138-1764-4 (alk. paper)
  ISBN-10: 0-8138-1764-1 (alk. paper)
  1. Alternative veterinary medicine.   2. Livestock—
Diseases—Alternative treatment.   3. Livestock—Health.
I. Keilty, Michael T.   II. Title.
SF745.5M67 2006
636.089′55—dc22   2005024520

The last digit is the print number: 9 8 7 6 5 4 3 2 1

Contents

Contributors

Sheila M. Andrew PhD   Associate Professor and Extension Dairy Specialist, Department of Animal Science, University of Connecticut, 3636 Horsebarn Road Ext., Storrs, CT 06269

Robin R. Rastani PhD   Research Associate, Department of Dairy Science, University of Wisconsin-Madison

Mark J. S. Miller PhD   Center of Cardiovascular Sciences, MC8, Albany Medical College, 47 New Scotland Avenue, Albany, NY 12208

Palmer J. Holden PhD   Professor of Animal Science and Extension Equine Specialist, Iowa State University, 109 Kildee Hall, Ames, IA 50011-3150

Lisa McCrory   NOFA-VT Dairy and Livestock Advisor, PO Box 697, Richmond, VT 05477

John Barlow   DVM Department of Animal Science, University of Vermont, Terrill Hall, Burlington, VT 05405

Cindy Engel BSc, PhD   Clover Forge Farm, Cratfield Road, Huntingfield, Halesworth, Suffolk IP190QB

R.W. Godfrey PhD   Associate Professor – Animal Science, Agricultural Experiment Station, University of Virgin Islands, RR 2 Box 10,000, Kingshill, St. Croix USVI 00850

R. E. Dodson   Assistant Director, Agricultural Experiment Station, University of Virgin Islands, RR 2 Box. 10,000, Kingshill, St. Croix USVI 00850

Jennifer K. Ketzis   R&D Manager, BV Natural Medicinal Products, Novartis Animal Health, Post Office Box CH-4002, Basel, Switzerland

Jerry Brunetti   c/o Agri-Dynamics, PO Box 735, Easton, PA 18044

Hubert J. Karreman VMD   Penn Dutch Cow Care, 1272 Mt. Pleasant Road, Quarryville, PA 17566

Joyce C. Harmon DVM MRCVS   Harmany Equine Clinic, Ltd., PO Box 488, Washington, VA 22747

Stephen J. DeVincent DVM, MA   Director of Ecology Program, APUA, 76 Kneeland Street, Boston, MA 02111

Alan H. Fredeen PhD   Professor, Haley Institute of Animal Science and Aquaculture, Nova Scotia Agricultural College, Box 550, Truro, NSS Canada B2N5E3

Randy Kidd DVM PhD   16879 46th Street, McLouth, KS 666054

Gary L. Valen   Director of Operations, Glynwood Center, Box 157, Cold Spring, NY 10516

Introduction

Thomas F. Morris

Producing nutritious and tasty food in a plentiful manner that does not pollute planet Earth and minimizes the potential long-term degradation of natural resources, including antibiotics, should be the goal of all societies. Current methods of food production do not meet all of these goals. This book is our small effort to provide information about methods of livestock production that meet these goals better.

The idea that current methods of food production are not sustainable in the long term is a controversial topic. There are two main views on this topic. The conventional view is the amount of food needed by a rapidly increasing world population can only be produced using every technique and chemical available to farmers, and the environmental effects of producing food using conventional methods are minimal (Avery, 2000). Some have detailed problems with our current methods of food production (Manning, 2004, 2001), and some have detailed problems with past uses of the land for food production (Diamond, 2004). We agree more with the views held by authors Diamond and Manning, and many of the authors in this book also hold similar views, but Avery's arguments for the efficiency and abundance of food produced using current methods are noteworthy. We hope this book will stimulate discussion about our current methods of livestock production, and provide information that will advance a form of livestock production that meets the long- and short-term goals of human food production.

We have divided the book into four sections. The first section is the largest and contains a diverse set of ideas about the science of alternative health care practices for livestock. There has been little applied research to rigorously evaluate alternative therapies. We report the results of three experiments in Chapters 1, 3, and 4. A homeopathic treatment for mastitis was tested by Andrew and Rastani, a homeopathic nosode treatment for calf scours and mastitis was tested by McCrory and Barlow, and the ability of various herbal remedies to replace antibiotics was tested by Holden. None of the experiments had conclusive results, but all showed that the treatments had some effect, and further study is warranted. Obtaining conclusive results when testing alternative therapies can be problematic due to many factors. McCrory and Barlow use their experimental design and results to discuss the factors every researcher has to solve if they plan to rigorously evaluate alternative therapies.

Biochemical science is the topic of Miller's chapter (Chapter 2) on the mode of action of two plants from the Amazon used for livestock and human therapies. Reading this chapter is challenging unless you have some knowledge of biochemistry, but we think the chapter is one of the most important in the book because biochemical descriptions of modes of actions of medicinal plants are urgently needed to understand which plants are effective therapies.

The chapters by Engel (Chapter 5), Godfrey and Dodson (Chapter 6), and Ketzis (Chapter 7) describe the current scientific literature for alternative therapies on three important topics: livestock self-medication, methods of controlling parasites in small ruminants, and medicinal plants for control of endo- and ecto-parasites. Engel's chapter on livestock self-medication is a thought-provoking document that reminds me of the arguments that occurred in the literature in the 1970s and 1980s about whether humans produced pheromones. Most scientists at that time did not believe humans produced pheromones, but in 1986 data were published that convinced most scientists that humans produced pheromones and that human behavior is affected by the pheromones (Preti et al., 1986). Engel's chapter has almost convinced me that livestock have unexplained abilities to find minerals deficient in their diet by seeking plants that contain higher than normal amounts of the deficient minerals.

Some of the more potent pesticides are used to control parasites in livestock. The chapter by Ketzis shows the need for more research on the mechanisms of action of medicinal plants traditionally used to treat parasites of livestock. Methods of performing the research and results of recent research on the use of medicinal plants to control parasites are also described by Ketzis. Parasites are especially troublesome for farmers in developing countries who produce food using small ruminants. The chapter by Godfrey and Dodson explains how comparatively little research has been completed on alternative methods of controlling parasites in small ruminants. The authors then provide a review of the literature for alternative control of one of the most difficult parasites to control; gastrointestinal nematode parasites. More work similar to Miller's chapter on the mode of action of Amazonian plants is needed to sort the many plants traditionally used to treat parasites in livestock.

Section 2 of this book contains three chapters written by veterinarians. These chapters contain the practitioners' view of alternative methods from the grass roots. The chapter by Brunetti (Chapter 8) has data from the author's own research about the mineral content of nontraditional forage plants, or weeds as most people call them. It would be helpful if more rigorous research was conducted on the nutritional and phytonutritional content of weeds. There are a little or no research data in scientific journals about the phytonutritional content of traditional and nontraditional livestock feed; we need more information about this topic. Research on the content of phytonutrients in plants consumed by humans is in its infancy. More programs such as the one at the University of New Hampshire's Carotenoid Project, that has the objective "to investigate ways to increase the phytonutrient content of food crops" for human consumption (UNH, 2004), are needed for livestock feed.

The chapter by Karreman (Chapter 9) is a history buff's delight. Karreman gives us a perspective on the history of livestock health care, and provides a link to today's treatments and attitudes about livestock health care. Much of the livestock in the past were draft animals such as horses. Chapter 10 by Harman is a holistic discourse on the care of horses using herbs and alternative methods. Horses are not considered livestock by the USDA, but many societies depend on horses for draft power and our society invests heavily on horses for recreation and as work animals.

Sections 3 and 4 contain two chapters each. Section 3 describes concerns of two scientists about two conventional health care therapies for livestock. DeVincent makes a strong and well-documented case for reducing the amount of antibiotics used for prophylactic purposes during livestock production, and for developing alternatives for the prophylactic use of antibiotics. This is a controversial topic. Fredeen discusses another controversial topic; the use of rBST in the dairy industry. Conclusions drawn by scientists and citizens about these types of difficult topics are usually greatly affected by whether they emphasize the ideas embodied in the "Precautionary Principle" (Precautionary Principle, 2004) or more conventional ideas about the use of scientific and technological information.

The authors in Section 4 describe ways to promote alternative methods of health care for livestock. Kidd details the steps necessary to obtain funding for research and education projects concerning alternative topics. The information is concise and valid for obtaining funding for all types of projects, not only alternative projects. Information in our final chapter by Valen provides a blueprint for promotion of foods from livestock that are grown using alternative methods. The market for meat, milk, and other livestock products grown and processed using alternative methods is small, but it is growing rapidly. The choice of consumers in the future will determine the size of this market.

We thank the authors for their energy, time, and thoughts. We hope this book proves interesting to many readers, and that we have attained our goal of providing more people with information about methods of livestock production that can enhance our planet.

Michael T. Keilty

On October 20–21 2000, The University of Connecticut College of Agriculture and Natural Resources at Storrs, Connecticut, held a conference entitled "Alternative and Herbal Livestock Health Practices, A Scientific Review of Current Knowledge." Sixty-four individuals attended the conference with numerous others requesting conference abstracts. Twelve veterinarians attended along with farmers, extension educators, and university professionals. The conference drew a wide range of participants from across the United States from Maine and Pennsylvania to Ohio, and as far as Kansas. The conference was sponsored by The Northeast Region Sustainable Agriculture Research and Education (SARE) program, and the University of Connecticut College of Agriculture and Natural Resources. Many of the attendees felt such a symposium offered a way to address the growing questions about excess antibiotic, hormone, and steroid uses, biotechnology and genetic modification, and food safety which concern the public and to which scientists, clinicians, and agricultural professionals must find answers. Additionally, many felt that there are practically no programs or texts on alternative health for large animals to be used by livestock producers, veterinarians, and extension educators. Finally, most felt the need for more work to offer validated scientific assessments of many alternative and herbal therapies that are becoming increasingly attractive to livestock producers, veterinarians, and extension educators.

Important concerns regarding food safety, particularly antibiotic and chemical residues in meat, milk, and other livestock foods, have stimulated a renewed interest in alternative methods of promoting livestock health. This parallels the resurgent interest in alternative medical practices in human health. An example is the National Institute of Health's establishment of a National Center for Complementary and Alternative Medicine. The lack of a good source-referenced compilation of alternative practices for livestock seriously limits communication among experts in alternative medicine, veterinarians, agriculture extension educators, and livestock producers.

We are what we eat, and with this in mind a new understanding of ancient and novel methods of developing alternative livestock medicine is slowly being developed as increased research funding becomes available and traditionally trained field veterinarians and farmers experiment with alternative methods. These methods include such items as holistic medicine, botanical medicine, and homeopathy. The nomenclature in alternative human and veterinary medicine is changing as practice and research move forward. Many of the older alternative methods are being used with new advances in conventional methods. This volume is not a training manual but an overview of some alternative livestock practices compiled by researchers, practicing veterinarians, and extension specialists.

Organically produced livestock are regulated under the National Organic Program (NOP). No substance, synthetic or natural, that is prohibited on the National List can be used for health care if the animal is to remain certified. Many alternative livestock health practices have been found safe and are accepted in organic production. One of the most important health practices for organic producers and others who raise livestock in nonconventional systems is access to the outdoors: shade, shelter, exercise areas, fresh air, and direct sunlight suitable to the species and its stage of development. Livestock's access to an appropriate environment is an important cultural livestock health practice. Many of the chapters in this volume combine these cultural practices with various alternative practices.

Farming has been my life's work. I was born and raised on a farm, studied agricultural education in post-secondary school, taught agriculture with an emphasis on environmental issues in secondary and post-secondary levels, and currently work in the sustainable agriculture research programs at the University of Connecticut College of Agriculture and Natural Resources. In 1974 I purchased a farm and began employing biodiversity principles in farming practices, combining livestock (sheep, cattle, and poultry), gardens (vegetables and herbs—wholesale and retail) with an emphasis on rotating all farming components, including livestock and crop production. Soon it was the farmer learning from the livestock as I observed them seeking out their own medicine through grazing and browsing on various forages that have medicinal qualities. If livestock are allowed the opportunity to forage in forests, wetlands, hedgerows, and other areas on the farm that have significant biodiversity in plants, instead of consuming the standard pasture/forage seed mixtures sold to farmers, livestock will seek their own medicine. Some of these farm areas sought by livestock may be the least important production areas, at least as we were taught to understand. Many medicinal plants with significant active properties grow in poor soils.

Livestock in confinement have no opportunity to seek out medicinal plants, as their food is brought to them, with little thought about the healing power of the plants. My hope is that this volume will help all who are nurturing, tending, learning, and caring for agricultural livestock to understand better some of the many alternative health practices currently being examined by farmers, researchers, and veterinarians.

References

Avery, D. 2000. *Saving the Planet with Pesticides and Plastic: The Environmental Triumph of High-Yield Farming*, 2nd edn. Hudson Institute, Washington, DC.

Diamond, J. 2004. *Collapse: How Societies Choose to Fail or Succeed*. Viking Books, New York, NY.

Manning, R. 2001. *Food's Frontier: The Next Green Revolution*. University of California Press, Berkeley, CA.

Manning, R. 2004. *Against the Grain: How Agriculture Has Hijacked Civilization*. North Point Press, New York, NY.

Precautionary Principle. 2004. Information from four Web sites with different views of the concept: Available at: http://www.gdrc.org/u-gov/precaution-3.html. http://www.pprinciple. net/. http://www.biotech-info.net/precautionary.html. http://www.reason.com/9904/fe.rb.precautionary.shtml. Accessed Dec. 29, 2004.

Preti, G., W.B. Cutler, A. Krieger, G.R. Huggins, C.R. Garcia, and R. Lawley. 1986. Human axillary secretions influence women's menstrual cycles: the role of donor extract from women. *Hormones Behav.* 20:463–473.

UNH, 2004. The carotenoid project. Available at: http://luteinlab.unh.edu/index.html. Accessed Dec. 29, 2004.

Section I
Science of Alternative Methods

Chapter 1
Evaluation of a Homeopathic Therapy for Subclinical Mastitis in Lactating Holstein Cows

Sheila M. Andrew and Robin R. Rastani

Introduction

The production of high-quality milk for human food consumption is a priority for the dairy industry and necessary for maintaining safety of the human food supply. The use of antibiotics for eliminating infections due to pathogens is an important component of dairy cattle management. The efficacy of antibiotics is dependent on many factors. These include the animal, the disease, the pathogen, and the environment. Although the food supply is protected by strict regulations, antibiotic residues are a risk factor associated with antibiotic therapy that can result in financial losses for dairy producers (Smucker, 1996). In addition, there is the potential for antibiotic residues in animal-based foods to have a negative impact on human health. Therefore, identifying alternative therapies that are both effective and reduce the risk of antibiotic residues in milk would be beneficial to dairy producers and consumers. In this chapter we will discuss mastitis and the conventional treatments used to eliminate the pathogens. In addition, we will discuss various alternative treatments, and we will present the results of a research study to evaluate a homeopathic treatment.

Mastitis

Mastitis is the most common disease occurring in dairy cattle and has been estimated to cost the United States dairy industry two billion dollars per year (Blosser, 1979). Mastitis can be present in either a clinical or a subclinical form. Clinical mastitis is characterized by udder inflammation, abnormal milk, increased milk somatic cell counts (SCC), and usually the presence of a pathogen in the udder. The cow may exhibit systemic effects, such as elevated body temperature and decreased feed intake, but in most cases symptoms of the disease are confined to the mammary gland. Subclinical mastitis is defined as the presence of a pathogen in the udder and elevated SCC without visual signs of the disease. Depending on the type and severity of clinical mastitis, intramammary antibiotic therapy is administered under the guidance of a valid veterinarian–client relationship (Boeckman and Carlson, 2003). Although antibiotic treatment is not generally used to control subclinical mastitis, this form of mastitis is more insidious and can result in decreased milk production over the lactation period (Bartlett et al., 1990; Jones et al., 1984).

Somatic cells are leukocytes, a component of the immune system, that are present in milk at concentrations of less than 200,000 cells/ml in uninfected glands (Schalm et al., 1971). The SCC increase markedly with inflammation primarily due to the influx of polymorphonuclear neutrophils with a primary function of phagocytosis. There is a linear relationship between whole herd SCC and the percent of infected quarters within a herd. For bulk tank SCC of 200,000, 400,000, and 750,000 cells/ml, the percent quarters infected were estimated to be 6.2%, 12.8%, and 24.3%, respectively (Eberhart et al., 1982). For individual cows, estimates suggest for every 100,000 SCC/ml increase there is a corresponding decrease of 1.5 pounds of milk per day over the 305 day lactation period. This can result in a loss of 450 pounds of milk per cow per lactation (Eberhart et al., 1982). Therefore, SCC both within a cow and within a herd are useful indicators of the infection status of the mammary gland.

Antibiotic therapy for mastitis

Establishing a comprehensive mastitis control program is the most effective means for controlling mastitis. Mastitis control programs that are the most successful focus on prevention of mastitis through good management practices and the judicious use of antibiotics under the guidance of a veterinarian (Boeckman and Carlson, 2003). Prevention strategies aimed at decreasing the risk of infection are preferred over treatment for three reasons: prevention strategies are more cost effective, they reduce the need for antibiotic use, and they result in a healthier herd.

Antibiotics have been available for use in food producing animals since 1948 (Mitchell et al., 1998) and will continue to be considered necessary to treat infections to promote animal well-being. Although antibiotics are used to treat a variety of infections, mastitis is the most common reason for antibiotic use in dairy cattle (Sundlof et al., 1995), and there are a variety of antibiotics that have been approved for use in treating clinical mastitis. Results from a survey of food animal practitioners indicated that the most common class of antibiotics used therapeutically is beta-lactams, including penicillin G, ceftiofur sodium, cloxacillin, cephapirin, and ampicillin (Sundlof et al., 1995). When antibiotic therapy is warranted, the goal is to return the gland and milk to normal conditions and to eliminate the pathogen.

The success of antibiotic therapy is variable and depends on many factors. These include factors associated with the animal, the pathogen, and the environment. For example, the efficacy of antibiotic therapy can be compromised in glands that are severely swollen or in cases of a long established infection due to *Staphylococcus aureus* (Timms, 2001). Estimates of cure rates from mastitis due to *S. aureus* range from 20 to 75% cure (Eberhart et al., 1987), whereas, cure rates for mastitis due to *Streptococcus agalactiae* can approach 90% or greater. The variable success rate for curing infections with antibiotics underscores the need for alternative effective methods to reduce the incidence of this disease.

Avoiding antibiotic residues in milk and dairy products is a fundamental aspect of quality food production. The risk of an antibiotic residue contamination of bulk milk increases with an increase in the rate of mastitis within a herd in addition to other factors, such as lack of record-keeping and not identifying treated cows (McEwen, et al., 1991). Violative concentrations of antibiotics in commingled milk affect the marketability of the milk and will result in regulatory actions, which may include financial penalties and possible suspension of license for food production. In addition, there is the potential for antibiotic residues in animal-based foods to have a negative impact on human health. Therefore, reducing the need for antibiotic therapy will be beneficial for both maintaining animal health and promoting human food safety.

Antibiotic residues from animal-based foods can potentially impact microflora in the human gastrointestinal tract. The primary areas of concern are alterations in microbial functions, populations, and antimicrobial resistance patterns that may develop when human intestinal microflora are exposed to antibiotic residues from consumed meat and milk (USFDA, 2001). Therapeutic concentrations of orally administered antibiotics have temporarily increased the growth of resistant bacteria for several classes of antibiotics (Nord et al., 1984). However, the significance and long-term effect of these alterations on the functioning of the gastrointestinal tract are unknown. In contrast, Elder et al. (1993) compared the frequency of antibiotic resistant bacteria found in the stool microflora between vegetarians and nonvegetarians over a 12-month period and no treatment difference in prevalence of resistant organisms was observed.

Another concern for antibiotic residues is the potential for allergenic immune response by sensitive individuals to an antibiotic that may be present as a residue in consumed animal tissue and milk (Huber, 1986). This risk is small because it is unlikely that antibiotic residues would be immunogenic due to the low dose, the fact that the residue is taken orally. Evidence that the risk is small is shown by the extremely small number of immunogenic responses reported over a 25-year period (Dowdney et al., 1991).

Although the research does not conclusively implicate a link between antibiotic residue in animal-based foods and antibiotic resistance in human microflora, continued vigilance is warranted. In addition, the goal of reducing antibiotic residues in the human food supply is vital to ensure high quality food.

Alternative therapies for mastitis treatment

Development of novel, nontraditional methods for treating infections has the potential for significantly impacting animal health and human food safety. There has been considerable interest in a variety of complementary and alternative therapies for food-producing animals that focus on reducing the use of antibiotics. These therapies cover a wide variety of treatments and products, ranging from compounds with known antimicrobial activities to therapies that are not easily evaluated using currently established scientific methods.

Several compounds found in milk or associated with pathogenic bacteria have documented antimicrobial activities and have been evaluated for mastitis therapy with varying results. One such compound is the lantibiotic, nisin, which has antibacterial activity against Gram positive bacteria and has been used in the food industry (Breukink and de Kruijff, 1999). Nisin has the classification "Generally Regarded As Safe" by the US Food and Drug Administration (FDA) and, therefore, is not subject to human health regulations. This product has the potential to be used in treating Gram positive infections in animals and has recently been evaluated for use as a mastitis treatment; however, the results have been equivocal (Mantovani and Russell, 2001; Sears, 2001). Lactoferrin is another compound with antimicrobial activity that is present in milk and other body tissues. The concentration of this protein increases in milk during an infection and has been shown to bind to particular mastitis pathogens (Harmon et al., 1975). Lactoferrin has been used in other biological systems; however, similar to nisin, its effectiveness as a mastitis treatment has not been fully developed.

Another class of complementary and alternative treatments that have gained prominence in both human and animal health have been characterized as treatments not generally accepted as traditional therapies in the medical community (Loken, 2001). In the veterinary community these "nontraditional" therapies include botanical supplements and therapies, acupuncture, mind–body techniques, chiropractic, and homeopathy (Fontanarosa, 2001). Several of these alternative therapies, such as acupuncture, have had a long history of use in Asia and Europe and have more recently gained prominence in the United States for both human and animal therapies (Loken, 2001). A recent survey indicated that 7 of the 27 veterinary medical schools that responded to the survey include educational and research programs in complementary and alternative veterinary medicine (Schoen, 2000). In addition, there was strong interest for many of the other schools to establish programs in this area. Thus, the interest in these therapies is increasing for food animal and companion animal veterinary medicine. However, there is a lack of a good body of scientific knowledge on the safety and efficacy of these therapies. Much of the information is based on case studies and testimonials. While there is some evidence of efficacy of several types of alternative therapies, a rigorous evaluation of these therapies is needed for these products to be useful to animal agriculture.

Published reports on alternative treatments for mastitis have primarily focused on homeopathic treatments (Egan, 1995; Garbe, 2003; McCrory, 1997; Merek et al., 1989). In particular, homeopathic therapies present a challenge for evaluating effects attributable to the test compounds for several reasons that will be elaborated in the next section.

Homeopathic therapy for mastitis

Homeopathy is a collection of therapies that are based on a theory of "similars" and "like cures like" (Loken, 2001; Vockeroth, 1999). The claim for this type of therapy is that treatment with a compound (extremely diluted) that causes the pathology will effectively resolve the condition in the animal (Vockeroth, 1999). The compounds may be of plant origin or extracted from milk from infected animals. These compounds are then highly diluted by serial dilutions resulting in a final 10^{10} to 10^{100} dilution of the original compounds (Loken, 2001). A vigorous shaking at each dilution is required. The theory is that the compounds become more potent with each dilution (Vockeroth, 1999). Because of these dilutions, it is impossible to quantify the active ingredients in the final solution and, therefore, it can be difficult to attribute biological effects to the active compound using methodologies currently recommended for conventional scientific studies.

Several studies have evaluated the effect of homeopathic treatment on mastitis. However, only a small percentage of these studies would be classified as a controlled research study with the appropriate positive and/or negative controls. The majority of research comes from Europe, primarily Germany. A recent Ph.D. research dissertation from Germany described an evaluation of a homeopathic treatment for mastitis using a 300-cow dairy farm (Garbe, 2003). This research contained a negative control (placebo) and was a double-blinded study that evaluated the effect of a homeopathic treatment for maintaining the health of the mammary gland at the end of a lactation cycle and as a treatment for mastitis in the subsequent lactation. Individual quarters from cows that were not infected with a pathogen were treated at the end of a lactation cycle with either a homeopathic treatment developed specifically for the farm or a placebo. For those cows with an intramammary infection, an antibiotic was also administered in the affected quarter. In the subsequent lactation, cases of mastitis were treated with either the homeopathic product or conventional intramammary antibiotics. The results suggest that the homeopathic treatment was more effective for maintaining the health of the udder when used to treat healthy quarters at the cessation of lactation, whereas, during lactation, the homeopathic treatment of clinical mastitis was not as effective as treatment with antibiotics. These results agree with another study that determined that a homeopathic treatment was not successful in eliminating a chronic *S. aureus* clinical mastitis infection (Spranger, 1998). Also, Egan (1995) evaluated a homeopathic treatment for subclinical mastitis and found no significant differences in the prevalence of contagious mastitis pathogens before and after 28 days of treatment.

A positive result for a homeopathic treatment was reported by Merek et al. (1989). They determined that a series of two treatments with a homeopathic treatment resolved clinical mastitis caused by the coliform *Escherichia coli*. However, mastitis due to *E. coli* is generally of short duration and is eliminated by the host immune system unless it is of a severe nature and the animal may not survive (Erskine et al., 1991). Therefore, it may not be appropriate to attribute the positive effects reported by Merek et al. (1989) to the homeopathic treatment.

A placebo-controlled double-blind study in the United States evaluated nosode homeopathic treatments for the prevention and treatment of mastitis on organic and conventional dairy farms (McCrory, 1997). The study included over 1,000 cows across 11 dairy farms. No differences in new intramammary infections between the homeopathic treatment used on organic farms and antibiotic therapy used on conventional farms were reported. Of these controlled studies, only one of the five studies showed a benefit of the homeopathic treatment for clinical mastitis. However, the results of Garbe (2003) were interesting, because their study indicated a benefit from the homeopathic treatment for maintaining healthy udders. Further studies are needed to fully evaluate homeopathic treatments.

Study objective

The objectives of our study were to evaluate the effects of a homeopathy therapy on somatic cell counts, immunoglobulin response, and new subclinical intramammary infections in lactating dairy cows.

Study overview

Animals and treatments

Twenty-four Holstein dairy cows from a 450-cow commercial dairy herd were paired by days in lactation, milk production, parity, SCC, and intramammary pathogen prevalence, and the animals were assigned to one of two treatments in a double-blind study. The treatments were a homeopathic therapy consisting of plant extracts and compounds derived from mastitis pathogens and diluted to approximately 10^{65} or a placebo. The compounds contained in the homeopathy therapy were all listed as "Generally Regarded As Safe" compounds by the US FDA. The treatments were applied as a spray on the nasal membranes, following the manufacturer's directions for administration. The Animal Care and Use Committee of the University of Connecticut approved the use of animals for this study.

Cows were housed in a freestall facility, milked twice daily, and separated into two groups by treatment. This was required, since the manufacturer of the product indicated that if cows from the placebo treatment came into contact with the treated cows, then effects of the treatment may be observed in the placebo group. Cows were fed, free choice, a total mixed ration balanced to meet nutrient requirements and they had free access to drinking water (NRC, 1989).

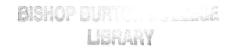
BISHOP BURTON COLLEGE
LIBRARY

Study methodology

The study was 60 days in length. At day −1, foremilk was aseptically collected from each quarter of all cows and analyzed for mastitis pathogens at the University of Connecticut Mastitis Laboratory and bacteriological status of milk samples was determined by diagnostic procedures recommended by the National Mastitis Council (1987). Milk was then sampled from the total milking of each cow on day –1 and analyzed for SCC (Marshall, 1992) and for the immunoglobulins G_1 (IgG_1) using ELISA quantitation kits (Bethyl Laboratories, Inc; Montgomery, TX). These values provided baseline nonspecific estimates of the intramammary infection status of each quarter and the immune system status.

On day 1 through day 10, the homeopathic therapy and the placebo were administered twice daily before each milking. On days 3, 7, 10, 13, 16, 22, 28, 35, 42, 49, and 56 milk was sampled and analyzed for SCC. On days 3, 13, 22, 28, 35, 42, 49, and 56 the milk samples were also analyzed for IgG_1. In addition, on days 28 and 56, foremilk from each quarter for all cows was aseptically collected and analyzed for mastitis pathogen as described earlier. If a cow developed clinical mastitis, the data from that cow were removed from the analysis due to marked increases in SCC and immunoglobulins due to clinical mastitis that may bias the analysis. In this study, the sample size was not large enough to accurately determine treatment differences for clinical mastitis, because clinical mastitis is usually a low incidence disease.

Statistical analysis

Treatment differences over time were tested for SCC, and IgG_1 using the mixed model of SAS with day as a repeated measure (SAS, 1997). Differences in pathogen prevalence were analyzed by logistic regression (SAS, 1997). Treatment differences were declared significant at $P < 0.05$ and trends were discussed at $P = 0.05$ to $P < 0.10$.

Study results

During the 60-day study, three cows treated with the placebo were excluded from the study. One cow developed fever and milk production decreased markedly, and two cows developed clinical mastitis. In the pretreatment aseptic sample of milk, 41.6% of quarters from cows treated with the homeopathic treatment and 44% of quarters from cows treated with the placebo were infected with a mastitis pathogen and did not significantly differ (Table 1.1). The exclusion of these animals from the analysis did not affect the final results.

The most prevalent intramammary pathogens present were *Streptococcus dysgalactiae* and coliforms. The level of mastitis pathogens present in cows at our study farm was higher than what was observed in two other studies (Eberhart et al., 1982; Bartlett, et al., 1990). This corresponded to 9 out of 12 cows for the homeopathic group and 5 out of 9 cows for the placebo group that were identified with an intramammary infection before the treatment period (Table 1.2). The major pathogens present in this herd were *S. dysgalactiae, Streptococcus uberis, S. aureus,* and coliforms. There were no treatment differences in SCC and IgG_1 in milk sampled during the pretreatment period (Figures 1.1 and 1.2).

Table 1.1 The number of infected quarters and the classification of pathogens within quarters infected with subclinical mastitis at three time points: 1 day pretreatment (d-1), day 28 (d28), and day 56 (d56) of study for cows treated for 10 days with a homeopathic treatment (H) or a placebo (P)

	d-1		d28		d56	
Pathogen	H	P	H	P	H	P
n	48	36	48	36	48	36
Total number of quarters infected						
All pathogens	20	16	21	13	28	14*
Streptococcus dysgalactiae	5	5	3	2	21	8*
Streptococcus uberis	3	2	3	1	0	0
Staphylococcus aureus	0	5	0	3	0	2
Coliforms	7	2	2	2	0	1
Minor pathogens	5	2	13	5	7	3

*Significant treatment difference for all pathogens and *S. dysgalactiae* at d56 ($P < 0.05$).

The number of cows infected or quarters infected did not differ at day 28 compared with the infection rate during the pretreatment period (Tables 1.1 and 1.2). At day 56, there was an increase in quarters infected with major pathogens and *S. dysgalactiae* for cows administered the homeopathic treatment compared with the infection rate for cows treated with the placebo (Table 1.1). The increase in pathogens for treated cows was due solely to new intramammary infections caused by *S. dysgalactiae* (Table 1.2). It is important to note that the overall prevalence rate of infections due to *S. dysgalactiae* was markedly, but not statistically, increased at day 56 across both treatments compared with the prevalence rates at day -1 and day 28, and that the treated cows were affected to a greater degree by this intramammary pathogen (Table 1.1).

During the 10-day treatment period, SCC in milk from cows treated with the placebo increased, while SCC in those treated with the homeopathic treatment remained the same (Figure 1.1). The concentration of IgG_1 did not change during this time for both treatments (Figure 1.2). In contrast, the SCC for cows treated with the homeopathic treatment increased after day 25 and then decreased

Table 1.2 The number of cows infected with a mastitis pathogen, one or greater major pathogens and one or greater minor pathogens at one day pretreatment (d-1) and number of cows with new intramammary infections at day 28 (d28) and day 56 (d56) of study for cows treated for ten days with a homeopathic treatment (H) or a placebo (P)

	d-1		d28		d56*	
Pathogen	H	P	H	P	H	P
n	12	9	12	9	12	9
			Number of new infections			
Total number of cows infected	9	5	8	4	9	5**
Number of cows infected with:						
One or greater major pathogens	8	5	3	1	9	5
One or greater minor pathogens	4	2	6	4	5	1

* Trend for a time by treatment effect ($P < 0.10$).
**All new infections due to major pathogens during time d56 were due to *Strep. dysgalactiae*.

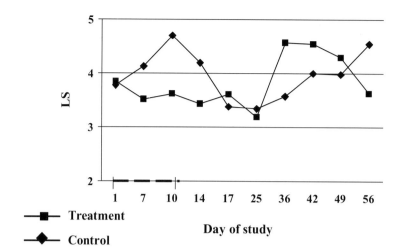

Fig. 1.1 The effect of homeopathic treatment or placebo on linear score of SCC in milk from Holstein cows. Treatment was administered twice daily from day 1 to day 10.

by day 56, and the SCC of cows treated with the placebo decreased by day 25 and then increased up to day 56. These opposing changes in SCC by treatment resulted in no significant treatment differences across the 60-day period. The milk IgG_1 concentrations for the cows treated with the homeopathic treatment spiked at week 5 and week 8 of the study. The first peak at week 5 corresponded with the increase in SCC at the same time for the homeopathic treated cows. The lower concentration on SCC and IgG_1 at 25 days and week 4, respectively, occurred when there was a lower prevalence of *S. dysgalactiae* for both treatments.

Immunoglobulin G_1, an antibody that is part of the acquired immunity system, increases in milk in infected quarters (Sordillo et al., 1997). Likewise, SCC increases due to intramammary infection. The marked increases in these two components, IgG_1 and SCC, were observed for the cows treated

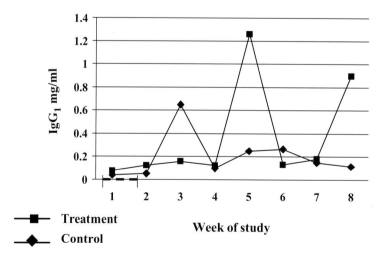

Fig. 1.2 The effect of homeopathic treatment on IgG_1 concentrations in milk from Holstein cows. Treatment was administered twice daily from day 1 to day 10.

with the homeopathic therapy before the milk culture, showing a greater increase in infection with *S. dysgalactiae*. Some possible explanations for these effects are as follows: 1. There may have been an increase in intramammary infection across the whole herd at this time. However, the SCC of the bulk tank milk did not differ during this time, suggesting that this was not a herd event. The intramammary infection status of the herd at that time was not available. 2. Since the cows were housed separately (as per the study design), there may have been different environmental conditions that resulted in a greater infection rate for the treated cows. 3. The homeopathic treatment may have affected the immune system of the cows resulting in an increased susceptibility to intramammary infection. 4. During the 10-day treatment period, the SCC of the treated group did not differ, whereas the SCC for cows treated with a placebo increased during this time period (Figure 1.1). This may indicate that the homeopathy therapy was effective during the 10-day period of treatment, but that this time period was too short in duration to provide a long-term benefit.

We recommend that it would be useful to conduct homeopathic studies using the solutions containing the active compounds over a range of the serial dilutions. Using this approach, it is expected that any treatment effects would be observed as the product becomes more dilute, as suggested by homeopathic practitioners. This method would also provide a more rigorous evaluation of the homeopathic methodologies and provide evidence of the effectiveness of homeopathic compounds.

Conclusions

Mastitis is a significant health concern for the dairy industry. Conventional treatments for clinical mastitis are based on antibiotic therapy and will continue to be a component of a successful mastitis control program that is focused on prevention of mastitis. However, due to variable effectiveness of antibiotics and human health concerns, identifying safe, effective alternatives to antibiotic therapies would be beneficial for animal health and human food safety. Many alternative therapies have not been adequately evaluated. In particular, homeopathic therapies are difficult to evaluate using conventional research methods. In this study, treatment effects were noted for a homeopathic therapy that may be due to the alternative treatment. Additional (albeit, expensive) studies are needed to definitively determine if these compounds are useful for the control of mastitis.

Acknowledgments

The authors would like to acknowledge the commercial farm for the use of their cows and their active support and labor for this project. Also, the authors thank Lynn Hinckley and the Connecticut Mastitis Laboratory for pathogen analysis and Dr. Larry Silbart for technical advice.

References

Bartlett, P.C., G.Y. Miller, C.R. Anderson, and J.H. Kirk. 1990. Milk production and somatic cell count in Michigan dairy herds. *J. Dairy Sci.* 73:2794.

Blosser, T.H. 1979. Economic losses from the national research program on mastitis in the United States. *J. Dairy Sci.* 62:119.

Boeckman, S. and K.R. Carlson. 2003. *Milk and Dairy Beef Residue Prevention Protocol*. Agri-Education, Inc., Stratford, IA.

Breukink, E. and B. de Kruijff. 1999. The lantobiotic nisin, a special case or not. *Biochim. Biophys. Acta.* 1462:223.

Dowdney, J.M., L. Maes, J.P. Raynaud, F. Blanc, J.P. Scheid, T. Jackson, S. Lens, and C. Verschueren. 1991. Risk assessment of antibiotic residues of beta-lactams and macrolides in food products with regard to their immuno-allergenic potential. *Food Chem. Toxicol.* 29:477.

Eberhart, R.J., R.J. Harmon, D.E. Jasper, and R.P. Natzke. 1987. *Current Concepts of Bovine Mastitis.* National Mastitis Council, Arlington, VA.

Eberhart, R.J., L.J. Hutchinson, and S.B. Spencer. 1982. Relationships of bulk tank somatic cell counts to prevalence of intramammary infection and to indices of herd production. *J. Food Prot.* 45:1125.

Egan, J. 1995. Evaluation of homeopathic treatment for sub-clinical mastitis. *Vet. Rec.* 137:48.

Elder, H.A., I. Roy, S. Lehman, R.L. Phillips, and E.H. Kass. 1993. Human studies to measure the effect of antibiotic residues. *Vet. Human Toxicol.* 35:31.

Erskine R.J., J.W. Tyler, M.G. Riddell, Jr., and R.C. Wilson. 1991. Theory, use, and realities of efficacy and food safety of antimicrobial treatment for coliform mastitis. *J. Am. Vet. Med. Assoc.* 198:980.

Fontanarosa, P.B. 2001. Publication of complementary and alternative medicine research in mainstream biomedical journals. *J. Altern. Complement. Med.* 7:S139.

Garbe, S. 2003. Investigation of the effect of homeopathic treatment on the improvement of udder health in health in dairy cows. Ph.D. Dissertation. Fachbereich Veterinarmedizin, Freie Universitat Berlin.

Harmon, R.J., F.L. Schanbacher, L.C. Ferguson, and K.L. Smith. 1975. Concentration of lactoferrin in milk of normal lactating cows and changes occurring during mastitis. *Am. J. Vet. Res.* 36:1001.

Huber, W.G. 1986. Allergenicity of antibacterial drug residues. In *Drug Residues in Animals* (ed. A.G. Rico), pp. 33–49. Academic Press, Toronto, Ontario.

Jones, G.M., R.E. Pearson, G.A. Clabaugh, and C.W. Heald. 1984. Relationships between somatic cell counts and milk production. *J. Dairy Sci.* 67:1823.

Loken, T. 2001. Alternative therapy of animals—homeopathy and other alternative methods of therapy. *Acta Vet. Scand.* 95(Suppl. 1):47.

Mantovani, H.C. and J.B. Russell. 2001. Nisin resistance of *Streptococcus bovis. Appl. Environ. Microbiol.* 67:808.

Marshall, T.R. 1992. *Standard Methods for Examination of Dairy Products,* 16th edn. American Publication Health Association, Inc., Washington, DC.

McCrory, L. 1997. Evaluation and documentation of homeopathic nosodes in organic and conventional dairy production. USDA Northeast SARE Project no. LNE97-086.

McEwen, S.C., W.D. Black, and A.H. Meek. 1991. Antibiotic residue prevention methods, farm management, and occurrence of antibiotic residues in milk. *J. Dairy Sci.* 74:2128.

Merek, C.C., B. Sonnenwald, and H. Rollwage. 1989. The administration of homeopathic drugs for the treatment of acute mastitis in cattle. *Berl Munch Tierarztl Wochenschr.* 102:266.

Mitchell, J.M., M.W. Griffiths, S.A. McEwen, W.B. McNab, and A.J. Yee. 1998. Antimicrobial drug residues in milk and meat: causes, concerns, prevalence, regulations, tests, and test performance. *J. Food Prot.* 61:742.

National Mastitis Council, Inc. 1987. *Laboratory Field Handbook of Bovine Mastitis.* W. D. Hoard & Sons Co., Fort Atkinson, WI.

National Research Council (NRC). 1989. *Nutrient Requirements of Dairy Cattle.* 6th rev. edn. National Academy of Science, Washington, DC.

Nord, C.E., A. Heimdahl, and L. Kager. 1984. The impact of different antimicrobial agents on normal gastrointestinal microflora of humans. *Rev. Infect. Dis.* 6(Suppl. 1):S270.

SAS® User's Guide: Statistics, Version 7 Edition. 1997. SAS Institution, Inc., Cary, NC.

Schalm, O.W., E.J. Carroll, and N.C. Jain. 1971. Number and types of somatic cells. In *Bovine Mastitis*, pp. 113–123. Lea and Febiger, Philadelphia, PA.

Schoen, A.M. 2000. Results of a survey on educational and research programs in complementary and alternative veterinary medicine at veterinary medical schools in the United States. JAVMA 216:502.

Sears, P. 2001. Use of antimicrobial nisin to treat *Streptococcus agalactiae* mastitis. In *Proc. 2nd International Symp. on Mastitis and Milk Quality,* pp. 251–253. National Mastitis Council, Vancouver, BC, Canada.

Smucker, J.M. 1997. Results of the national tanker monitoring program. In *Natl. Mastitis Counc. Ann. Mtg. Proc.*, Albuquerque, NM, pp. 185–186. National Mastitis Council, Inc., Madison, WI.

Sordillo, L.M., K. Shafer-Weaver, and D. DeRosa. 1997. Immunobiology of the mammary gland. *J. Dairy Sci.* 80:1851.

Spranger, J. 1998. Guidelines for prevention and therapy in ecological animal farms as in the example of bovine mastitis. *Dtsch Tierarztl Wochenschr.* 105:321.

Sundlof, S.F., J.B. Kaneene, and R. Miller. 1995. National survey on veterinarian-initiated drug use in lactating cows. *J. Am. Vet. Med. Assoc.* 207:347.

Timms, L. 2001. Evaluation of recommended and extended pirlimycin therapy strategies in four high somatic cell count herds. In *Proc. Second Intl. Mastitis Milk Quality Symp.*, p. 534.

U.S. Food and Drug Administration (USFDA). 2001. Assessment of the effects of antimicrobial drug residues from food of animal origin on the human intestinal tract. USFDA, Center of Veterinary Medicine Draft Guidance Document #52, December 19, 2001.

Vockeroth, W.G. 1999. Veterinary homeopathy: an overview. *Can. Vet. J.* 40:592.

Chapter 2
Potential Role of Amazonian Medicinal Plants for Health Maintenance in Livestock

Mark J.S. Miller

Introduction

Health maintenance in developing countries often involves a mixture of western medicine and ethnomedicine, with the exact blend varying from condition to condition, fiscal constraints, and the influence of tradition. At the same time in developed countries there is growing concern over the presence of pharmaceuticals, hormones, and xenobiotics in the food chain. This has led to the search for alternative approaches to maintain livestock health and integrity, especially the growing trend of organic and free-range farming. One possible solution is the use of traditional ethnomedicines, sometimes referred to as alternative or complementary medicine, as a means of enhancing and maintaining livestock health. However, our vista of ethnomedicines, botanicals, and natural products is usually restricted to a European experience, with little exploration into other cultures and approaches that are currently in use.

We have been exploring the Amazon River basin as a source of unique medicinal plants, with a focus on mechanisms of action and verification of their applicability and interpretation of the traditional information. Here we focus on two medicinal plants and their potential use in livestock as a source of therapeutics and health maintenance. These plants are ethnomedically known as sangre de grado (or sangre de drago) and cat's claw (or una de gato). Sangre de grado is a tree sap or resin (*Croton palanostigma*, and *Croton lechleri*) and una de gato is a vine whose bark and roots (*Uncaria tomentosa*) are made into tea (Duke and Vasquez, 1994). Both possess remarkable actions and applications to organic farming and livestock that should be explored.

Sangre de grado: ethnomedical background

Sangre de grado is found throughout Amazonia but the highest quality resin is derived from Ecuador and Peru. It is usually wild-crafted but it has been successfully farmed in a number of countries. The trees are fast growing, reaching a height of 40 feet in 3 years and production is based on felling the trees to collect the sap from incisions made every 20 cm along the trunk. About 1–1.5 liters of resin can be collected from each tree, with trees cultivated in a 2–3 year cycle.

Table 2.1 Applications of sangre de grado or extracts

Topical	Gastrointestinal	Generalized
Wound healing	Ulcer healing	Antimicrobial
Hemostasis	Diarrhea	Antiviral
Erythema/swelling	Cramping	
Itch	Vomiting/nausea	
Pain	Pain	

A remarkable characteristic of sangre de grado in ethnomedical use is the diversity of conditions for which it provides benefits (Table 2.1) (Duke and Vasquez, 1994; Miller et al., 2000, 2001b). It is applied topically for wounds, skin irritations, hemostasis, insect bites, and stings and it is also taken orally for numerous gastrointestinal complaints including diarrhea, ulcer healing, nausea, cramping, and severe gastrointestinal distress. There have been reports of its effectiveness as an antiviral agent (rhinovirus, herpes) and cancer applications (Chen et al., 1994; Pieters et al., 1993; Sandoval et al., 2002a; Ubillas, 1994).

Sangre de grado: proposed active chemicals

While there are numerous unique chemicals that have been identified in sangre de grado, there has been a lack of consensus as to the "active chemicals" because of the diversity of actions exhibited by the ethnomedicine. Hence, certain actions are mediated by some chemical constituents and other applications reflect different components. This is typical of complex natural substances, and while the variety of chemical entities within sangre de grado restricts development as a drug, it opens up more therapeutic opportunities as a natural product. Certainly extracts, which concentrate specific chemical elements, may be developed for more focused purposes and applications.

Nevertheless, the predominant chemical classes in sangre de grado are proanthocyanidins and anthocyanidins, which are largely responsible for the intense color of the resin (Phillipson, 1995). Proanthocyanidins are oligomers, chemically related to anthocyanins and catechins, and are very effective antioxidants. Indeed, one commercial product, Progrado™, that is enriched proanthocyanidins, has an ORAC (oxygen radical absorption capacity) value of 4,459 which is about 10 times higher than ORAC values for powders from fruits that are naturally vitamin C enriched, and over 100 times higher than those for fresh cranberries.

Phillipson (1995) noted the presence of crolechinol, crolechinic acid, korberin A and B, $3'4'-O$-dimethylcedrusin, and taspine. The latter along with polyphenolic rich fractions have been postulated to be responsible for wound healing as they enhance the activity of fibroblasts (Cai et al., 1991; Chen et al., 1994; Perdue et al., 1979; Porras-Reyes et al., 1993; Vaisberg et al., 1989). However, the ability of sangre de grado to inhibit neurogenic inflammation is also likely to contribute to wound healing (Miller et al., 2001b).

Sangre de grado has also been shown to have antimicrobial actions in vitro and in vivo (Chen et al., 1994; Miller et al., 2001b; Phillipson, 1995), although with dilution this effect is diminished. There are benefits evident in cancer (Chen at al. 1994; Sandoval et al. 2002a) although it is not clear as to whether catechins, like that found in green tea, are the primary source of these anticancer actions. There are certainly similarities with sangre de grado causing cancer cells to undergo programmed cell death (apoptosis) and losing cytoskeletal integrity (Sandoval et al., 2002a).

Nevertheless, we have determined that a central action is responsible for the primary therapeutic applications of sangre de grado in skin and gastrointestinal health, an action that is both unique and a key to its remarkable therapeutic potential. Sangre de grado at extraordinarily low concentrations limits the ability of sensory afferent nerves to be activated (Miller et al., 2000, 2001b). This effect is not mediated by any known pathway e.g., vanilloids, cannabinoids, anti-histamine, anesthetic, but in simplistic terms it has characteristics of an anti-chili pepper as the pungent chemical capsaicin is the prototypical activator of sensory afferent nerves.

Sensory afferent nerves and neurogenic inflammation

Sensory afferent nerves, sometimes called C fibers or primary afferents, serve a protective role, alerting the central nervous system that there has been a breach of barrier—skin, gut, and lung. Once activated, not only do the nerves identify the location of the breach but they also initiate and maintain a local response focused on limiting the extent of the barrier dysfunction. They are responsible for a range of annoying symptoms as shown in Figure 2.1. When excessive or sustained these symptoms can become major concerns, and an over-active neurogenic response can maintain and exacerbate a minor condition and lead to secondary problems. For example, a profound itch may lead to a significant infection if scratching is uncontrolled, and diarrhea may lead to wasting, dehydration, and poor nutrition if allowed to persist.

While sensory afferent nerves can be activated by several chemical pathways, including capsaicin, proteases (tryptase or bee stings), prostaglandin E2, and bradykinin, sangre de grado is capable of suppressing neural activation independent of the activator involved (Miller et al., 2001b). Here

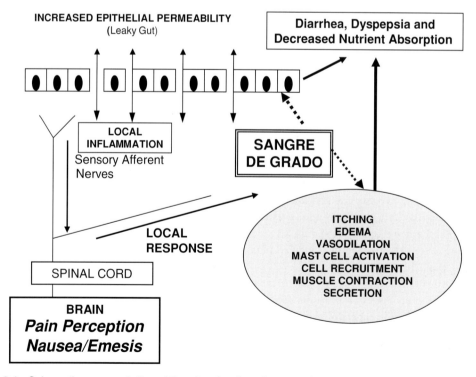

Fig. 2.1 Schematic representation of the site of action of sangre de grado on intestinal dysfunction.

sangre de grado defies current classification, but the most likely interpretation is that sangre de grado activates a novel receptor that is inhibitory in function, stabilizing the neural membrane potential thereby reducing the ability of the nerve to fire an action potential. In other words, sangre de grado can offer relief from a large variety of initiating events because its actions are not dependent upon blocking a single stimulatory process.

As mentioned above, an easy way to conceptualize how sangre de grado works is to consider it as an anti-chili pepper. Capsaicin, the prototypical stimulant of these nerves, induces localized secretion, vasodilation, and pain, which are readily blocked by sangre de grado (Figure 2.2). Capsaicin activates vanilloid receptor 1 (VR1 or the chili pepper receptor), a deletion of this nerve from the genome prevents mice from exhibiting the hyperalgesia evident in inflammation (Caterina et al., 2000; Davis et al., 2000), indicating that this pathway is a critical process for inflammatory pain. Sangre de grado is currently the only therapeutic option (cannabinoids like marijuana can achieve similar goals but are unlikely to meet regulatory demands and are associated with significant complications) that prevents the neural response to vanilloid receptor activation, indicating the uniqueness and value of this medicinal plant.

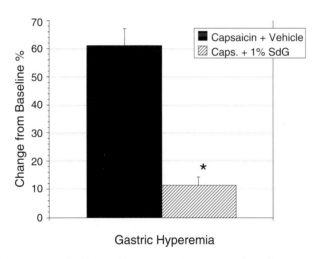

Fig. 2.2 Suppression of capsaicin-induced hyperemia by sangre de grado.

Nevertheless, the benefits of sangre de grado go beyond vanilloid receptors. Subsets of sensory afferent nerve exist, for example the nerves that sense itch and nausea are distinct from those that sense pain (Schmelz, 2001). Further activation of pain pathways is sometimes seen with capsaicin when used to stop itching, which only swaps one troublesome symptom for another. Opioids are excellent analgesics but they promote itch and emesis, effects that are blocked by sangre de grado. Sangre de grado is unique in that it possesses anti-itch, analgesia, and inhibitory actions on erythema and edema (Miller et al., 2001b); its breadth and potency of actions across numerous conditions is unique amongst therapeutic agents (Table 2.1).

Sangre de grado and gastrointestinal applications

The ulcer healing attributes of sangre de grado were investigated in rats (Miller et al., 2000) when they consumed the sangre de grado latex present in drinking water at great dilutions (1:1,000 and 1:10,000). The rate of healing of gastric ulcers was found to be comparable to that seen with a combination of antibiotics (penicillin and streptomycin) but with additional advantages in that sangre de grado substantially reduced the inflammation in the floor of the ulcer bed (Miller et al., 2000). Sangre de grado therapy was also associated with a substantial reduction in the gene expression of proinflammatory cytokines (IL-1, IL-6, TNFα) and enzymes (COX2 and iNOS). Similarly, neurogenic secretory mechanisms that underlie diarrhea are also abrogated by sangre de grado (Miller et al., 2000). Others have suggested that an anti-secretory action may involve an inhibition of cAMP-mediated epithelial secretion (Gabriel et al., 1999; Holodniy et al., 1999), which may be operative independent of neurogenic mediated responses.

A sangre de grado extract has been shown to possess anti-emetic actions, blocking the induction of vomiting and retching produced by morphine. This opioid-induced response is often seen post-surgically and is thought to be mediated by a spinal pathway involving withdrawal of pain pathways that normally exert a tonic influence of the symptoms of nausea and itch. The benefits of sangre de grado, however, seem to be totally mediated at a peripheral nervous system level, there is no evidence of central nervous system actions, e.g., there is no sedation or hypothermia as would be expected with cannabinoids.

Applications to livestock

Given this background there are a number of conditions where sangre de grado offers therapeutic options in the treatment of livestock. Certainly as liquid bandage for treating wounds, lacerations, and abrasions it is remarkably effective. The proanthocyanidins polymerize with exposed connective tissue, forming a seal that looks like a natural scab but has the added advantages of being a powerful antioxidant, antibiotic, inhibitor of itch, analgesic, and retarding bleeding and promoting healing. The suppression of neurogenic responses that are associated with sangre de grado allows for symptom-free healing and reduced likelihood of recurrence of the wound.

A similar application is insect bites and stings. We demonstrated that a sangre de grado balm produced relief from redness, swelling, pain, itch, and discomfort within minutes of application in response to fire ants, bees, wasps, and plant reactions (Miller et al., 2001b). Under some circumstances, geographical and seasonal, these conditions can produce serious consequences and compromise the quality of the livestock health. Rapid and sustained relief from these events is highly desirable.

For gastrointestinal perturbations the ability of sangre de grado to convey significant relief from numerous initiating events makes it quite attractive. It is readily applicable as it can simply be added to drinking water or applied by simple gavage. It can be used in conjunction with other approaches against specific pathogens offering significant symptomatic relief.

Finally, cost is not an issue that hinders its use and application. It is inexpensive, especially given its potency. The difficult problem is its availability. It has not been commercialized for these purposes in western countries. Indeed, it was the focus of one biotechnology company where a proanthocyanidin-enriched fraction was developed as a prescription drug treatment for diarrhea (Holodniy et al., 1999); however, it did not advance beyond phase III trials. Other approaches based on extracts for oral and topical uses are being explored and may have cross-over potential. However, access to material at a reasonable price may be constrained by companies not establishing a unique selling position and competitive edge. Thus, it is not the inability of sangre de grado to offer benefit that will limit its commercial success in livestock, it is whether businesses are prepared to invest in developing a product that has no barriers to competitors and copycats. Validated proprietary extracts assist in establishing a competitive market position, but the cost of these products will have to be compatible with market forces, especially costs appropriate for livestock applications, for use to become widespread. Certainly, the therapeutic opportunities exist but getting a meaningful product into commerce will require an appreciation of these constraints.

Cat's claw—una de gato

Cat's claw is a vine that is common throughout South American rainforests (Duke and Vasquez, 1994). A decoction or tea is made from the bark or roots, although it is not necessary to kill the vine to harvest the bark. So we advocate only using bark and cutting the vine above ground level to foster regrowth. Cat's claw has suffered from significant confusion as to its purpose and ethnomedical use. Internet searches will confirm this, but the only clear action that is consistent with the relevant science and traditional use is the application of cat's claw as an anti-inflammatory agent. The proposed actions of cat's claw as an immune stimulant are poorly supported and reflect a pre-occupation that oxindole alkaloids are the active chemical species in cat's claw (Laus et al., 1997). Those contentions can be readily dismissed by comparing the effects of the subspecies *Uncaria guianensis*, which is naturally devoid of oxindole alkaloids, with the actions of *Uncaria tomentosa*. In this case, *U. guianensis* is a more potent inhibitor of tumor necrosis factor alpha (TNFα) production, antioxidant, and anti-inflammatory agent (Sandoval et al., 2002b). Furthermore, a double blind placebo controlled trial demonstrated that *U. guianensis* is highly effective in relieving the pain and symptoms of osteoarthritis in humans at the remarkably low dose of less than 2 mg/kg per day for freeze dried extract (Piscoya et al., 2000).

Mechanism of action

Cat's claw offers the most potent inhibition of TNFα for a natural product yet described (Sandoval et al. 2000, 2002b). This is achieved by the suppression of the transcription factor nuclear factor–kappa B (NF-κB), which regulates the full spectrum of inflammation (Sandoval-Chacon et al., 1998)—chemokines, adhesion molecules, enzymes, and cytokines (Figure 2.3). TNFα is one of the primary targets of NF-κB, and its importance in chronic inflammation has become clear after the outstanding success of absorbing antibodies—Remicade® in neutralizing intractable diseases like rheumatoid arthritis, Crohn's disease, and psoriasis. However, while Remicade® has provided "proof of principle" that TNFα is a major contributor of chronic inflammation, it is not applicable to livestock based on cost and its humanized antibody construct; it does help place the potential use of cat's claw in perspective.

Cat's claw is a highly effective antioxidant but its true potential lies in its ability to modify cellular responses to oxidative stress and immune activation, which goes beyond the mere annihilation of oxidant and radical species (Miller et al., 2001a, Yepez et al., 1991). Redox based events can dictate whether cells decide to repair damage, commit apoptosis, or contribute to the production of inflammatory mediators to eliminate threats, real or perceived.

The classic antioxidants like vitamin C possess bioactivities that are more akin to chemical–chemical annihilation, where they protect cells from an extracellular locus by quenching oxidants and radicals before they have access to the critical regulatory centers. By way of contrast, catechins that are present in high concentrations in green tea, and curcumin, the transcriptional inhibitory chemical from the spice turmeric, along with cat's claw are examples of phytonutrients that have

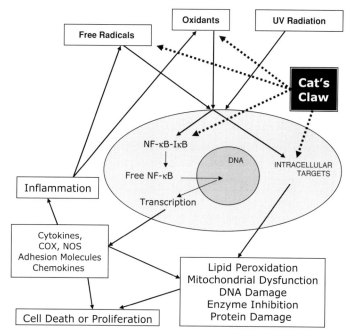

Fig. 2.3 Schematic representation of the site of action for cat's claw.

far greater effects on cellular events. These antioxidants possess actions on cellular decision-making and activity that are not explained by simple quenching but rather by actions on intracellular signal transduction mechanisms (Miller et al., 2001a). For this reason they are more potent as cytoprotective agents and modifiers of disease activity.

Chronic inflammation

Cat's claw has been shown to be effective in several chronic states of inflammation, with greatest benefits seen in those that are driven by TNFα or other type 1 immune responses. Examples are arthritis (Piscoya et al., 2000), chronic gut inflammation (Sandoval-Chacon, 1998; Sandoval et al., 2002b), as well as chronic skin inflammation. Consistent with a mechanism of action that is based on regulating gene expression, benefits are evident within 3–7 days. Benefits from chondroitin and glucosamine therapy in arthritis, however, require 4–12 weeks because the inflammatory process is not interrupted as when regulating gene expression, but rather the therapy is based on enhancing repair. However, that is self-limiting if damage continues unabated.

In many ways the activity of cat's claw resembles glucocorticoids like prednisone, because of the actions on gene expression and in particular NF-κB. However, cat's claw does not exhibit the side effects and complications of glucocorticoids. Part of the gentleness (safety) that is associated with cat's claw is attributable to its incomplete suppression of TNFα production, in that maximal responses plateau at 80%. Therefore cat's claw modulates rather than obliterates immune activity. As a result immune system balance can be achieved without secondary oscillations and compensations in regulatory processes.

Applications to livestock

Cat's claw has numerous applications for conditions of inflammation independent of the organ involved. This therapy may allow conditions of healing which would encourage farmers not to abandon ill animals. Cat's claw comes in a variety of formulations but the least expensive form is where the bark is ground into a powder (micropulverized). This form is less bioavailable yet effective, and can be readily added to feeds, as a preventative measure or as a therapy. Cat's claw can also be added to the drinking water with this micropulverized formulation although more highly processed formulations are generally more soluble. Cat's claw does not present taste problems and so administration in feeds or water is a remarkably easy way to deliver effective doses to livestock. Ethnomedically it is consumed as a tea.

Cost considerations are minimal as it is quite potent. Considering the cost of pharmaceuticals, and even other medicinal plant approaches, cat's claw is an effective, reliable alternative to treating inflammatory conditions. Access to veterinary specific products is limited, but kilogram quantities are available from bulk natural product stores or importers. Cost effective alternative formulations that are more highly processed are not yet available for the livestock market.

Summary

Amazonian ethnomedicines like sangre de grado and cat's claw possess important and unique biological properties that offer therapeutic options in the livestock industry. Their benefits are similar if not superior to those of pharmaceuticals, depending on the application, yet are natural substances that are consistent with the desire to limit the introduction of drugs and xenobiotics in the food chain. These medicinal plants are easy to apply to a livestock setting and are pluripotential, allowing for significant therapeutic flexibility. Their characteristics could make them valuable and safe alternatives to pharmaceuticals in maintaining livestock health. The current hurdles lie in availability in a format suitable for this application.

References

Cai, Y., F.J. Evans, M.F. Roberts, J.D. Phillipson, M.H. Zenk, and Y.Y. Gleba. 1991. Polyphenolic compounds from *Croton lechleri*. *Phytochemistry* 30:2033–2040.

Caterina, M.J., A. Leffler, A.B. Malmberg, W.J. Martin, J., Trafton, K.R. Petersen-Zeitz, M. Koltzenburg, A.I. Basbaum, and D. Julius. 2000. Impaired nociception and pain sensation in mice lacking the capsaicin receptor. *Science* 288:306–313.

Chen, Z.P., Y. Cai, and J.D. Phillipson. 1994. Studies on the anti-tumor, anti-bacterial, and wound-healing properties of Dragon's blood. *Planta Med.* 60:541–545.

Davis, J.B., J. Gray, M.J. Gunthorpe, et al. 2000. Vanilloid receptor-1 is essential for inflammatory thermal hyperalgesia. *Nature* 405:183–187.

Duke, J. and R. Vasquez. 1994. *Amazonian Ethnomedical Dictionary*. CRC Press, Boca Raton, FL.

Gabriel, S.E., S.E. Davenport, R.J. Steagall, V. Viaml, T.R. Carlson, and J. Rozhon. 1999. A plant-derived inhibitor of cAMP-mediated fluid and chloride secretion. *Am. J. Gastrointest. Liver Physiol.* 276:G58–G63.

Holodniy, M., J. Koch, M. Mistal, J.M. Schmidt, A. Khandwala, J.E. Pennington, and S.B. Porter. 1999. A double blind, randomized, placebo-controlled phase II study to assess the safety and efficacy of orally administered SP-303 for the symptomatic treatment of diarrhea in patients with AIDS. *Am. J. Gastroenterol.* 94: 3267–3273.

Laus, G., D. Brossner, and K. Keplinger. 1997. Alkaloids of Peruvian *Uncaria tomentosa. Phytochemistry* 45:855–860.

Miller, M.J.S., F.M. Angeles, B.K. Reuter, P. Bobrowski, and M. Sandoval. 2001a. Dietary antioxidants protect gut epithelial cells from oxidant induced apoptosis. *BMC Complement. Altern. Med.* 1:11.

Miller, M.J.S., W.K. MacNaughton, X.-J. Zhang, J.H. Thompson, R.M. Charbonnet, P. Bobrowski, J. Lao, A.M. Trentacosti, and M. Sandoval. 2000. Treatment of gastric ulcers and diarrhea with the Amazonian herbal medicine sangre de grado. *Am. J. Physiol. Gastrointest. Liver Physiol.* 279:G192–G200.

Miller, M.J.S., N. Vergnolle, W. McKnight, R.A. Musah, C.A. Davison, A.M. Trentacosti, J.H. Thompson, M. Sandoval, and J.L. Wallace. 2001b. Inhibition of neurogenic inflammation by the Amazonian herbal medicine sangre de grado. *J. Investig. Dermatol.* 117:725–730.

Perdue, G.P., R.N. Blomster, D.A. Blake, and N.R. Farnsworth. 1979. South American plants: taspine isolation and anti-inflammatory activity. *J. Pharm. Sci.* 68:124–125.

Phillipson, J.D. 1995. A matter of sensitivity. *Phytochemistry* 38:1319–1343.

Pieters, L., T. De Bruyne, M. Claeys, A. Vlietink, M. Calomme, and D. Vanden Berghe. 1993. Isolation of dihydrobenzofuran lignan from South American Dragon's blood (*Croton* spp.) as an inhibitor of cell proliferation. *J. Nat. Prod.* 56:899–906.

Piscoya, J., Z. Rodriguez, S. Bustamante, M.J.S. Miller, and M. Sandoval. 2000. Efficacy and safety of freeze dried cat's claw in osteoarthritis of the knee: mechanisms of action of the specie *Uncaria guianensis. Inflamm. Res.* 50:442–448.

Porras-Reyes, R.H., W.H. Lewis, J. Roman, L. Simchowitz, and T.A. Mustoe. 1993. Enhancement of wound healing by the alkaloid taspine: defining mechanisms of action. *Proc. Soc. Exp. Biol. Med.* 203:18–25.

Sandoval, M., R.M. Charbonnet, N.N. Okuhama, J. Roberts, Z. Krenova, A.M. Trentacosti, and M.J.S. Miller. 2000. Cat's claw inhibits TNFα production and scavenges free radicals: role in cytoprotection. *Free Radic. Biol. Med.* 29:71–78.

Sandoval, M., N.N. Okuhama, M. Clark, F.M. Angeles, J. Lao, S.A. Bustamante, and M.J.S. Miller. 2002a. Sangre de grado Croton palanostigma induces apoptosis in human gastrointestinal cancer cells. *J. Ethnopharmacol.* 80:121–129.

Sandoval, M., N.N. Okuhama, X.-J. Zhang, L.A. Condezo, J. Lao, F.M. Angeles, P. Bobrowski, and M.J.S. Miller. 2002b. Anti-inflammatory and antioxidant activities of cat's claw (*Uncaria tomentosa* and *Uncaria guianensis*) are independent of their alkaloid content. *Phytomedicine* 9:325–337.

Sandoval-Chacon, M., J.H. Thompson, X. Liu, E.E. Mannick, H. Sadowska-Krowicka, R. Charbonnet, D.A. Clark, and M.J.S. Miller. 1998. Anti-inflammatory actions of cat's claw: the role of NF-κB. *Aliment. Pharmacol. Ther.* 12:1279–1289.

Schmelz, M. 2001. A neural pathway for itch. *Nature Neurosci.* 4:9–10.

Ubillas, R. 1994. SP-303, an antiviral oligomeric proanthocyanidin from the latex of *Croton lechleri* (sangre de drago). *Phytomedicine* 1:77–106.

Vaisberg, A.J., M. Milla, M.C. Planas, J.L. Cordova, E. Rosas de Augusti, R. Ferreyra, M.C. Mustinga, L. Carlin, and G.B. Hammond. 1989. Taspine is the cicatrizant principle in sangre de grado extracted from *Croton lechleri. Planta Med.* 55:140–143.

Yepez, A.M., O.L. de Ugaz, C.M. Alvarez, V. De Feo, R. Aquino, F. De Simone, and C. Pizza. 1991. Quinovic acid glycosides from *Uncaria guianensis. Phytochemistry* 30:1635–1637.

Chapter 3
Botanicals for Pigs

Palmer J. Holden

Introduction

Most drugs used in food animals have specific well-established purposes: to treat or prevent infections, to enhance growth, or to fight parasites. Antibiotics are among the few classes of drugs used in food animals both therapeutically to treat disease and subtherapeutically to enhance performance and efficiency of feed utilization (National Academy Press, 1999). Since their introduction in the early 1950s, commercial antimicrobial products have been widely utilized by U.S. livestock producers at subtherapeutic rates in feed to enhance growth rate and feed efficiency. Although the mechanism(s) of action of antibiotics has not been conclusively determined, repeated experiments have demonstrated continued effectiveness of these compounds at subtherapeutic levels in swine feeds (Hayes and Black, 1981; Zimmerman, 1986). The 1995 National Animal Health Monitoring System (NAHMS, 1995) survey reported that 92.7% of growing-finishing swine received growth promotant products in their feed. As a result of their enhanced specificity and predictability, synthetic pharmaceutical products have replaced traditional herbal remedies as the mainstay therapeutic regimens in modern human and animal medicine although alternative remedies are making a comeback.

Widespread usage of human therapeutic antimicrobials at subtherapeutic levels in animal feeds has been criticized (Holmberg, et al., 1984; May, 1994). Development of antibiotic resistant microbial populations in animals, which could be transferred to humans by contact or through the food chain, has been a concern investigated by two National Academy of Science (NAS) committees. Although the studies showed that no link between antibiotic resistant microbes in animals and transference to humans could be proven, concerns still exist in the medical community about this potential risk. Not medicating animals also poses the risks of the animals developing diseases, increased loss or morbidity, and decreased growth rate and efficiency.

Concerns regarding the development of resistant bacteria in animals have encouraged interest in finding alternatives to feed additives. This issue has resulted in a segment of consumers who prefer to eat meat from animals that have not been fed or treated with antibiotics. Thus, there is an impetus to find other "natural" products that can be used in pork production to encourage performance yet not develop resistant organisms.

The use of botanical products (herbs) for inclusion in swine diets to improve growth rate, feed efficiency, and carcass characteristics has not been investigated, although the known pharmacological properties of selected botanicals make them candidates for improvement of growth rates and feed utilization.

Historically, a wide range of cultures have used herbal remedies. Prior to the development of sulfonamides and penicillin at the beginning of the 20th century, botanically based products represented a major source of medication against a wide range of infectious and chronic diseases. Selected herbs are known to possess natural antimicrobial activity and other characteristics that could be useful in value-added (natural) animal protein production. This area of investigation has not undergone substantive examination because commercial antimicrobial products are relatively of low cost, have proven effectiveness, and are readily available. The possibility of developing significant antibiotic resistant bacteria through the use of human drugs in animals and subsequent transfer of resistance to human pathogens has caused concerns within the medical community. Inclusion of herbs in animal feeds as alternative growth promotion and efficiency stimulating strategies can address some of these concerns while producing a more holistically grown pork product.

Some researchers have maintained an interest in botanicals for inclusion in "holistic" preventative regimen (Ellingwood, 1983). These characteristics have been researched and reported in several texts chronicling herbal medical applications (Tyler, et al., 1976). The effectiveness of botanical products in conjunction with modern livestock production practices has not been reported. Table 3.1 lists a variety of plants and the potential response of the plant parts to ingestion by livestock.

Alternative products are available that may possess growth enhancing activity similar to that of current subtherapeutic antibiotics. And these likely would not produce antibiotic resistance to human therapeutic agents while offering pork producers an alternative mechanism to maintain production efficiency and to alleviate consumer and the medical community fears about antibiotic resistance development. Based on historical data and human medicinal experiences, selected botanicals afford such a potential substitution opportunity. Limited information about use of botanicals in livestock production ('de Bairacli Levy, 1991) makes this evaluation timely and potentially beneficial.

Studies were undertaken to evaluate the use of four botanicals, which can be effectively grown in Iowa, for swine production as substitutes for commercial, synthetic growth promotants in swine diets. These botanicals are garlic (*Allium sativum*), Echinacea (*Echinacea purpurea*), peppermint (*Mentha piperita*), and goldenseal (*Hydrastis canadensis*).

Echinacea (purple coneflower)

Echinacea species are perennial herbs capable of being grown throughout the Midwestern United States. There are nine species, but *Echinacea augustifolia*, *E. purpurea*, and *Echinacea pallida* are most commonly considered for medicinal purposes (McGregor, 1968). The whole plant, including aerial portions and taproots, has been utilized. Additionally, pressed juice from the aerial portion of *E. purpurea* and aqueous and alcohol extracts of the roots have viral inhibition characteristics in cell culture (Wacker and Hilbig, 1978). The German government has approved oral use of Echinacea for respiratory and urinary tract infections in humans and topically for improving wound healing. Liquid preparations have been shown to have immune-stimulating activity and enhance several white blood cell types as well as phagocytes, cells that can destroy bacteria and protozoa (Burton Goldberg Group, 1999).

Garlic (*A. sativum*)

Garlic, a member of the lily family, is a perennial plant cultivated worldwide. Garlic bulbs, either fresh or dehydrated, are used for medicinal purposes. The bulbs contain volatile oils composed of allicin, diallyl disulfide, and diallyl trisulfide, which are considered the reservoirs for most pharmacological

Table 3.1 Plant parts and the potential responses to ingestion of the parts by livestock

Plant	Parts	Increase appetite	Increase digestion	Decrease diarrhea	Decrease inflammation	Antiseptic	Antioxidant	Antibacterial
Basil	Leaf		•			•		•
Cinnamon	Bark	•	•			•	•	•
Garlic	Bulb		•			•	•	•
Mustard	Seed		•			•		•
Parsley	Leaf		•			•		
Peppermint	Leaf	•	•	•	•	•		•
Rosemary	Leaf		•			•	•	•
Sage	Leaf		•			•	•	•
Thyme	Whole plant	•	•				•	•

BISHOP BURTON COLLEGE
LIBRARY

properties attributable to garlic. Garlic demonstrates a broad spectrum of antimicrobial activity against many bacteria, viruses, parasites, and fungi (Hughes and Lawson, 1991). Garlic has also shown an ability to aid certain immune functions, particularly increasing natural killer cells' activity (Foster, 1991).

Goldenseal (*H. canadensis*)

Goldenseal, native to eastern North America, is a perennial herb. The most pharmacologically active isoquinolone alkaloid, berberine, is concentrated in the rhizome and roots. Berberine has been demonstrated to possess antimicrobial, immunostimulatory, anticonvulsant, sedative, hypotensive, choleretic, and carminative properties. This antimicrobial property has been demonstrated against a wide range of bacteria, protozoa, and fungi (Duke, 1985). Berberine and berberine-containing plants are generally considered nontoxic. The LD50 for berberine in rats was reported as greater than 1,000 mg per kilogram body weight (Hladon, 1975).

Peppermint (*M. piperita*)

Peppermint grows under a wide range of conditions. The most popular varieties are black peppermint (*M. piperita var. vulgaris*) and white peppermint (*M. piperita var. officinalics*). The major medicinal components of peppermint are the volatile oils found predominantly in the aerial portions of the plant. The principal components of these oils are terpenoids, menthol, methone, and menthyl acetate. Other components that may have pharmaceutical properties include polyplenols, flavonoids, and betaine.

Menthol possesses carminative (gas relieving), antispasmodic, and cholerectic properties. Peppermint and other members of the mint family have demonstrated significant antiviral capability including treatment of common cold (Kerman and Kucera, 1967). Peppermint also inhibits antimicrobial activity against *Streptococcus pyogenes*, *Staphylococcus aureus*, *Pseudomonas aeruginosa*, and *Candida albicans* (Sanyal and Varma, 1969). The LD50 of menthol in rats is 3,280 mg/kg and a fatal dose for humans was reported as 1 g/kg. Hypersensitivity reactions (skin rashes) have also been reported (Briggs, 1993).

Experimental design

These experiments were conducted at the Iowa State University Swine Nutrition and Management Center in temperature-regulated nursery rooms. Graded levels of these botanicals were fed to weanling pigs and compared to a standard nursery diet containing 45 parts per million (ppm) Mecadox (Carbadox, Phibro Animal Health). Pigs were weaned at an average of 18 days (14–21) and 6.25 kg (5.15–7.85) and allotted at random to pens by litter and initial weight immediately after weaning. There were 20 or 24 pens of five pigs each, providing 4–6 replications of the dietary treatments. Each pen received a prestarter treatment diet of 16 kg per pig and then the pigs werer switched to the starter treatment diet for the remainder of the 5-week study (Tables 3.2 and 3.3). The positive control diet contained 45 ppm of Mecadox. Botanical treatments consisted of the same diet without Mecadox and increasing levels of botanicals replaced corn, with the 0% level considered the negative control.

Table 3.2 Example diets (%)

Ingredient	Prestarter	Starter
Corn, yellow	36.43	51.57
Whey, dried	25.00	10.00
Appetein	5.00	0.00
Soybean meal, dehulled	29.20	33.50
Dicalcium phosphate	1.65	2.19
Limestone	0.90	0.78
Salt	0.00	0.25
Lysine, synthetic	0.20	0.20
Methionine, DL	0.10	0.10
Vitamins, trace minerals	0.52	0.41
Animal fat, stabilized	1.00	1.00
Mecadox 2.5/botanical	–	–
Total	100.00	100.00

Pigs were grown in 1.2×1.2 meter raised-deck pens and the average room temperature was $24 \pm 2°C$. Heat mats supplied supplemental heat. Pigs were weighed and feed disappearance measured weekly for 5 weeks. In the first year (1997) of studies the project was completed at the end of the nursery phase. In 1999–2000, when the Echinacea, garlic, and peppermint studies were repeated, upon completion of the nursery phase pigs were fed the standard farm grower feed containing Tylan at 36 ppm (Tylosin, Elanco Animal Health) and finisher containing bacitracin methylene dislicylate (BMD) at 27 ppm (Alpharma, Inc.) diets. Grower-finisher medications were included because of an ileitis infection present on the farm. Post-nursery weights were recorded every 4 weeks to evaluate long term effects of the nursery treatments. We measured the average daily gain (ADG), average daily feed (ADF), and feed efficiency (F/G), which is the amount of feed consumed by the pigs divided by the amount of weight gain (F/G) of the pigs every week.

Where appropriate, one pig at the end of the nursery phase from each botanical treatment was taken to the ISU Meat Laboratory, slaughtered, and various muscles evaluated for sensory and quality characteristics. Pigs fed Mecadox were not slaughtered at this time because of a 42-day withdrawal requirement.

Between the first set of trials (1997–1998) and the second set (1999–2000) the farm was depopulated and repopulated. The herd has a high health status, including porcine respiratory and reproductive syndrome (PRRS) free. This health status may have reduced the need for medications in the nursery.

The ADG, ADF, and F/G data were analyzed using a statistical procedure called the general linear models procedure in the statistical analysis system (SAS, 1996) with the pen as the experimental unit. We report the least square means for the measured variables in the tables. Unless the reader is

Table 3.3 Calculated analysis of example diets (%)

Nutrient	Prestarter	Starter
Lysine	1.46	1.28
Methionine+cystine	0.88	0.66
Calcium	0.79	0.79
Phosphorus, total	0.72	0.70

familiar with statistical analysis of replicated experiments, the tables and the interpretation of the data can be confusing.

Given below is a brief layperson's guide to the statistics and interpretation of our data. We include this to help the reader understand the experimental results. There is much natural variation in the rate of weight gain and feed consumption among pigs. This variation is the reason we have four to six replications of our feed treatments for each experiment. We need the replications so we can distinguish between natural variation in weight gain and feed consumption, and the effect of our medicinal treatments on weight gain and feed consumption. Because of the natural variation among pigs, we often need the average weight gain value for a feed treatment be at least 10% different than the average weight gain of another feed treatment before we can declare that a particular feed treatment is significantly better or worse than another treatment. The reader will notice that many of the results for ADG, ADF, and F/G shown in the tables later in the chapter were not considered statistically significant. For example, in Table 3.4 in weeks 0–2, the ADG varied from a high of

Table 3.4 Effect of Echinacea on ADG, ADF consumption, and F/G or feed to weight gain ratio for pigs in experiment I

	Mecadox (0.0045%)	Echinacea levels (%)			
		0.0	0.1	0.5	2.0
		Week 0–1			
ADG, kg	0.11	0.11	0.10	0.11	0.10
ADF, kg	0.21	0.23	0.21	0.20	0.19
F/G	2.06	2.08	1.98	1.85	2.04
		Weeks 0–2			
ADG, kg	0.20	0.16	0.17	0.18	0.17
ADF, kg	0.33	0.31	0.29	0.29	0.29
F/G[a,b]	1.62	1.93	1.71	1.62	1.65
		Weeks 0–3			
ADG, kg[c]	0.25	0.22	0.23	0.24	0.24
ADF, kg	0.41	0.39	0.38	0.38	0.39
F/G[d]	1.66	1.79	1.65	1.57	1.59
		Weeks 0–4			
ADG, kg[e]	0.32	0.29	0.30	0.30	0.31
ADF, kg	0.51	0.49	0.48	0.48	0.50
F/G[e,f]	1.60	1.71	1.62	1.58	1.58
		Weeks 0–5			
ADG, kg	0.38	0.35	0.35	0.36	0.37
ADF, kg	0.64	0.61	0.59	0.60	0.61
F/G[g]	1.65	1.73	1.68	1.65	1.66

[a] Mecadox had significantly greater F/G than 0.0% Echinacea.
[b] 0.0% Echinacea had significantly lower F/G than 0.1%, 0.5%, and 2.0% Echinacea.
[c] Mecadox had significantly greater ADG than 0.0% Echinacea.
[d] 0.0% Echinacea had significantly lower F/G than 0.5% and 2.0% Echinacea.
[e] Mecadox had significantly greater F/G than 0.0% Echinacea.
[f] 0.0% Echinacea had significantly lower F/G than 0.1%, 0.5%, and 2.0% Echinacea.
[g] Mecadox had significantly greater F/G than 0.0% and 0.1% Echinacea.
There was no significant difference in ADG, ADF, and F/G values for treatments without a superscript. No significant difference indicates that the natural variation of the weight gain, feed consumption, and feed efficiency of the pigs was as great as the variation caused by the feed treatments.

0.20 kg per day for the Mecadox treated feed to a low of 0.16 kg per day for the feed treated with no added Echinacea, but there were no statistically significant differences in ADG for any of the treatments because the differences in ADG that we measured were not greater than the natural variation in the weight gained for the individual pigs in each treament.

Results of the experiments

Echinacea I

We show all the data for the first Echinacea experiment in Table 3.4. At the tested inclusion levels (0, 0.1, 0.5, and 2.0%) no statistical advantage existed when compared with the diet containing 45 ppm Mecadox or with a "negative" control containing no antimicrobial or botanical inclusions (Table 3.4). The results showed that in weeks 0–3 and 0–4 the higher levels of Echinacea (0.5 and 2.0%) were significantly more efficient but daily gain and feed intake were not statistically affected. Total performance for the entire experiment, weeks 0–5, was not statistically different. These data suggest higher levels of Echinacea enhanced feed efficiency compared to the 0% Echinacea during the first 2 weeks and were greater than the Mecadox diet during the weeks 0–3 and 0–4. Echinacea-treated pigs exhibited a slight, but not objectionable, off-flavor when compared to pigs fed noninclusion levels. Overall, the performance was similar, suggesting minimal subclinical stress during this experiment. Higher levels of Echinacea may be required to enhance growth rate and feed efficiency.

Echinacea II

Our second trial evaluated lower levels than were used in the Echinacea I experiment. The objective was to reduce the cost of the Echinacea additive and potentially maintain some of the observed feed efficiencies. Mecadox or Echinacea (0, 0.10, 0.25, and 0.50%) replaced corn. One pig was removed during the nursery phase and one during the finishing phase. Reported data are cumulative from the start of the experiment (Table 3.5). In week 1 there were no statistical differences, indicating similar performance between the treatments. Subsequent performance indicated no advantage for feeding Echinacea with the exception of Weeks 0–2 and 0–3 when a significant quadratic observation was made for the Echinacea levels for feed/gain. The Mecadox diet had significantly better performance than the treatment levels of Echinacea in weeks 0–2, 0–3, 0–4, and 0–5. Growth rate during the postnursery phase was not affected by nursery treatments. These lower levels of Echinacea failed to enhance performance.

Echinacea III

This third Echinacea trial was initiated to explore higher levels of Echinacea. Mecadox (45 ppm) or Echinacea (0, 1.5, and 3.0%) replaced corn. No pigs were removed during the nursery phase. During the grow-finish phase one poor-doer was removed from the Mecadox treatment and a ruptured pig was removed from the 3% Echinacea treatment. There were few treatment differences (Table 3.6). Mecadox generally increased daily gain in weeks 0–3 and 0–5. Echinacea additions depressed feed/gain in weeks 0–2 and 0–3. However, 3% Echinacea enhanced overall gain in the week 0–5 nursery period when compared to 0 and 1.5% levels and supported gains equal to the Mecadox diet. No significant gain responses were observed postnursery although the highest level of Echinacea

Table 3.5 Effect of Echinacea on ADG, ADF consumption, and F/G or feed to weight gain ratio for pigs in experiment II

	Mecadox (0.0045%)	Echinacea levels (%)			
		0.00	0.10	0.25	0.50
		Week 1			
ADG, kg	0.12	0.14	0.11	0.12	0.10
ADF, kg	0.18	0.22	0.19	0.18	0.17
F/G	1.59	1.52	1.67	1.64	1.64
		Weeks 0–2			
ADG, kg[a]	0.17	0.16	0.12	0.15	0.16
ADF, kg	0.24	0.24	0.24	0.23	0.23
F/G[b,c]	1.39	1.52	2.08	1.59	1.49
		Weeks 0–3			
ADG, kg[b]	0.30	0.27	0.23	0.26	0.27
ADF, kg	0.39	0.37	0.36	0.36	0.36
F/G[c]	1.32	1.35	1.52	1.39	1.33
		Weeks 0–4			
ADG, kg	0.38	0.32	0.31	0.33	0.32
ADF, kg	0.53	0.48	0.48	0.48	0.46
F/G[b]	1.39	1.49	1.52	1.43	1.47
		Weeks 0–5			
ADG, kg[b]	0.45	0.41	0.40	0.40	0.39
ADF, kg	0.65	0.60	0.60	0.59	0.58
F/G[b]	1.45	1.45	1.52	1.49	1.49
ADG, kg					
Weeks 0–9	0.60	0.59	0.58	0.54	0.58
Weeks 0–13	0.68	0.65	0.67	0.66	0.65
Weeks 0–17	0.77	0.75	0.77	0.75	0.73

[a] Mecadox had significantly greater ADG than the average value for 0.10%, 0.25%, and 0.50% Echinacea.
[b] Mecadox had significantly greater ADG or lower F/G than average value for 0.0%, 0.10%, 0.25%, and 0.50% Echinacea.
[c] Echinacea produced a significant increase and then a significant decrease (quadratic response) in F/G.

fed during the nursery supported gains equal to those of the Mecadox pigs. Neither Mecadox nor Echinacea was fed after the nursery period.

Garlic I

At the tested garlic inclusions (0, 0.5, 2.5, and 5%), increasing levels of garlic generally depressed feed intake and average daily gain in nursery pigs and depressed performance compared to the Mecadox diet (Table 3.7). The overall summary, weeks 0–5, indicated the Mecadox diet significantly improved daily gain compared to the garlic treatments; generally the higher the level of garlic, the poorer the daily gain. Mecadox ADF was significantly greater than the 5% level of garlic. Overall feed efficiency favored the 0% garlic diet, but was statistically different only from the 2.5% garlic treatment.

The 5.0% level of garlic significantly reduced feed intake in weeks 0–2, 0–3, and 0–5 when compared to Mecadox. Additionally, in weeks 0–3 as the level of garlic increased, feed intake decreased.

Table 3.6 Effect of Echinacea on ADG, ADF consumption, and F/G or feed to weight gain ratio for pigs in experiment III

	Mecadox (0.0045%)	Echinacea levels (%)		
		0.0	1.5	3.0
		Week 0–1		
ADG, kg	0.09	0.09	0.06	0.07
ADF, kg	0.15	0.16	0.15	0.15
F/G	1.82	1.82	2.70	2.22
		Weeks 0–2		
ADG, kg	0.16	0.15	0.14	0.13
ADF, kg	0.22	0.23	0.22	0.22
F/G[a]	1.41	1.56	1.61	1.64
		Weeks 0–3		
ADG, kg[b,c]	0.25	0.23	0.22	0.24
ADF, kg	0.34	0.34	0.32	0.33
F/G[b,c]	1.33	1.43	1.47	1.39
		Weeks 0–4		
ADG, kg	0.30	0.29	0.27	0.29
ADF, kg	0.43	0.42	0.41	0.42
F/G	1.39	1.45	1.52	1.43
		Weeks 0–5		
ADG, kg[c]	0.37	0.35	0.34	0.37
ADF, kg	0.53	0.53	0.5	0.54
F/G	1.45	1.52	1.47	1.47
		Weeks 0–9		
ADG, kg	0.54	0.53	0.52	0.56
		Weeks 0–13		
ADG, kg	0.63	0.61	0.60	0.65
		Weeks 0–17		
ADG, kg	0.73	0.71	0.71	0.75

[a] Echinacea produced a significant linear increase in F/G.
[b] Mecadox had significantly greater ADG or lower F/G than average value for 0%, 1.5% and 3.0% Echinacea.
[c] Echinacea produced a significant increase and then a significant decrease (quadratic response) in ADG or F/G.

Muscle samples from all slaughtered pigs had "very objectionable" or "extremely objectionable" off-flavors (Table 3.8). This suggests that the garlic odor was sufficiently strong in the room that it also flavored muscle samples of pigs not fed garlic. A visitor's first observation was that the room and adjacent hallway had a very strong, objectionable odor of garlic combined with hog manure throughout the nursery phase.

Garlic II

The second garlic trial fed inclusion levels of 0.00, 0.10, 0.25, and 0.50% garlic, levels that we hoped would be low enough not to depress performance or alter meat flavors. Pigs fed diets without Mecadox demonstrated significantly poorer performance (Table 3.9). Based upon this and the 1997

Table 3.7 Effect of garlic on ADG, ADF consumption, and F/G or feed to weight gain ratio for pigs in experiment I

	Mecadox (0.0045%)	Garlic levels (%)			
		0.0	0.5	2.5	5.0
		Week 0–1			
ADG, kg	0.11	0.07	0.09	0.09	0.03
ADF, kg	0.19	0.17	0.18	0.18	0.15
F/G	1.84	0.88	3.04	−0.50	4.19
		Weeks 0–2			
ADG, kg[a]	0.27	0.23	0.21	0.21	0.17
ADF, kg[a]	0.36	0.32	0.31	0.30	0.25
F/G	1.34	1.42	1.51	1.56	1.45
		Weeks 0–3			
ADG, kg[b,c]	0.34	0.24	0.26	0.24	0.22
ADF, kg[d]	0.50	0.44	0.42	0.41	0.35
F/G	1.48	1.90	1.66	1.80	1.65
		Weeks 0–4			
ADG, kg	0.38	0.32	0.31	0.51	0.27
ADF, kg	0.61	0.53	0.53	0.96	0.47
F/G[e]	1.60	1.67	1.72	1.91	1.74
		Weeks 0–5			
ADG, kg[f]	0.45	0.39	0.38	0.34	0.35
ADF, kg[g]	0.74	0.61	0.68	0.62	0.58
F/G[h]	1.66	1.56	1.81	1.88	1.65

[a] Mecadox had significantly greater ADG and ADF than 5.0% garlic.
[b] Mecadox had significantly greater ADG than average value for 0.0%, 0.5%, and 2.5% garlic.
[c] Mecadox had significantly greater ADG than 5.0% garlic.
[d] Mecadox had significantly greater ADF than 2.5% and 5.0% garlic and 0.0% garlic was significantly greater than 5.0% garlic.
[e] Mecadox had a significantly lower F/G than garlic at 2.5%.
[f] Mecadox had a significantly greater ADG than 0.5%, 2.0%, and 5.0% garlic.
[g] Mecadox had a significantly greater ADF than 5.0% garlic.
[h] Garlic at 0.0% had a significantly greater F/G than 2.5% garlic.

Table 3.8 Effect of garlic on the flavor of pig muscle in experiment I[a]

	Garlic levels (%)			
	0.0	0.5	2.5	5.0
Flavor score	1.33	1.00	1.33	1.00
Off-flavor score	4.33	5.33	7.00	9.33
Off-flavors[b]	Sour	VO	VO	EO

[a] Flavor score is from 1 to 10 with low scores indicating less flavor. Off-flavor score is from 1 to 10 with low values indicating no or small off-flavors.
[b] VO = very objectionable; EO = extremely objectionable.

Table 3.9 Effect of garlic on ADG, ADF consumption, and F/G or feed to weight gain ratio for pigs in experiment II

	Mecadox (0.0045%)	Garlic levels (%)			
		0.00	0.10	0.25	0.50
Initial weight, kg	7.0	6.7	6.8	7.0	7.1
5-week weight, kg	22.9	20.5	21.0	21.2	20.3
17-week weight, kg	96.4	95.2	97.1	97.1	93.6
Week 0–1					
ADG, kg	0.15	0.13	0.16	0.12	0.14
ADF, kg	0.23	0.21	0.24	0.22	0.21
F/G	1.49	1.64	1.54	1.85	1.52
Weeks 0–2					
ADG, kg	0.18	0.15	0.16	0.16	0.13
ADF, kg	0.30	0.26	0.28	0.29	0.26
F/G	1.67	1.82	1.75	1.82	1.96
Weeks 0–3					
ADG, kg[a]	0.31	0.26	0.26	0.26	0.24
ADF, kg[a]	0.44	0.38	0.39	0.41	0.37
F/G[b]	1.41	1.45	1.52	1.56	1.54
Weeks 0–4					
ADG, kg[a]	0.39	0.33	0.34	0.33	0.30
ADF, kg[a]	0.58	0.49	0.51	0.51	0.48
F/G[c]	1.47	1.49	1.49	1.54	1.56
Weeks 0–5					
ADG, kg[a]	0.46	0.40	0.41	0.41	0.38
ADF, kg[a]	0.68	0.57	0.61	0.62	0.57
F/G	1.49	1.47	1.52	1.52	1.52
ADG, kg					
Weeks 0–9	0.59	0.55	0.57	0.58	0.52
Weeks 0–13	0.68	0.66	0.67	0.69	0.63
Weeks 0–17	0.77	0.76	0.78	0.78	0.75

[a] Mecadox had a significantly greater ADG or ADF than average value for 0.0%, 0.10%, 0.25%, and 0.50% garlic.
[b] Mecadox had a significantly lower F/G than average value for 0.0%, 0.10%, 0.25%, and 0.50% garlic.
[c] Garlic had a significant linear increase in F/G.

study, pigs fed diets with Mecadox performed better. The addition of garlic did not enhance pig performance. Because of the garlic flavoring of the pork in the first garlic study (Table 3.8) muscle samples were tested at the end of the nursery period and again 2 weeks later. At the end of the nursery phase, a slight garlic flavor was detected in muscle but after 2 weeks on a garlic-free diet no garlic flavor was detected (Table 3.10).

Goldenseal I

This study evaluated four levels of goldenseal (0.0–1.0%) to a diet containing Mecadox (Table 3.11). Although not performing to the level of the Mecadox-fed pigs, those fed 0.25% and 1.00% goldenseal diets performed numerically better than those fed 0.00% and 0.05% goldenseal diets.

Table 3.10 Effect of garlic on flavor of pig muscle in Experiment II[a]. End of nursery trial results

	Garlic (%)			
	0.00	0.10	0.25	0.50
Flavor score	1.0	1.0	1.0	1.0
Off-flavor score	5.0	4.7	3.7	3.3
Off-flavor	Sour liver,	Sour liver,	Sour liver,	Sour, metallic
Garlic score	1.0	1.0	2.0	1.0
After 2 weeks of no garlic in diet[a]				
Garlic, %	0.00			0.50
Flavor score	1.7			1.3
Off-flavor score	3.3			4.0
Off-flavor	Sour, liver, metallic			Sour, liver
Garlic score	1.0			1.0

[a] Flavor score is from 1 to 10 with low scores indicating less flavor.
Off-flavor score is from 1 to 10 with low values indicating no or small off-flavors.

Table 3.11 Effect of goldenseal on ADG, ADF consumption, and F/G or feed to weight gain ratio for pigs in experiment I

	Mecadox (0.0045%)	Goldenseal (%)			
		0.00	0.05	0.25	1.00
		Week 0–1			
ADG, kg[a]	0.12	0.08	0.09	0.11	0.10
ADF, kg	0.19	0.20	0.22	0.21	0.20
F/G	1.60	7.14	3.62	1.96	2.22
		Weeks 0–2			
ADG, kg[a]	0.27	0.21	0.22	0.22	0.21
ADF, kg[b]	0.39	0.36	0.33	0.34	0.33
F/G[c]	1.22	1.85	1.89	1.61	1.70
		Weeks 0–3			
ADG, kg[d]	0.32	0.26	0.24	0.28	0.26
ADF, kg[a,e]	0.51	0.47	0.43	0.45	0.43
F/G[f]	1.38	1.92	2.09	1.66	1.69
		Weeks 0–4			
ADG, kg[c]	0.37	0.32	0.31	0.33	0.33
ADF, kg	0.60	0.56	0.53	0.54	0.53
F/G[g]	1.46	1.88	2.00	1.65	1.63

[a] Mecadox had a significantly greater ADG or ADF than 0.00% goldenseal
[b] Mecadox had a significantly greater ADF than 0.05%, 0.25%, and 1.00% goldenseal
[c] Mecadox had a significantly greater ADG or lower F/G than 0.00% and 0.05% goldenseal
[d] Mecadox had a significantly greater ADG than 0.00%, 0.25%, 0.05%, and 1.00% goldenseal
[e] Mecadox had a significantly greater ADF than 0.05%, 0.25%, and 1.00% goldenseal
[f] Mecadox had a significantly lower F/G than 0.00% and 0.05% goldenseal
[g] Mecadox had a significantly lower F/G than 0.00%, 0.25%, 0.05%, and 1.00% goldenseal

Mecadox-fed pigs generally performed statistically better than the other treatments. Increasing levels of goldenseal did not influence the muscle characteristics evaluated.

Some F/Gs appear unreasonable because of an occasional pen with very poor gains with normal or high feed intakes. The Mecadox diet in week 1 produced daily gains greater than the 0.00% goldenseal diet and feed intake greater than the 0.05% goldenseal. This suggests additions of goldenseal produced performance comparable to the Mecadox pigs during the first week. During weeks 0–2 the Mecadox diet ADG was significantly greater than the 0.00% diet and tended to be greater than the three higher levels of goldenseal. Mecadox F/G was improved over the 0.00% and 0.05% goldenseal but not statistically different from the higher levels.

Weeks 0–3 had significantly greater ADG and ADF for the Mecadox pigs over the other treatments. The ADF of the two highest levels of goldenseal tended to be greater than the 0.00% negative control. F/G for Mecadox-fed pigs was not statistically different from the two highest levels of goldenseal and significantly greater than the 0.00 and 0.05% diets, with the two highest levels also having improved efficiency compared to the 0.05% diet. During weeks 0–4 the Mecadox diet ADG was significantly higher than the 0.00% and 0.05% goldenseal diets ($P < 0.05$). Overall feed efficiency was lowest for the Mecadox diet when compared to the 0.00% and 0.05% treatments but not statistically different from the two highest level. The two highest levels tended to be more efficient than the 0.00% and 0.05% goldenseal diets.

Peppermint I

Nursery pigs fed inclusion levels of peppermint (0, 0.5, 2.5, and 5.0%) failed to respond to the added levels (Table 3.12). Pigs on all treatments (including the Mecadox and 0% peppermint) performed similarly over the entire experimental period. The pigs fed the 5% peppermint diet in week 1 required significantly more feed per pound of gain than the pigs fed Mecadox, probably because of the bulkiness of that diet. During weeks 0–2 the pigs on the control diet (0%) required significantly more feed than the pigs fed Mecadox and 2.5% peppermint. Generally the pigs fed both Mecadox and peppermint performed similarly during this period. No statistical differences were observed after the first 2 weeks.

Peppermint II

This experiment evaluated Mecadox and 0, 0.5, and 1.0% peppermint levels under a similar feeding regimen plus a 12-week postnursery to observe any carry-over effects (Table 3.13). Peppermint failed to elicit a positive nursery response and those pigs performed more poorly statistically when compared to the Mecadox-fed pigs. Pigs fed Mecadox maintained their advantage when cumulative performance was evaluated for the additional 12 weeks, but performance within each weighing period was not statistically different after the nursery phase. Under the conditions of this experiment peppermint, as in the Peppermint I experiment, was not an efficacious addition to swine nursery diets.

Summary

The historic use of herbal remedies to treat and prevent infectious disease has been supplanted with the emergence of specific man-made chemotherapeutic and antibacterial agents. However, selected herbs are known to naturally possess antibacterial and other characteristics, which could

Table 3.12 Effect of peppermint on ADG, ADF consumption, and F/G or feed to weight gain ratio for pigs in experiment I

	Mecadox (0.0045%)	Peppermint (%)			
		0.00	0.50	2.50	5.00
		Week 1			
ADG, kg	0.12	0.10	0.10	0.09	0.07
ADF, kg	0.22	0.24	0.22	0.20	0.17
F/G[a]	1.85	2.54	2.22	2.46	3.18
		Weeks 0–2			
ADG, kg	0.18	0.16	0.18	0.18	0.15
ADF, kg	0.30	0.31	0.34	0.29	0.27
F/G[b]	1.68	1.98	1.83	1.67	1.76
		Weeks 0–3			
ADG, kg	0.23	0.20	0.23	0.24	0.21
ADF, kg	0.41	0.39	0.44	0.41	0.40
F/G	1.82	1.95	1.95	1.76	1.94
		Weeks 0–4			
ADG, kg	0.27	0.26	0.29	0.27	0.26
ADF, kg	0.50	0.48	0.54	0.49	0.51
F/G	1.85	1.88	1.88	1.77	1.92
		Weeks 0–5			
ADG, kg	0.33	0.30	0.33	0.32	0.30
ADF, kg	0.62	0.58	0.64	0.58	0.62
F/G	1.89	1.91	1.94	1.81	2.04

[a] Mecadox had a significantly lower F/G than 5.0% peppermint.
[b] Mecadox had a significantly lower F/G than 0.0% goldenseal and goldenseal at 2.5% had a significantly lower F/G than 0.0%.

be useful in animal protein production. The possibility of significant antibiotic-resistant bacteria development through the use of human drugs in animals and subsequent transfer of this resistance to human pathogens has caused concerns within the medical community. Inclusion of herbs in animal feeds as alternative growth promotion and efficiency stimulating strategies can address these concerns.

The pharmacological properties of some herbs provide an opportunity for growth rate and feed efficiency advantages, and to reduce the potential for selection of microbes resistant to therapeutics used in human medicine. Garlic, Echinacea, and goldenseal possess known antibacterial properties. Peppermint demonstrates carminative (intestinal gas relieving) and cholerectic (acute diarrhea) effects that may improve the digestive process. Such characteristics make these herbs potentially effective in improved feed utilization and growth stimulation in young swine.

A goal of this project is the development of value-added pork products, which can be grown by Iowa producers utilizing homegrown, naturally occurring, environmentally friendly feed additives. The four selected herbs are capable of being grown effectively in Iowa. These alternative crops can be grown with minimal capital investment and are unaffected by many common agronomic pests. Such characteristics would enable Iowa swine producers to grow their own natural growth promotants for inclusion in swine diets. The benefits of reduced synthetic growth promotant usage and of the potential for development of a differentiable retail pork make the examination of these botanicals of

Table 3.13 Effect of peppermint on ADG, ADF consumption, and F/G or feed to weight gain ratio for pigs in experiment II

	Mecadox (0.0045%)	Peppermint levels (%)			
		0.00	0.25	0.50	1.00
		Week 0–1			
ADG, kg	0.06	0.04	0.03	0.03	0.04
ADF, kg[a]	0.14	0.14	0.11	0.11	0.13
F/G	2.38	3.57	4.17	3.45	3.45
		Weeks 0–2			
ADG, kg[b]	0.18	0.13	0.14	0.13	0.12
ADF, kg[b]	0.25	0.23	0.20	0.19	0.20
F/G[a,c]	1.43	1.72	1.43	1.52	1.67
		Weeks 0–3			
ADG, kg[b]	0.29	0.24	0.23	0.21	0.22
ADF, kg[b]	0.40	0.35	0.31	0.30	0.33
F/G[a]	1.35	1.47	1.39	1.43	1.49
		Weeks 0–4			
ADG, kg[b]	0.36	0.29	0.28	0.28	0.27
ADF, kg[b]	0.52	0.44	0.41	0.42	0.43
F/G	1.45	1.52	1.49	1.52	1.61
		Weeks 0–5			
ADG, kg[b]	0.43	0.38	0.36	0.36	0.35
ADF, kg[b]	0.64	0.58	0.54	0.54	0.56
F/G	1.49	1.52	1.47	1.52	1.61
ADG, kg					
Weeks 0–9[b]	0.53	0.49	0.48	0.48	0.46
Weeks 0–13[b]	0.61	0.57	0.57	0.55	0.55
Weeks 0–17[b]	0.70	0.68	0.67	0.65	0.61

[a] Mecadox had a significantly greater ADF than the average value for 0.00%, 0.25%, 0.50%, and 1.00% peppermint.

[b] Mecadox had a significantly greater ADG or ADF than the average value for 0.25%, 0.50%, and 1.00% peppermint.

[c] Peppermint produced a significant increase and then a significant decrease (quadratic response) in F/G.

significant scientific and economic interest. In addition they offer the potential for flavoring the pork of treated swine to produce a distinctive value-added product.

These four botanical products, garlic (*A. sativum*), Echinacea (*E. purpurea*), peppermint (*M. piperita*), and goldenseal (*H. canadensis*), have been selected for inclusion in swine feeds based on their pharmacological properties and their agronomic characteristics.

Garlic, a botanical that grows in Iowa, was compared to a standard antibacterial nursery dietary regimen. At the tested inclusion levels (0.5, 2.5, and 5%) increasing levels of garlic generally depressed feed intake and average daily gain in nursery pigs and depressed performance compared to the positive control diet with Mecadox. Muscle samples from the garlic-fed pigs all had "very objectionable" or "extremely objectionable" off-flavors.

Echinacea, a botanical that grows in Iowa, was compared to a standard antibacterial nursery dietary regimen. At the tested inclusion levels (0.1, 0.5, and 2.0%) no statistical advantage existed when compared with a "positive" control diet with 50 g/ton Mecadox or with a "negative" control containing no antibacterial inclusions. Echinacea treated pigs exhibited a slight, but not objectionable, off-flavor when compared with noninclusion levels. Higher levels of Echinacea inclusions may be required to enhance growth rate and feed efficiency swine production.

Goldenseal (0.0–1.0%) was compared to a standard antibacterial nursery dietary regimen. Although not performing to the level of the Mecadox control, pigs on the 0.25% and 1.00% goldenseal diets generally performed better than the 0.00% and 0.05% goldenseal diets and were often not statistically different from the Mecadox control pigs. Increasing levels of goldenseal did not influence the muscle characteristics evaluated.

Peppermint, a botanical that grows in Iowa, was compared to a standard antibacterial nursery dietary regimen. Performance of pigs on all treatments was similar, including the positive and negative controls. At the tested inclusion levels (0, 0.5, 2.5, and 5.0%) no statistical advantage existed over the 5-week study when compared with a "positive" control diet with 50 g/ton Mecadox or with a "negative" control containing no antibacterial inclusions. Increasing levels of peppermint did not influence the muscle characteristics evaluated.

Acknowledgment

These research projects were supported through grants from the Leopold Center for Sustainable Agriculture, Iowa State University, Ames, IA 50011.

References

Briggs, C. 1993. *Can J. Pharm. Sci.* 28:89–92.
Burton Goldberg Group. 1999. *Alternative Medicine, the Definitive Guide*, p. 263. Future Medicine Publishing, Inc., Tiburon, CA.
'de Bairacli Levy, J. 1991. *The Complete Herbal Handbook for Farm and Stable*. Faber and Faber Limited, London, UK.
Duke, J.A. 1985. *Handbook of Medicinal Herbs*, pp. 78, 238–239, 287–288. CRC Press, Boca Raton, FL.
Ellingwood, F. 1983. *America Motica Medica, Therapeutics and Pharmacognosy*. Eclectic Medical Publications, Portland, OR.
Foster, S. 1991. Botanical Series 311. American Botanical Council, Austin, TX.
Hayes, V. and C. Black. 1981. *Antibiotics in Animal Feeds*. Report 88. Council for Agricultural Science and Technology, Ames, IA.
Hladon, B. 1975. *Acta Pol. Pharm.* 32:113–120.
Holmberg, S., et al. 1984. Drug-resistant Salmonella from animals. *Fed. Antimicrobials* 311(10): 617–622.
Hughes, B.G. and L. Lawson. 1991. *Phytother. Res.* 5:154–158.
Kerman, E.C. and L. Kucera. 1967. *Proc. Soc. Exp. Biol. Med.* 124:874–875.
May, 1994. Joint Hearing: Center for Veterinary Medicine and Antibacterial Use Committees. Washington, DC. Anti Infective Drugs: Advisory as Reported in: *JAVMA* 205:19–20.
McGregor, R.L. 1968. The taxonomy of the genus *Echinacea* (Compositae). *Univ. Kansas Sci. Bull.* 48:113–142.

NAHMS (National Animal Health Monitoring System). 1995. Part II: *Reference of 1995 U.S. Grower/Finisher Health & Management Practices*. USDA-APHIS-CEAH, Fort Collins, CO.

National Academy Press. 1999. *The Use of Drugs in Food Animals: Benefits and Risks*. Committee on Drug Use in Food Animals, Washington, DC.

Sanyal, A. and K.C. Varma. 1969. *Indian J. Microbiol.* 9(1):23–24.

SAS. 1996. *The SAS System for Windows*, volume 6.12, 6th edn. SAS Institution Inc., Cary, NC.

Tyler V.F, L.R. Brader, and J.E. Robbers. 1976. *Pharmacognosy*, 7th edn. Lea and Febiger, Philadelphia, PA.

Wacker, A. and W. Hilbig. 1978. *Planta Med.* 33:89–102.

Wagner, H. and A. Proksch. 1985. *Econ. Med. Plant Res.* 1:113-115.

Zimmerman, D. 1986. Role of subtherapeutic levels of antimicrobials in pig production. *J. An. Sci.* 62:318–332.

Chapter 4

Evaluation of Homeopathic Nosodes for Mastitis and Calf Scours: Lessons from the Vermont Nosode Project

Lisa McCrory and John Barlow

Introduction

Mastitis continues to be considered the most costly disease of dairy cows (Fetrow et al., 2000). Mastitis also has numerous detrimental effects on milk quality and composition. Unfortunately, the use of antibiotics has not proven completely effective in curing all types of existing udder infections during lactation and increases the risk of residues in milk and dairy products (Hady et al., 1993). Alternative treatments and preventative measures should be evaluated as methods to reduce the incidence of new mastitis cases and to eliminate existing cases.

Neonatal diarrhea is a major cause of dairy calf morbidity and mortality and can result in significant financial loss on dairy farms. Eliminating neonatal diarrhea can be labor intensive and frustrating. Neonatal diarrhea caused by enterotoxigenic *Escherichia coli* is of particular concern on many dairy farms, as it typically occurs in calves less than 1 week of age and frequently results in high mortality if calves are not treated promptly (Navarre et al., 2000).

Homeopathic medicines, including nosodes, have been recommended as an alternative to conventional therapies for the prevention and treatment of bovine mastitis and *E. coli* calf scours. It has been suggested that homeopathic nosodes function in a manner similar to conventional vaccines, in that they act to increase the natural resistance mechanisms of the cow, and thus prevent occurrence of new infections and enhance the cure rate of existing infections (Day, 1986, 1995; Macleod, 1991; Stopes and Woodward, 1990). However, a limited number of clinical field trials have been conducted for the evaluation of the efficacy of homeopathic treatments in dairy cattle. There were three objectives to the homeopathy project conducted in Vermont: (1) to evaluate homeopathic nosodes in the prevention and treatment of bovine mastitis and calf scours, (2) to document the use of homeopathy on Vermont dairy farms, and (3) to facilitate information exchange on the use of homeopathy on dairy farms. In this review, we provide a description of the research methods for the nosode field trials, some preliminary results of these trials, and a review of some of the factors that should be considered in the design of future clinical studies to evaluate the efficacy of homeopathic medicines for the treatment of mastitis in dairy cattle.

Methods

A research project evaluating the effectiveness of nosodes for mastitis and calf scours was initiated in September 1997 with the enrollment of 11 dairy farms, including over 1,000 lactating cows and 300 calves. Table 4.1 contains descriptive information on the original 11 farms participating in this study. The field trial was conducted from January 1998 to July 1999 by the Northeast Organic Farming Association of Vermont with the collaboration of the University of Vermont Quality Milk Research Laboratory, and was funded under a grant awarded through the USDA Northeast Sustainable Agri-culture Research and Education (SARE) initiative. The months from September 1997 to December 1997 were spent meeting with participating farmers to educate them about the research process and establish protocols. Time was devoted to training of farmers on proper milk sampling and nosode treatment procedures. This was critical to assure compliance by the participating farmers.

Ten of the original 11 farms completed the 18-month study period, with farm 3 (Table 4.1) being removed from the study due to evidence of improper treatment administration and poor milk sampling practices.

Nosode preparation and administration

The *E. coli* nosode was a commercially available product obtained from Washington Homeopathic Products, Inc., Bethesda, MD. Farmers who agreed to participate in the *E. coli* study gave newborn calves one of two treatments, the nosode or a placebo control that were identical in appearance. Treatments used on each farm were randomly labeled as "A" or "B" so that both farmers and researchers were blinded to the treatments. Treatments were given to all new-born calves once daily

Table 4.1   Summary of herds enrolled in study

Herd	Breed[a]	Herd size	Housing and feed source[b]	Antibiotic use for mastitis[c]	Homeopathy for clinical mastitis[d]	Number of cows treated	Number of cows control
1	H	130	F C	Y	Never	94	97
2	H	50	T P	Y	Never	38	35
3[e]	H/DB/J	75	F P	N	Never	NA	NA
4	J	65	F P	N	Sometimes	31	33
5	J	22	F P	N	Frequently	17	14
6	J	40	T P	N	Frequently	36	31
7	J	20	T P	N	Frequently	13	20
8	H/J	140	F C	Y	Never	101	107
9	J	30	T P	N	Frequently	18	21
10	H	250	F C	Y	Never	171	170
11	J	60	T P	N	Frequently	41	40
					Total cows	560	568
					Certified organic	156	159
					Conventional	404	409

[a] H = Holstein; J = Jersey; DB = Dutch Belt.
[b] F = Freestall; T = Tiestall; P = Pasture based; C = Confinement fed total mixed ration.
[c] Based on dry treatment practices (e.g., dry treat all).
[d] Never, sometimes, or frequently treat clinical cases using homeopathy.
[e] Herd 3 was dropped from the study due to poor treatment and sampling compliance.

for the first 3 days of life. The calves were alternately assigned to a treatment group at birth in an attempt to randomize treatments, and to assure equal numbers of animals in each treatment group. Producers recorded all health problems of the treated calves during the first 3 weeks of the calves' life.

A mastitis nosode was prepared commercially (Washington Homeopathic Products, Inc.) from six common mastitis pathogens isolated from cows within the participating herds. Lactating cows in these herds were stratified by lactation number, days in milk, and composite milk somatic cell count (SCC), prior to being randomly assigned to one of two treatment groups. Heifers entered the study before the expected calving date and were alternately assigned to a treatment group. Each treatment group was given either the mastitis nosode or the placebo as an aerosol spray applied to the vaginal mucosa at recommended time intervals throughout the trial. As a double-blind experimental design, treatment groups within farms were randomly assigned to receive the placebo or the nosode, and the key to the treatments was maintained in a sealed envelope until the completion of the trial.

The mastitis nosode was prepared from quarter milk samples obtained from cows with clinical mastitis from the participating farms during November 1997. Milk samples from these individual cases were cultured to identify the pathogen causing mastitis. Thus clinical milk samples were obtained from cows where a single mastitis pathogen was identified to be causing an intramammary infection (IMI). The nosode was prepared as a 30C potency from clinically abnormal milk samples infected with the following mastitis pathogens: *Staphylococcus aureus, Staphylococcus chromogenes, Streptococcus uberis, Streptococcus dysgalactiae, E. coli*, and *Klebsiella* spp. Milk samples, obtained from two farms per pathogen, were selected randomly for inclusion in the final mastitis nosode preparation. Milk samples infected with the specific pathogens were obtained from the following farms: farms 2 and 6, *S. aureus;* farms 4 and 9, *S. chromogenes*; farms 2 and 9, *S. uberis*; farms 1 and 4, *S. dysgalactiae*; farms 3 and 8, *E. coli*; and farms 1 and 8, *Klebsiella* spp. (Table 4.1).

Treatment procedures: In all herds, the mastitis nosode and placebo were diluted in a solution of 50% alcohol and administered as an aerosol spray applied to the vaginal mucosa of dry cows, lactating cows, and bred heifers. Treatments were administered initially for five consecutive days, and then once every 2 months for the remainder of the study in all animals, plus at calving and at dry off for all lactating animals.

Farmers were instructed to manage all animals that developed clinical disease (including mastitis or calf scours) according to established practices for each farm. Farmers were asked to record all disease events, treatments, and the outcomes, although no formal criteria and protocols for recording clinical disease events were established in this study.

Measures of efficacy: Effect of treatment on mastitis rates was evaluated by bacteriological culture of milk samples from all cows collected at: calving, 30 days postpartum; dry off, the onset of clinical mastitis prior to any treatment; and 30 days following the onset of clinical mastitis. Duplicate individual quarter milk samples were collected aseptically by cooperating farmers. Samples were either refrigerated and delivered to the laboratory within 24 hours, or were stored frozen and delivered to the laboratory 2–3 weeks after collection. Milk samples (0.01 ml) were streak-plated on quadrants of tryptose-blood agar containing 5% washed bovine red cells and 0.1% esculin. Plates were incubated at 37°C for 48 hours and presumptive diagnosis of isolates made. Species identification was done by methods recommended by the National Mastitis Council. A quarter was diagnosed as affected by one of the following factors: (1) both milk samples contained 500 cfu/ml, or more, of the same bacterial isolate; or (2) a clinical sample contained at least 100 cfu/ml of an isolate. Somatic cell counts of all individual quarter milk samples were determined using a Fossomatic 90. In addition, all herds enrolled in the study were either on monthly DHIA testing for individual cow milk production and composite SCC (eight of ten herds), or obtained monthly milk production and SCC data by an alternative means (two of ten herds).

Differences between treatment groups in prevalence of all IMI, prevalence of new IMI, rates of clinical mastitis, and spontaneous cure rates of IMI were examined. Spontaneous cure of an IMI was defined as an infected milk sample that was negative for the same species (or a closely related species, in the case of coagulase negative staphylococci) on two subsequent samples. Also, differences in SCC of infected quarters were compared between treatment groups. A modified Student t test was used to compare differences in proportions for prevalence of IMI and spontaneous cure between treatment groups. Control and treatment groups were compared for differences in distribution of cows by lactation number and DIM throughout the study, and for SCC prior to initiation of the treatments. Treatment effects were tested within parities (lactation number). Between the treatment groups, differences in SCC of individual infected quarters, SCC of individual bacteriological negative quarters, SCC of composite milk samples of cows, and monthly milk production of cows were examined by analysis of variance. Season and month of year were included as dependent variables affecting milk production and composite SCC.

Cases of clinical mastitis were identified by each farmer. Clinical mastitis was defined as the presence of abnormal milk secretions, or abnormal swelling of the gland, or both. Clinical mastitis may be accompanied by systemic signs of illness such as loss of appetite or fever. Farmers collected milk samples from all quarters of cows with clinical mastitis, prior to initiation of any mastitis treatments. Farmers or veterinarians treated clinical cases as commonly practiced on each farm, and all treatments were recorded. The overall and the pathogen specific incidence rates of clinical mastitis were compared between treatment groups on individual farms and on all farms. The incidence rate of clinical mastitis was expressed as the number of quarter cases per 1,000 cow-days at risk. Only lactating cow-days were considered in the calculation of total number of cow-days at risk for treated and control cows on each farm. The number of lactating days at risk for each cow was determined using individual cow DHIA records. Differences in rates of clinical mastitis were tested by Fisher's exact probability test.

Bulk tank milk samples were collected weekly and frozen for subsequent analysis. Bulk tank milk samples were analyzed by bacteriological culture and somatic cell count. Changes in bulk tank somatic cell count and bacteriology were examined for the 6 months before, for the 18 months during, and for the 6 months after the study.

Results

Anecdotal information, including case histories, provided by veterinary practitioners using homeopathy, suggest that homeopathic remedies may be useful in effectively preventing and treating mastitis. To the best of our knowledge, this project involved the largest sample size for a placebo-controlled, double-blind, clinical field trial of nosode efficacy for the prevention of mastitis among dairy cattle. This study was conducted on ten different farms that used either conventional or organic production practices and ranged in size from 20 to 250 lactating cows. Collaborating farms used a range of management practices, including intensive seasonal rotational grazing systems feeding strictly grass forages and a small amount of grain for 6 months of the year, and year-round confinement systems feeding a total mixed ration to maximize year-round milk production.

One important outcome of this project was the documentation of the use of homeopathic remedies on farms and the development of a resource for information on how different remedies may be used.

Table 4.2   Summary of calf scours cases for all farms

Treatment	Number of calves	Number of calves with scours[a]	Number of calves with scours between days 0 and 7
Nosode	142	8 (5.6)	5 (3.5)
Placebo	145	10 (6.9)	2 (1.4)
Total	287	18 (6.3)	7 (2.4)

[a] Values in parentheses are percent of calves with scours.

A range of homeopathic and conventional treatment practices were used by the farmers in this study. All farmers in this study had established relationships with a veterinary practitioner for emergency and consultative services. Many of the farmers also enlisted the service of a veterinarian specializing in homeopathic medical practice. In addition, all farmers frequently made treatment decisions for individual animal health problems, such as clinical mastitis, independent of veterinary input. A resource directory on the use of homeopathic medicines in dairy production has been developed by one of the authors (L. M.) as a result of this project, and is available through the Northeast Organic Farming Association of Vermont, Richmond, VT.

E. coli nosode efficacy

A total of 287 calves were enrolled in this portion of the project. Approximately 6% of all calves were observed by farmers to have scours, and approximately 2.5% of all calves developed scours in the first 7 days of life (Table 4.2). No information was available on specific diagnosis of calf gastrointestinal diseases among these calves. No calf deaths due to scours were reported by farmers during the duration of this study, although at least two of the farms had reported historic problems with mortalities associated with calf scours. Rate of scours in the nosode treated group did not differ from the control group for either calves with scours at all ages, or calves with scours between days 0 and 7 postpartum (Table 4.2). However, given an apparent low rate of calf scours morbidity and mortality observed in this study, the ability to identify a significant reduction in risk of scours in the treated group may not be practical due to the sample size. For the current sample size, and an observed 7% disease incidence in the control group, the disease rate in the nosode treated group would need to be $\leq 1\%$ to show significant efficacy of the nosode treatment (95% confidence, 80% power). In other words, near complete elimination of scours in the nosode treated group would have been required to find a significant positive effect for the treatment for a study population of this size.

Mastitis nosode efficacy

Rates of new IMI among primiparous and multiparous cows treated with the homeopathic nosode did not differ from those of cows in the control group (Table 4.3 and Figure 4.1). These results are consistent with what might be expected if mastitis nosodes function in a manner analogous to that of an autogenous vaccine. Rates of new infections would most likely be affected by changes in management practices that affect either the prevalence of pathogens in the environment or the susceptibility of cows in the herd. A vaccine administered to a host is likely to have limited effect on environmental prevalence of many mastitis pathogens. For example, the *E. coli* J-5 vaccine (and similar bacterins commonly used in the dairy industry) has been shown in field trials to have no effect

Table 4.3 Number of new intramammary infections among multiparous cows

Sample time	Treatment group	Number of eligible quarters	S. aureus	S. chromogenes	S. uberis	S. dysgalactiae	E. coli	Klebsiella spp.	Sum of six species in the nosode	Negative quarters
Fresh	Nosode	1,471	29	32	52	8	7	9	137	938
	Control	1,457	28	40	45	9	9	1	132	912
Fresh + 30	Nosode	775	7	4	3	4	1	3	22	599
	Control	844	3	15	7	1	5	1	32	639
Dry	Nosode	965	5	4	9	0	3	3	24	721
	Control	985	4	4	2	0	1	3	14	679
All	Nosode	3,211	41	40	64	12	11	15	183	2,258
	Control	3,286	35	59	54	10	15	5	178	2,230

BISHOP BURTON COLLEGE
LIBRARY

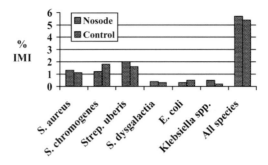

Fig. 4.1 New intramammary infections among multiparous cows.

on the rate of new IMI, but to effectively decrease the severity and duration of *E. coli* clinical mastitis (Hogan et al., 1992). If mastitis nosodes function in a manner analogous to a vaccine, then there may be no effect on IMI rates; however, differences in spontaneous cure rates and rates of clinical mastitis might be observed. Based on power calculations it may be predicted that the sample size of treatment and control groups (3,200 eligible quarters, Table 4.3) was large enough to identify a biologically plausible difference in the quarter level new infection rates between treatment groups, assuming a new infection rate in the control group of 5 to 10% (95% confidence, 80% power).

Discussion

We present here some preliminary results of separate placebo controlled double-blind studies conducted in Vermont to assess the efficacy of mastitis and *E. coli* nosodes used in dairy cattle. These studies might be considered a starting point for the critical evaluation of alternative therapies used in food animal medicine. No difference in calf scours morbidity was observed between calves treated with an *E. coli* nosode and a placebo control; however, the study was limited by a small sample size. No difference in percent of new mammary infections was observed between the nosode treated group and the placebo control group. Sample size for evaluation of the mastitis nosode was predicted to be adequate to identify a biologically plausible reduction in new infection rate for the treated group compared with the placebo control group, yet no difference in infection rates were observed.

To further stimulate discussion and further study we present some comments on the challenges with the study design, and some issues that have been brought to our attention concerning the study of homeopathy. We conclude with a review of the considerations for the design of field trials to study homeopathy.

Challenges with the design of the study

Herd selection

In general, the herds involved in this study were run by good or excellent managers. This is supported by the relatively low rates of calf morbidity and mortality (Table 4.2), the relatively low rates of clinical mastitis, and low bulk tank somatic cell counts (data not shown). For example, the percent of unweaned dairy heifer deaths due to scours, diarrhea, or other digestive problems has been reported to be approximately 6.5% nationally (National Animal Health Monitoring System, USDA, 1996), and deaths in herds in this study were well below this level with no reports of calf mortalities due to scours. The high health quality of these herds likely reduced the opportunity to observe a significant reduction in either calf scours or mastitis. However, this potential limitation must be weighed against the possibility of poor compliance of managers who demonstrate a lower standard of milk quality and udder health. Barkema et al. (1999) studied management style and the association with bulk tank milk somatic cell count, and found that there was a strong relationship between a "quick and dirty" management style and a high bulk milk SCC, and that the farmers with a high bulk tank SCC implemented mastitis prevention measures less often and for shorter periods. Selection of participating herds may influence the outcome of future studies. Adequate characterization of the study population is an important criterion for interpretation of results.

Effect of study participation

By participating in a study, farmers may become more aware of their mastitis prevention practices, and improvements in overall udder health and milk quality might be expected.

Compliance with study protocols

Cooperator herds were not always good at taking milk samples on time. For example, samples may have been taken a few days postfresh instead of on the day of calving. This should not be a significant problem, as few samples were taken outside an acceptable range of days. Constant (monthly) review of protocols and methods to assess compliance are necessary within long term field trials.

Standardization of clinical observations

Some farmers were more observant and treated cows for situations that may have been overlooked on other farms. For example, a number of organic herds recorded clinical mastitis cases in the early dry period, which raises the question of whether this was a measure of better observation of dry cows by these farmers, or the result of no dry cow therapy use on organic farms. Regardless, the number of "clinical" cases reported for a herd depended on farmer observation.

Nosode preparation

There is some controversy regarding the appropriate clinical samples to be obtained for nosode preparation. In the Vermont study it was decided to prepare a "pooled" nosode from a small number of selected milk samples from clinical cases caused by major mastitis pathogens obtained across a few selected herds participating in the study. It might be suggested that nosodes be herd specific, prepared from cases of mastitis observed in a single herd, and applied to that herd. Further, the number of cases represented may range from a selected number of cases to all observed cases. However, the issues of potential changes in mastitis strain diversity within a herd over time and in differences in clinical case presentation suggest that the selection of samples for nosode preparation is complex and dynamic (as is mastitis). This implies that nosode preparations may have a limited efficacy over time if strain types causing mastitis in a population change over time to differ from the strain originally used in the preparation of the nosode. Therefore, some practitioners suggest it is optimal to prepare an individualized nosode from a single milk sample and apply that product only to that individual case. However, this individualized use of a nosode preparation deviates from the objective of using homeopathic nosodes in mastitis prophylaxis. The potential of applying individualized therapies in a split herd randomized controlled field trial needs further consideration.

Nosode administration

Much preliminary discussion on appropriate methods of nosode administration took place, and two experienced large animal homeopathic vets, Dr. Steve Woodard and Dr. Edgar Sheaffer, were consulted. It is important for the nosode to come in contact with the mucous membranes and choices were the mouth, nose, eye, or vulva. Because the study design required individual animal treatment, it was decided that the best way to administer the treatments was through vulvar mucous membranes. The farms involved had various management styles, including 100% confinement in freestalls, tie barn housing with access to pasture, and freestall housing with access to pasture. Alternative routes of administration were considered, such as individual oral treatments, or group treatments via water sources; however, management constraints made both of these unacceptable. Management constraints on many farms would not allow separation into two groups for treatment via separate water sources. Oral administration of individual treatments was considered unacceptable, especially for farmers using freestall housing. Administration of the treatments via the vulvar mucous membranes was relatively easy on most farms and was typically done while cows were restrained at milking.

Timing of administration

Dr. Steve Woodard reported from personal experience that when using a mastitis nosode on other farms, it is necessary to give the nosode to all the animals a minimum of every 5 months. It was decided to booster animals every 2 months to ensure no reduction in the effects of the treatment. In addition it was decided that, since the animal was being handled at calving and dry off and since there tends to be a certain amount of stress at these times, it would be good to give the animals a booster at these times as well.

Nosode potency

The mastitis nosode is a 30 C potency in a 50% alcohol solution. The alcohol solution is believed to give the nosode a longer shelf life making it effective for at least 5 months provided it is stored in a cool and dry place. Potency and administration methods are variables that should be considered in future studies.

Study design

A randomized placebo controlled split herd design was applied in this study. However, one potential limitation is that treated and control animals were comingled within herds. This has two possible effects. First, even if the nosode treatment reduced the prevalence of mastitis among the treated individuals, the spread of mastitis pathogens within the herds might be driven by the higher prevalence among individuals in the control group. That is, the study design allowed for possible contamination of the treated group by exposure to the higher pathogen prevalence of the control group, and thus possible reduction in observed efficacy of the treated group. Second, and conversely, as has been suggested by some practitioners, treatment of an individual may be transferred to other individuals in the population by exposure to that treated individual (e.g. nose–nose contact, etc.). If such indirect transfer of a treatment is possible, then comingling of treated and control individuals would allow for transfer of treatment effects to the control group. In either of these two situations, comingling of treated and control individuals would result in an observation of no apparent treatment effect in the treated group compared to the control group. Alternatives for split herd study designs might be considered; however, the number of farms with facilities to house two isolated groups of lactating cattle managed under identical conditions is likely limited.

What response to a nosode is normal or expected

The response to the nosode is suggested to be very fast. A first response can be a discharge of infectious tissue (aggravation) as part of a homeopathic treatment. This is interpreted as the animal's response of cleaning itself out and is looked upon as a favorable response. In the case of mastitis, this may include an acute inflammatory response such as a rapid elevation in somatic cell count. Such a response has been reported after the use of an intramammary homeopathic preparation (Lafi and Hassan, 2000). In that study the authors reported the number of leukocytes increased dramatically following infusion of the product; however, the composition of the excipient was not described, and the researchers did not evaluate the response to an excipient control.

Many of the above issues (especially those concerning nosode preparation methods, and administration regimens) highlight the diversity of opinion and the limited research available to support clinical decisions regarding use of nosodes for infectious disease control in populations. The use of nosodes is controversial, with many homeopathic practitioners not recommending their use, and relying on only application of classical homeopathic principles and preparations. A consensus on product preparation methods and application is an important consideration for design of future field trials.

Other issues

Can we really study homeopathy?

One of the participating farmers pointed out, "since we know so little about how homeopathy works, is it possible that the cows getting the placebo are actually getting 'treated' by the other cows just by rubbing noses, sharing the same space, grazing the same ground?" "There is so little that we know about how homeopathy works. Is it possible to study its effects in a conventional, reductionist design when it may work in a more holistic, energetic way?" How do we measure such effects? Why look at bacteriologic outcomes, when homeopathy may be acting in a more holistic way? It is the belief of one of the authors (Barlow) that the answers to these questions lie in how advocates recommend the use of homeopathic preparations.

The use of homeopathic remedies is being promoted for the treatment and prevention of mastitis. Therefore, it seems appropriate to test a hypothesis that homeopathic nosodes are significantly better than untreated ones for the prevention of mastitis. To test this hypothesis it seems reasonable to use a discrete outcome for mastitis occurrence, such as differences in prevalence and incidence of bacteriologic infections, or bacteriologic cure rates. Homeopathy is being promoted as a treatment alternative for mastitis, so discrete measures of mastitis risk and occurrence are indicated—if homeopathy were being promoted only as a method to enhance the vitality of the whole farm system, then outcome measures of a more holistic nature would be more appropriate. Therefore, in anticipation of a call for additional studies on the efficacy of homeopathic treatments used in food animal medicine, a review of the design and critical features of clinical field trials is provided.

Design and critical features of field trials

Practitioners and producers require information about the effectiveness and safety of treatments and preventatives such as pharmaceuticals, vaccines, and alternative therapies. Information may come from numerous sources including anecdotal clinical experience (personal and collective), laboratory studies, and clinical field trials. Information obtained from well-designed clinical field trials may provide some of the strongest evidence of the efficacy of specific therapeutic options. But such information is often lacking for both conventional and alternative therapies in veterinary medicine. Elbers and Schukken (1995) described the critical features of veterinary field trials in their review of veterinary field trials of drug and vaccine efficacy published in the *Veterinary Record* from 1988 to 1992. This review provides a list of criteria for the evaluation of field trials (Table 4.4). In this review it was noted that a considerable number of papers lacked details of the study design and a formal analysis of the data. Of particular concern were the number of papers that: (1) used small numbers of animals in treatment groups (46% with ≤ 10 animals per group), (2) did not state that treatment

Table 4.4 Criteria and features for assessing the quality of clinical field trials

Feature	Schukken and Deluyker (1995)	Elbers and Schukken (1995)	Kleijnen et al. (1991)	Linde et al. (1997)
Characterize the patient population or case adequately (describe symptoms, duration, severity)	Yes[a]	No	Yes	Yes
Number of treatment groups and the inclusion of a control group	Yes	Yes	Yes	Yes
Numbers of animals in each treatment group relative to the number in the control group	Yes	Yes	Yes	Yes
Random allocation of animals to the treatment and control groups (confounders eliminated)	Yes	Yes	Yes	Yes
Intervention (treatment) well described (repeatability of trial)	Yes	No	Yes	Yes
Single or double blinding	Yes	Yes	Yes	Yes
Outcome well defined (measurable)	Yes	No	Yes	Yes
Descriptions of statistical analysis applied	Yes	Yes	Yes	Yes
Calculation of the type II error and statistical power	Yes	Yes	Yes	No
Potential problems associated with clustering of patients due to housing or grouping for management	Yes	Yes	No/NA	No/NA

[a] Yes, if authors included the feature or criteria in their review. No, if the feature or criteria were not mentioned in the reference. NA = may not be directly applicable in human trials; however, clustering within treatment groups may be possible.

allocation was random (50%), (3) did not use or state whether treatments were blinded (94%), or (4) did not make a formal statistical analysis of results (25%). Similar reviews of study design quality have been completed for published clinical trials of homeopathic therapies used in human medicine (Kleijnen et al., 1991; Linde et al., 1997). The same types of concerns were raised in these reviews, with issues of study population size, appropriate control groups, randomization, double blinding, and adequate statistical analysis being of particular concern (Table 4.4). Kleijnen et al. (1991) found a surprisingly small number of published human clinical trials on homeopathy that are of high methodological quality. Despite these results, these authors stated they were surprised by the amount of positive evidence in favor of homeopathy, even among the trials with higher methodological quality. Based on the number of positive results the authors stated they "would be ready to accept that homeopathy can be efficacious, if only the mechanisms of action were more plausible." Similar, positive trends were observed by Linde et al. (1997) in their meta-analysis of the human clinical trial literature. In summary, both reviews of the human literature suggest that the evidence from clinical trials of homeopathy "is positive, but not sufficient to draw definitive conclusions because most trials are of low methodological quality" (Kleijnen et al., 1991). In addition to the issue of methodological quality of clinical trials, two other issues are raised by these reports with regard to the study of homeopathy. First is the possible effect of publication bias on a review of the literature, and second is the question of conducting research on a treatment modality where the mechanism of action is not completely understood.

With regard to publication bias, the extent to which this bias affected the conclusions of homeopathy efficacy in the reports by Linde et al. and Kleijnen et al. is unknown. The journal of publication and the bias of scientific reviewers for a particular journal may affect the publication of a clinical trial on alternative therapies. This was recently illustrated in a publication by Resch et al. (2000). These authors submitted two versions of an invented report describing a randomized, placebo controlled, trial of appetite suppressants to reviewers of scientific medical journals. Resch et al. compared the review of conventional "questionable" appetite suppressant (hydroxycitrate) with an unorthodox controversial drug (homeopathic sulfur), where the only difference in the two manuscripts was the name of the therapeutic. They identified a significant bias among reviewers in favor of the conventional version of the manuscript for the invented "research trial." They concluded "studies incongruent with a priori beliefs tend to be rated by outside reviewers as incompetently conducted." But the authors noted that while the bias observed "may put authors of unconventional papers at a disadvantage," they suggested "the disadvantage was not large enough to preclude publication in peer-reviewed conventional journals." They concluded that reviewer bias "does not explain the scarcity of methodologically sound papers on unconventional treatments in peer reviewed journals."

It has been suggested that it may be inappropriate to conduct research on treatment modalities where the mechanism of action is unknown or does not conform to current theories. Yet defenders or enthusiasts of alternative treatments typically suggest that there are many conventional therapies in common clinical use where the mechanism of action is incompletely understood. This may be true, and examples of efficacious conventional therapies where the mechanism of action is poorly defined may be presented; however, the understanding of these therapies is typically supported by accepted pharmacological mechanisms. Perhaps, a more relevant question may be that proposed by Kleijnen et al. (1991), "Are results of randomized double-blind trials less convincing because there is no plausible mechanism of action?" The answer to this question may be no, as Wynn (1998) seemed to suggest, since the theories on the homeopathy's mechanism of action are speculative. And while the reports of electromagnetic differences or unique energetic frequencies of homeopathic preparations might provide some vague clues to possible mechanisms of action, these reports do little to suggest a physiological cause and effect relationship between the treatment and the outcome. Therefore, it is likely appropriate that researchers concentrate on trying to detect a clinical effect of treatment, especially given the increasing interest in, and the amount of emotional debate engendered by, homeopathy.

It is clear from these reviews that improvements in trial design and data analysis are necessary in clinical field trials of both conventional and alternative treatment modalities in veterinary and human medicine. There is no reason to believe the influence of publication bias, data massage, bad methodology, etc. is less in conventional medicine than in alternative medicine research. However, the unique nature of homeopathy suggests that rigorous attention to detail in study design and data analysis may be required for the publication of clinical research trials on homeopathy. While Wynn (1998) has provided a review of studies on homeopathy in veterinary medicine, no assessment of the methodological quality of veterinary homeopathy research has been made. In the future, it appears that a critical review of clinical trials of homeopathy in food animal species is warranted.

It also seems clear from these reviews that it is possible to perform trials on the efficacy of homeopathy in a way that is acceptable to both classical (i.e., skeptical) physicians, and enthusiastic homeopaths (Kleijnen et al., 1991). Schukken and Deluyker (1995) provided a summary of the design and analysis of field trials for the evaluation of the efficacy of products for treatment of bovine mastitis. The recommendations made in that paper may also be applied to the design and analysis of products recommended for mastitis prevention, including alternative treatments such as homeopathy nosodes. In addition, the features (or criteria) for design of field trials for the evaluation of mastitis therapies are similar to those suggested for the evaluation of human homeopathic therapeutics (Table 4.4), so it should be possible to design clinical field trials of high methodological quality for the study of alternative therapies for mastitis prevention and treatment. Key among these design features are defining the trial objectives and the hypothesis being tested, reducing bias and confounding influences, assuring appropriate randomization and blocking, selecting appropriate experimental units, reference populations, and study populations. Defining appropriate treatment regimens (including blinding), and relevant response measures or outcomes, is also a critical component of study design. Finally, appropriate statistical analysis and reporting of results must be planned prior to initiation of the study. One complication to be considered in the study of homeopathy is the consistent application of an individual treatment regimen for a clinical case, and different potencies of various remedies may need to be compared, as "virtually no evidence exists about the correct choice of remedy or potency" (Kleijnen, 1991). A related difficulty is the apparent disagreement among homeopathic practitioners concerning the efficacy of the various types of homeopathic preparations and practices, including disagreements on the efficacy of prophylactic use of nosodes, or on the use of combination preparations to treat an animal with a clinical disease, such as mastitis, based only on the presenting sign (e.g., abnormal milk or mammary gland), and not a larger spectrum of signs and symptoms.

Using the criteria in Table 4.4 it should be possible to complete a review of literature on the use of homeopathy to prevent and treat mastitis in dairy cattle. Such a study is currently being conducted, and approximately 50 publications on the use of homeopathy for treatment of mastitis have been identified. Similar to the findings reported in the human literature, few of these publications appear to be of high methodological quality. Therefore the criteria described by Schukken and Deluyker for the design of mastitis therapy trials must also be applied to future studies. If skeptical practitioners are asked to accept the results of clinical field trials of homeopathy in food animal medicine, then additional evidence must consist of well-performed controlled trials with large numbers of participants under rigorous double-blind conditions.

References

Barkema, H.W., J.D. van der Ploeg, Y.H. Schukken, T.J.G.M. Lam, G. Benedictus, and A. Brand. 1999. Management style and its association with bulk milk somatic cell count and incidence of clinical mastitis. *J. Dairy Sci.* 82:1655–1663.

Day, C.E.I. 1986. *J. Vet. Homeopath.* 1:15–19.

Day, C.E.I. 1995. *The Homeopathic Treatment of Beef and Dairy Cattle.* Beaconsfield Publishers Ltd., Beaconsfield, UK.

Elbers, A.R.W. and Y.H. Schukken. 1995. Critical features of veterinary field trials. *Vet. Rec.*136: 187–192.

Fetrow, J., S. Stewart, S. Eicker, R. Farnsworth, and R. Bey. 2000. Mastitis: an economic consideration. In *Proc. National Mastitis Council*, pp. 3–47.

Hady, P.J., J.W. Lloyd, and J.B. Kaneene. 1993. Antibacterial use in lactating dairy cattle. *JAVMA* 203:210–220.

Hogan, J.S., K.L. Smith, D.A. Todhunter, and P.S. Schoenberger. 1992. Field trial to determine the efficacy of *Escherichia coli* J5 mastitis vaccine. *J. Dairy Sci.* 75:78–84.

Kleijnen, J., P. Knipschild, and G. ter Reit. 1991. Clinical trials of homeopathy. *British Med. J.* 302:316–323.

Lafi, S.Q. and M.N. Hassan. 2000. The Mast-O-Test and Mastop-H in identification and treatment of subclinical bovine mastitis in dairy herds. *J. Am. Holist. Vet. Med. Assoc.* 18:25–29.

Linde, K., N. Clausius, G. Ramirez, D. Melchart, F. Eitel, L.V. Hedges, and W.B. Jonas. 1997. Are the clinical effects of homeopathy placebo effects? A meta-analysis of placebo controlled trials. *Lancet* 350:834–843.

Macleod, G. 1991. The role of homeopathy. In *Proc. 4th British Mastitis Conf.*, pp. 25–32.

National Animal Health Monitoring System, United States Department of Agriculture. 1996. *Dairy '96 Part 1: Reference of 1996 Dairy Management Practices.* Centers for Epidemiology and Animal Health, p. 31. USDA:APHIS:VS, Fort Collins, CO.

Navarre, C.B., E.B. Belknao, and S.E. Rowe. (2000) Differentiation of gastrointestinal diseases of calves. *Vet. Clin. North Am. Food Anim. Pract.* 16:37–57.

Resch, K.I., E. Ernst, and J. Garrow. 2000. A randomized controlled study of reviewer bias against an unconventional therapy. *J. R. Soc. Med.* 93:164–167.

Wynn, S.G. 1998. Studies on use of homeopathy in animals. *JAVMA* 212:719–724.

Schukken, Y.H. and H.A. Deluyker. 1995. Design of field trials for the evaluation of antibacterial products for therapy of bovine clinical mastitis. *J. Vet. Pharmacol. Ther.* 18:274–283.

Stopes, C. and L. Woodward. 1990. The use and efficacy of a homeopathic nosode in the prevention of mastitis in dairy herds: a survey of practicing users. *IFOAM-Bull. Org. Agric.* 10:6–10.

Chapter 5
Livestock Self-medication

Cindy Engel

Introduction

Living systems are inherently self-regulatory and behavior is one means by which animals regulate their physiological and psychological states. Livestock managers are familiar with simple examples of self-regulation: over-heated cattle move into the shade where it is cooler; dehydrated, they search for water. However, behavioral self-regulation is far more refined than this. Deprived of only one amino acid, rats increase their consumption of novel foods until they find a diet that is rich in that missing amino acid. Furthermore, they learn an aversion to foodstuffs that are deficient in only one amino acid (Rogers and Rozin, 1996; Feurte et al., 2000). Lambs monitor the carbohydrate and protein content of their diet and adjust their feeding accordingly. If deprived of phosphorus, sheep not only identify a phosphorous-rich diet but learn a preference for the foods that correct deficiency malaise (Villalba and Provenza, 1999; Provenza, 1995).

Reviewers conclude that such "nutritional wisdom" is achieved via a combination of postingestive and hedonic feedback, and individual learning, proposing that "behavior is a function of its consequences" (Provenza, 1995; Provenza, et al., 1998). This is true of health maintenance in general.

The cost to an individual for not maintaining health can be high. Consequently natural selection has honed a variety of behavioral "health maintenance" strategies reviewed most recently by Hart, (1990, 1994) and Huffman (1997). As Hart points out, behavior is often the first line of defense against attack by pathogens and parasites (Hart, 1990, 1994; Huffman, 1997). As a result, animals have behavioral strategies for avoiding, preventing, and therapeutically addressing threats to survival. When an animal attempts to remedy a health threat by consuming or using a substance not made by itself, the behavior can be described as self-medication (Hart, 1990; Rodriguez and Wrangham, 1993; Boppré, 1984).

Animal self-medication therefore requires nothing more complicated than the pursuit of pleasant sensations or the removal of unpleasant sensations, i.e., hedonic feedback. Mammalian and avian behavioral strategies that reduce unpleasant sensations are clearly demonstrated in laboratory experiments. Rats and chickens self-administer appropriate levels of analgesic medication when subjected to physical pain (Colpaert et al., 1980; Kupers and Gybels, 1995; Danbury et al., 2000). Emotional pain (induced by being forced to watch a conspecific endure physical pain) causes laboratory rodents to self-administer morphine and cocaine (Kuzmin et al., 1996; Ramsey and Van Ree, 1993). When poisoned, rats show the specific "illness-response behavior" of seeking and consuming clay, which binds the toxin preventing further absorption into the blood. So reliable is this response to poisoning that clay consumption is seen as an indicator of nausea in rats (Takeda et al., 1993).

Recent research reveals that a range of wild and domestic animal species are capable of self-medicating their discomforts with both natural and artificial substances (Engel, 2002; Huffman, 2001). The implications of acknowledging self-medication behaviors in livestock are not to be underestimated for they hold the key to improving health and welfare.

Geophagy

Geophagy (earth-eating) is common among mammals and birds. Although previously assumed to indicate mineral or trace element deficiency, recent research suggests geophagy is more often about self-medication.

Geophagy is most common among those species that rely on plant material for a large part of their diet. Herbivores and omnivores are often unable to avoid the defensive secondary compounds of plants whilst obtaining the nutrients they require. Geophagy is also more common in tropic and sub-tropic regions where plants are more strongly defended against pests and disease. For these reasons, recent reviewers suggest that plant-eaters have a greater need for clay because of its immediate soothing effects on gastrointestinal malaise rather like the digestive medicine kaopectate (Johns and Duquette, 1991; Krishnamani and Mahaney, 2000). Clay not only adsorbs and absorbs plant toxins such as alkaloids but environmental toxins as well as some pathogens and parasites. It also acts as an antacid. Potentially clay offers rapid relief from malaise from multiple sources.

In Peru, macaws eat a daily dose of clay from the river banks of their tropical forest habitat. James Gilardi and colleagues at the University of California, Davis, have shown that clay effectively prevents up to 60% of plant alkaloids being absorbed into the blood (Gilardi et al., 1999). Howler monkeys also eat termite mound clay soil primarily to counter the effects of toxic secondary compounds in their leafy diets (de Souza et al., 2002). Elephants clear large areas of forest in Central Africa to mine clay subsoils. Their consumption of clay shows seasonal correlations with dietary habits. While eating mainly chemically defended leaves, they also eat clay. When they switch to eating nondefended fruits, they stop eating clay (Klaus et al., 1998).

Sometimes the primary cause of gastrointestinal malaise is not dietary toxins but intestinal parasites. Here too geophagy is beneficial. Rhesus macaques on Cayo Santiago Island, Puerto Rico, have reportedly learned to mine clay for the beneficial effects against heavy infestations of intestinal parasites (Knezevich, 1998).

Cattle, sheep, and deer are known to dig and lick at subsoils. In free-ranging conditions in the mountains of Venezuela, hybrid Holstein cattle regularly dig for subsoils. The soils they lick are predominantly clays rather than a soil with any particular mineral or trace element. William Mahaney of the Geophagy Research Unit, York University, Ontario, postulates that the cattle are licking the clay soil for the clay's soothing effect on gastrointestinal malaise (Mahaney et al., 1996). Clay additions to cattle feed increase feed conversion efficiency by up to 20% (Kruelen, 1985). This beneficial effect is thought to result from improved gastrointestinal conditions. In addition to influencing pH and binding toxins, clay is effective at adsorbing bovine coronavirus and rotavirus (Clark et al., 1998). Research at the University of New England, Australia has shown that bentonite clay in the diet of sheep increases the flow of both dietary and microbial protein to the intestines and has a beneficial effect on wool production (Fenn and Leng, 1990).

Johns and Duquette (1991) conclude that the primary way geophagy enhances nutritional status is by countering dietary toxins and secondarily by countering the effects of gastrointestinal parasites.

Natural charcoal is also consumed by wild and domestic species. Primates, ponies, deer, camels and pigs are reported to consume charcoal and coal (Tyler, 1972; Engel, 2002). Like clay, charcoal is used in human medicine to counter the effects of toxins. Activated (highly absorptive) charcoal is used as a general panacea for unidentified poisoning in hospitals. Experiments reveal that charcoal consumed by one particular population of red colobus monkeys in Zanzibar is capable of protecting them against their dietary plant toxins. Furthermore, those monkey populations with the charcoal-eating habit are gaining a reproductive advantage over other groups (Struhsaker et al., 1997; Cooney and Struhsaker, 1997). Ash-eating is also reported in wild animals and domestic livestock. In the absence of experimental research, Kruelen (1985) postulates that ash most likely acts as an antacid.

Geophagy is no longer considered an aberrant behavior but rather an essential self-regulation strategy among omnivores and herbivores.

Mechanical scours

Across Africa gorillas, chimpanzees, and bonobos swallow carefully folded hairy leaves which scrape intestinal parasites through the gut, emerging undigested onto the forest floor. Leaf-swallowing is therefore described as a form of self-medication that relies on the action of mechanical or physical scours rather than chemical action (Huffman and Caton, 2001). Other animal species appear to be using a similar method of parasite control. Bears in Alaska eat rough sedge (*Carex* sp.) before hibernation and shed boluses of undigested sedge along with tapeworms. Canada snow geese shed worms before migration apparently using undigested grass scours in a similar way (Huffman and Caton, 2001).

What is fascinating is the possibility that mechanical scours are widely used by mammals in response to intestinal discomfort of parasites. If so, the chewing of timber and other rough dry fibrous materials by livestock mammals may play a more adaptive role than previously assumed.

Astringents

Tannins in plants usually deter mammals from eating plants because their astringency puckers and dries the tongue and impairs digestion by binding proteins. However, tannins are not avoided entirely. Dan Janzen described how the Asiatic two-horned rhinoceros occasionally eats so much of the tannin-rich bark of the mangrove *Ceriops candolleana* that its urine turns dark orange. He postulated that the rhinoceros may have been self-medicating pointing out that the common antidysentery formula Enterovioform consists of about 50% tannin (Janzen, 1978).

Support for the suggestion that tannins impact directly on intestinal parasites comes from more recent research. When domesticated goats were fed polyethylene glycol (PEG), which deactivates tannins, the goats had an increase in the numbers of intestinal parasites (Kabasa et al., 2000). Given a choice, deer do not select food with the lowest tannin levels, but instead those containing moderate amounts, suggesting that a certain amount of tannin is attractive to them (VerheydenTixier and Duncan, 2000). Sheep, goats, and cattle increase tannin consumption when fed the deactivating PEG. Alternatively, when fed high-tannin diets lambs increase PEG intake (Provenza et al., 2000; Rollin, 2004).

These results show that many animals attempt to self-regulate tannin consumption to an optimal level.

When commercially raised deer in New Zealand were grazed on forage containing tannin-rich plants such as chicory, farmers found they needed to administer less chemical de-wormer (Hoskin et al., 1999). Furthermore, given a choice, parasitized deer and lambs select the bitter and astringent Puna Chicory, and thereby reduce their parasite load (Schreurs et al., 2002; Scales et al., 1994). Tannin-rich plants such as this are commonly selected in moderate amounts by free-ranging animals. Researchers in Australia and New Zealand have found that certain types of forage such as *Hedysarum coronarium*, *Lotus cornicularus* and *Lotus pedunculatus* containing more useful condensed tannins can increase lactation, wool growth, and live weight gain in sheep, apparently by reducing the detrimental effects of internal parasites (Aerts et al., 1999; Niezen, et al., 1996). Tannin-rich pastures may also provide opportunities for ungulates to regulate bloat (McMahon et al., 2000).

Bitters

Many potentially toxic plants taste bitter because of the defensive secondary compounds they contain, and bitterness is therefore often deterrent to mammals. However, recent research suggests that (as with astringents) some mammals have a preference for moderate consumption of bitters.

In the laboratory, mice consume up to 20% of their fluids from bitter-tasting water even when fresh water is provided. This habit of "bitter-sampling" has been shown to protect mice from disease (Vitazkova, et al., 2001). Researchers suggest that a liking for a little bitterness—as an indicator of bioactive secondary compounds—may be adaptive (Koshimizu et al., 1994). It would be interesting to investigate whether mammalian tolerance of bitter tastes changes with health status because this would indicate one possible mechanism of self-medication. Chimpanzees for example have similar tastes to humans yet when sick will seek one of the most bitter plants in their environment and suck on its medicinal pith (Huffman and Seifu, 1989).

Topical anointing

In the wild, mammals and birds manage skin irritations by anointing themselves with aromatic skin rubs such as tree resins, fruits, leaves, flowers, and insect secretions (Engel, 2002). Many livestock mammals attempt to coat themselves with mud to protect themselves from biting insects. When they roll and rub on muddied coats, the abrasive action crushes skin pests. Birds similarly use dust to dry skin oils and abrade skin pests.

Many bird species bring aromatic herbs to the nest at hatching time. Experiments show that the selected pungent herbs contain volatile oils that enhance the health of chicks by reducing the impacts of ectoparasites (Gwinner et al., 2000; Clark and Mason, 1988).

Livestock mammals and birds retain a requirement for skin care opportunities.

Psychological welfare

Experiments show that laboratory animals self-regulate their psychological welfare. Mice and rats self-administer appropriate levels of morphine or cocaine to deal with emotional stress (Ramsey and Van Ree, 1993; Kuzmin et al., 1996). Laboratory rats also use bio-feedback to calm themselves. When stressed they learn to self-administer strobe lighting at certain frequencies that change electrical activity in the brain and thereby calm heart rhythm and lower blood pressure. The rats thereby ingeniously calm themselves, reducing the likelihood of heart attack (Shlyahova and Vorobyova, 1999). A feeling of anxiety is clearly unpleasant, and it is the animals' desire to feel better that drives the self-regulation strategies.

Broiler chickens can self-medicate stress. It has long been known that supplementing chicken feed with vitamin C (ascorbic acid) helps chickens cope better with heat stress, but producers have difficulty knowing when, and by how much, to supplement the feed. Professor Mike Forbes, and his colleagues at Leeds University, UK, solved the problem by allowing individual birds to self-medicate. To do this, though, the birds need some way of detecting the tasteless, colorless, and odorless vitamin C. Birds have acute color vision and readily learn color associations. By coloring food containing vitamin C the researchers revealed that the birds could learn the positive effects of colored food within 3 days and self-medicate as and when necessary.

Kutlu and Forbes suggest that vitamin C works by reducing the production of the stress hormone corticosterone thereby reducing other symptoms of chronic stress. They point out that self-medication with vitamin C could be applied to other forms of stress such as parasite infection, high humidity, and high production rates (Kutlu and Forbes, 1993).

Discussion

The many examples noted above of self-medication by livestock demonstrate that even after generations of artificial selection livestock retain an ability to self-regulate aspects of their health and to self-medicate some of their ills if given an opportunity. This is perhaps not surprising considering the fundamental importance of health maintenance to survival. Interestingly, the ability to self-medicate is not restricted to natural materials with which animals are familiar (as seen by the broiler chickens successful use of carprofen and Ascorbic acid) suggesting that post-ingestive and/or hedonic feedback are used to find relief from malaise with novel substances.

It is clear that a healthy diet contains more than nutrients and energy. Non-nutrients such as plant secondary compounds are often bioactive and therefore potentially toxic or medicinal. Forage plants are not as easily classified as "toxic" or "medicinal." They can be both. Individual tastes for such plants may change with health status and observations of changes in behavior of sick livestock may yield valuable management advice.

Other non-nutrients are also important to livestock: clays, charcoals, fibrous wood, or bark all play a vital role in health-maintenance, and free access to such materials should be considered. Pilot trials on organic farms in the U.K. indicate that provision of clay licks (as solid blocks) is keenly accepted by cattle both indoors and outside.

Acknowledging animal self-medication produces a radical change in health management. It becomes evident, for example, that it is not optimal or efficient to simply add herbal/natural medicines to feed. There is a new approach that respects an individual animal's ability to self-select appropriate quantities and qualities of feedstuffs/medicines. If self-medication strategies can be enabled and optimized, they potentially offer a more accurate way of providing the individual animal with what it needs to restore health.

Obviously, there are many limitations to this thesis and more research is urgently required. In particular, it is important to establish just how much experience an individual animal needs to successfully self-medicate. It is also critical to understand the selection criteria used in a particular context so that mistakes can be reduced. For example, in some cases, behavior motivated by hedonic feedback leads to addictions and overindulgences. Even so, there are steps that can be safely implemented with the limited knowledge currently available.

Livestock managers might consider the following:

- Encourage behavioral self-regulation by providing highly diverse forage appropriate for the adaptive spectrum of the species, i.e. another good reason for increasing biodiversity.
- Investigate the medicinal potential of native plants that are usually considered "toxic." Tolerating a few specimens may provide essential medicinal compounds to livestock.
- Provide access to rubbing posts, mud, and aromatic cherbs.
- Enable access to subsoils for clays and chalks or provide clay blocks to ruminant stock ad libitum.
- Allow access to chewing wood or barks.

Providing livestock with access to a broad spectrum of nutrients, non-nutrients, natural bioactive compounds, and skin rubs could potentially reduce feed supplement and drug costs while at the same time increase yields.

Such management systems will not eliminate the need for veterinary medication. When drugs are necessary, however, it may still be possible—desirable even—to enable an element of self-medication. Just as individual lame broiler chickens successfully self-administered appropriate levels of analgesic medication, other livestock species may be able to self-select appropriate analgesia if supplied with a choice of concentrations of medicated feedstuffs.

Although experiments on inexperienced domesticated species reveal an inherent self-medication ability, to enable the widest spectrum of self-medication behavior in adult animals, it will be vital to encourage developmental and experiential learning of such strategies.

The evidence for self-medication by livestock and other animals is substantial. Researchers, unfortunately, have performed only minimal investigations about the potential benefits of self-medication by livestock. The inherent health-maintenance strategies of livestock should be investigated thoroughly. Many benefits to society could result from a concerted effort to document self-medication strategies of livestock and to elicit the underlying mechanisms of the self-medication strategies.

References

Aerts, R.J., T.N. Barry, and W.C. McNabb. 1999. Polyphenols and agriculture: beneficial effects of proanthocyanidins in forages. *Agric. Ecosystems Environ.* 75(1–2):1–12.

Boppré, M. 1984. Redefining pharmacophagy. *J. Chem. Ecol.* 10(7):1151–1154.

Clark, L. and J.R. Mason 1988. Effects of biologically active plants used as nest material and the derived benefit to starling nestlings. *Oecologia* 77:174–180.

Clark, K.L., A.B. Sarr, P.G. Grant, et al. 1998. In vitro studies on the use of clay, clay minerals and charcoal to adsorb bovine rotavirus and bovine coronavirus. *Vet. Microbiol.* 63(2–4):137–146.

Colpaert, F.C., P. Dewitte, P.C. Maroli, et al. 1980. Self-administration of the analgesic suprofen in arthritic rats: evidence of *Mycobacterium butyricum*-induced arthritis as an experimental model of chronic pain. *Life Sci.* 27:921–928.

Cooney, D.O. and T.T. Struhsaker. 1997 Adsorptive capacity of charcoals eaten by Zanzibar red colobus monkeys: implications for reducing dietary toxins, *Int. J. Primatol.* 18(2)235–246.

Danbury, T.C., C.A. Weeks, J.P. Chambers, et al. 2000. Self-selection of the analgesic drug carprofen by lame broiler chickens. *Vet. Rec.* 146:307–311.

de Souza, L.L., S.F. Ferrari, M.L. da Costa, and D.C. Kern. 2002. Geophagy as a correlate of folivory in red-handed Howler monkeys *(Alouatta belzebul)* Eastern Brazilian Amazonia. *J. Chem. Ecol.* 28:1613–1621.

Engel, C. 2002. *Wild Health: How Animals Keep Themselves Well and what We Can Learn from Them.* Houghton Mifflin, Boston, MA.

Fenn, P. and R.A. Leng. 1990. The effect of bentonite supplementation on ruminal protozoa density and wool growth in sheep either fed roughage based diets or grazing. *Austr. J. Agric. Res.* 41: 167–174.

Feurte, S., S. Nicoladis, and K.C. Berridge. 2000. Conditioned taste aversion in rats for a threonine-deficient diet: demonstration by the taste reactivity test. *Physiol. Behav.* 68(3):423–429.

Gilardi, J.D., S.S. Duffey, C.A. Munn, et al. 1999. Biochemical functions of geophagy in parrots: detoxification of dietary toxins and cytoprotoective effects. *J. Chem. Ecol.* 25(4):897–919.

Gwinner, H., M. Oltronge, L. Trost, et al. 2000. Green plants in starling nests: effects on nestlings. *Anim. Behav.* 59(2)301–309.

Hart, B.L. 1990. Behavioral adaptations to pathogens and parasites: five strategies. *Neurosci. Biobehav. Rev.* 14:223–294.

Hart, B.L. 1994. Behavioural defence against parasites: interaction with parasite invasiveness. Parasitology 109:S139–151.

Hoskin, S.O., T.N. Barry, P.R. Wilson, W.A.G. Charleston, and J. Hodgson. 1999. Effects of reducing anthelmintic input upon growth and faecal egg and larval counts in young farmed deer grazing chicory *(Cichorium intybus)* and perennial ryegrass *(Lolium perenne)* white clover (*Trifolium repens*) pasture. *J. Agric. Sci.* 132(3):335–345.

Huffman, M.A. 1997. Current evidence for self-medication in primates: a multidisciplinary perspective. *Yearbook Phys. Anthropol.* 40:171–200.

Huffman, M.A. 2001. Self-medicative behaviour in the African Great apes: an evolutionary perspective into the origins of human traditional medicine. *Bioscience* 51(8):651–661.

Huffman M.A. and J.M. Caton. 2001. Self-induced gut motility and the control of parasite infections in wild chimpanzees. *Int. J. Primatol.* 22(3):329–346.

Huffman, M.A. and M.K. Seifu. 1989. Observations on the illness and consumption of a possibly medicinal plant *Vernonia amygdalina* by wild chimpanzees in the Mahale Mountains National Park, Tanzania. *Primates* 30(1):51–63.

Janzen, D.H. 1978. Complications in interpreting the chemical defences of trees against tropical arboreal plant-eating vertebrates. In *Ecology of Arboreal Folivores* (ed. G.G. Montgomeries), pp. 73–84. Smithsonian Inst. Press, Washington, DC.

Johns, T. and M. Duquette. 1991. Detoxification and mineral supplementation as functions of geophagy. *Am. J. Clin. Nutr.* 53:448–456.

Kabasa, J.D., J. OpudaAsibo, and U. terMeulen. 2000. The effect of oral administration of polyethylene glycol on faecal helminth egg counts in pregnant goats grazed on browse containing condensed tannins. *Trop. Anim. Health Prod.* 32(2):73–86.

Klaus, G., C. Klaus-Hugi, and B. Schmid. 1998. Geophagy by large mammals at natural licks in the rain forest of the Dzanga National Park, Central African Republic. *J. Trop. Ecol.* 14:829–839.

Knezevich, M. 1998. Geophagy as a therapeutic mediator of Endoparasitism in a free-ranging group of Rhesus Macaques (*Macaca mulatta). Am. J. Primatol.* 44(1):71–82.

Koshimizu, K., H. Ohigashi, and M.A. Huffman. 1994. Use of *Vernonia amygdalina* by wild chimpanzees: possible roles of its bitter and related compounds. *Physiol. Behav.* 56(6): 1209–1216.

Krishnamani, R. and W.C. Mahaney. 2000. Geophagy among primates: adaptive significance and ecological consequences. *Anim. Behav.* 59:899–915.

Kruelen, D.A. 1985. Lick use by large herbivores: a review of benefits and banes of soil consumption. *Mammal Rev.* 15(3):107–123.

Kupers, R. and J. Gybels. 1995. The consumption of fentanyl is increased in rats with nociceptive pain but not with neuropathic pain. *Pain* 60:137–141.

Kutlu, H.R. and J.M. Forbes. 1993. Self-selection of ascorbic acid in coloured foods by heat-stressed broiler chickens. *Physiol. Behav.* 53:103–110.

Kuzmin, A., S. Semenova, E. Zartau, et al. 1996. Enhancement of morphine self-administration in drug-naïve, inbred strains of mice by acute emotional stress. *Eur. Neuropsychopharmacol.* 6:63–68.

Mahaney, W.C., M. Bezada, R.G.V. Hancock, et al. 1996. Geophagy of holstein hybrid cattle in the Northern Andes, Venezuela. *Mountain Res. Dev.* 16(2):177–180.

McMahon. L.R., T.A. McAllister, B.P. Berg, et al. 2000. A review of the effects of forage condensed tannins on ruminal fermentation and bloat in grazing cattle. *Can. J. Plant Sci.* 80(3)469–485.

Niezen, J.H., W.A.G. Charleston, J. Hodgson, A.D. Mackay, and D.M. Leathwick. 1996. Controlling internal parasites in grazing ruminants without recourse to anthelmintics: approaches, experiences and prospects. *Int. J. Parasitol.* 26(8–9):983–992.

Provenza, F.D. 1995. Post-ingestive feedback as an elementary determinant of food preference and intake in ruminants. *J. Range Manage.* 48:2–17.

Provenza, F.D., E.A. Buritt, A. Perevolotsky, et al. 2000 Self-regulation of polyethylene glycol by sheep fed diets of varying tannin concentrations. *J. Anim. Sci.* 78(5):1206–1212.

Provenza F.D., J.J. Villalba, C.D. Cheney, and S.J. Werner. 1998. Self-organisation of foraging behaviour: from simplicity to complexity without goals. *Nutr. Res. Rev.* 11(2):199–222.

Ramsey, N.F. and J.M. Van Ree. 1993. Emotional but not physical stress enhances intravenous cocaine self-administration in drug-naïve rats. *Brain Res.* 608:216–222.

Rodriguez, E. and R.W. Wrangham. 1993. Zoopharmacognosy: the use of medicinal plants by animals, in recent advances in phytochemistry, 27: In *Phytochemical Potential of Tropical Plants* (eds. K.R. Downum, J.T. Romeo, and H. Stafford), pp. 89–105. Plenum Press, New York.

Rogers, W. and P. Rozin. 1996. Novel food preferences in thiamine-deficient rats. *J. Comp. Physiol. Psychol.* 61:1–4.

Rollin, B.E. 2004. Animal agriculture and emerging social ethics for animals. *J. Anim. Sci.* 82: 955–964.

Scales, G.H., T.L. Knight, and D.J. Saville. 1994. Effect of herbage species and feeding level on internal parasites and production performance of grazing lambs. *N Z J. Agric. Res.* 38:237–247.

Schreurs N.M., N. Lopez-Villalobos, T.N. Barry, A.L. Molan, and W.C. McNabb. 2002. Effects of grazing undrenched weaner deer on chicory or perennial ryegrass/white clover on the viability of gastrointestinal nematodes and lungworms. *Vet. Rec.* 151(12):348–353.

Shlyahova, A.V. and T.M. Vorobyova. 1999. Control of emotional behaviour based on biological feedback. *Neurophysiology* 31(1):38–40.

Struhsaker, T.T., D.O. Cooney, and K.S. Siex. 1997. Charcoal consumption by Zanzibar red colobus monkeys: its function and its ecological and demographic consequences. *Int. J. Primatol.* 18(1): 61–72.

Takeda, N., S. Hasegawa, S. Morita, et al. 1993. Pica in rats is analogous to emesis: an animal model in emesis research. *Pharmacol. Biochem. Behav.* 45(4):817–821.

Tyler, S.T. 1972. The behaviour and social organisation of the new forest pony. *Anim. Behav. Monogr.* 5:96.

VerheydenTixier, H. and P. Duncan. 2000. Selection for small amounts of hydrolysable tannins by a concentrate selecting mammalian herbivore. *J. Chem. Ecol.* 26(2):351–358.

Villalba, J.J. and F.D. Provenza. 1999. Nutrient-specific preferences by lambs conditioned with intraluminal infusions of starch, casein, and water. *J. Anim. Sci.* 77(2):378–387.

Vitazkova, S.E. Long, A. Paul, et al. 2001. Mice suppress malaria infection by sampling 'bitter' chemotherapy agent. *Anim. Behav.* 61(5): 887–894.

Chapter 6
Alternative Methods of Controlling Parasites in Small Ruminants

R.W. Godfrey and R.E Dodson

Introduction

Chemotherapeutic agents have been used for many years to treat diseases and parasites in small ruminant livestock. There are not as many chemotherapeutic agents or compounds approved for use with small ruminates compared with the number approved for large ruminants because of the small number of small ruminants. In many cases, even though products were not approved for use in small ruminants, they were widely used to treat diseases and parasites of small ruminants due to their high level of effectiveness. Using products approved for use for one disease or animal on another disease or animal is referred to as extra label use, and such use is usually only made under the guidance of a veterinarian. In recent years with the increase in the size of the small ruminant industry in the United States, and the already existing large industry worldwide, the demand for animal health support has also increased. There have been new approvals of compounds and new compounds developed specifically for use in small ruminates. These new chemotherapeutic agents have received widespread acceptance and have proven to be effective for treating many diseases and parasites in small ruminates.

Public concern over the perceived excessive use of antibiotics in livestock and the development and use of genetically modified plants and animals (GMOs) for food production have led to an increase in concern about the use of antibiotics and GMOs. One concern is that organisms will develop resistance to antibiotics and these resistant organisms would pose a risk to consumers of animal products. The resistant organisms could threaten the human population because the effectiveness of antibiotics used to combat these organisms would be compromised or completely wiped out. Another concern is over the safety of the GMOs as it pertains to human health, the food chain, and the environment. These are just some of the reasons that have led livestock producers and researchers to explore alternative methods of managing animal health.

There is a paucity of scientific studies on the use of alternative methods for treating health in small ruminants. The lack of published data on formulations, dosages, efficacy, and toxicity limits the use of these alternative methods by livestock farmers. There are a large number of anecdotal reports of the successful use of alternative methods, such as medicinal plants and herbs, for treating animal diseases. Due to the anecdotal nature of these reports it is difficult to cite them or interpret the results and what impact they may have on livestock production. Further research needs to be conducted to evaluate the efficacy, safety, formulation, route of administration, and dose of these materials if they are to gain widespread acceptance in the livestock industry.

One of the major areas of concern to small ruminant producers in many regions of the world is the control of gastrointestinal nematode parasites (GINPs). Many GINPs have developed resistance to the anthelmintics currently in use. The resistance developed by GINPs is a major concern of livestock producers in the tropical and subtropical regions of the world because GINPs are widespread and have a major impact on worldwide livestock production (Waller, 1997a). With the increase in the use of chemotherapeutic anthelmintics and the development of GINP resistance to them, concern over the future efficacy and utility has initiated research efforts to develop and evaluate alternative methods of control. This is partly driven by livestock producers who are seeking new and novel ways to combat strains of resistant parasites in livestock. There is a growing body of work in the scientific literature describing the development and implementation of many of these practices and methods. This chapter will provide a review of material in the literature on the use of alternative methods of managing health of small ruminants with a primary emphasis on the control of GINP. Some of the methods that will be presented are under development and do not have widespread use or commercial application, but they possess the potential to have a large impact on the small ruminant livestock industry throughout the world.

Control of internal parasites

Throughout many regions of the world the frequent use of pharmaceuticals to control GINP of small ruminants has led to the development of resistance by the parasites to these pharmaceuticals. Resistance is defined as an efficacy below 95% for an anthelmintic used on a regular basis (Coles et al., 1992). The primary way in which the resistance is developed in GINP is by selecting for the trait. This is usually the result of frequent treatment of animals and the use of improper (i.e., low) doses. When GINPs are exposed to low doses of the anthelmintics, a subpopulation survives after the treatment and will continue to reproduce. The subsequent generations of GINP will have been inadvertently selected to possess resistance to the anthelmintics.

The efficacy of the parasiticide ivermectin as a method of controlling GINPs in various formulations is well documented (Yazwinski et al., 1983; Swan et al., 1984; McKellar and Mariner 1987; Bogan et al., 1988; Taylor et al., 1990; Rehbein et al., 1998). Resistance of GINP to ivermectin is also well documented in many regions around the world (Table 6.1). Resistance has also been developed under laboratory conditions (Egerton et al., 1988). Different strains of ivermectin resistant *Haemonchus contortus* show different developmental characteristics in the laboratory (Echevarria et al., 1993). A number of excellent reviews have examined the development of resistance of gastrointestinal nematode parasites to ivermectin anthelmintics (Coles et al. 1992; Waller, 1997b; Sangster, 1999).

Due to the resistance of many species of GINP to commercially available anthelmintics, new areas of research have focused on alternative methods of control. The alternative products need to meet certain criteria if they are to be accepted by producers. First, they must be effective at eliminating GINP to the same degree and for the same duration as the chemical agents. Second, they must be easy to administer as either a drench or a feed additive. And finally, they must cost the same or less than the chemical anthelmintics. Products developed that meet these criteria will be readily accepted by the small ruminant production industry.

One nonchemical method currently being evaluated as a control of *H. contortus* and *Trichostrongylus colubriformis* in sheep is the use of nematophagous fungi. These fungi are effective in controlling

Table 6.1 Regions of the world that have reported resistance of gastrointestinal nematode parasites to ivermectin anthelmintics

Region	References
Australia	Waller et al. (1987)
	Swan et al. (1994)
	LeJambre et al. (1995)
US Virgin Islands	Panitz et al. (2002)
Brazil	Santiago et al. (1986)
	Echevarria and Trindade (1989)
	Vieira (1992)
	Farias et al. (1997)
Kenya	Waruiru (1997)
Malaysia	Chandrawathani et al. (1999)
South Africa	Van Wyck and Malan (1989)
	Van Wyk et al. (1997)
New Zealand	Pomroy and Whelan (1993)
Zimbabwe	Boersma and Pandev (1997)

populations of GINP because they interrupt the life cycle of the nematode by acting on the larval stages outside the body of the animal. The nematophagous fungus *Duddingtonia flagrans* traps nematode worms in its hyphae as they migrate through the soil. The efficacy of the nematophagous fungi *D. flagrans* and *Arthrobotrys* spp. in controlling the free-living stages of nematode parasites, specifically *T. colubriformis*, was studied by Faedo et al. (1997). They administered fungal spores orally in preinfected sheep and collected fecal samples to monitor effectiveness by egg counts and infective larval cultures. The results showed that *D. flagrans* had a better survival rate after passage through the gastrointestinal tract of sheep than did *Arthrobotrys* spp. The *D. flagrans* had the added benefit of causing a decrease in the development of *T. colubriformis* eggs to larvae in fecal cultures. They concluded that because of the low dose of spores needed ($1-5 \times 10^6$) for effective control and because only 50% of the spores need to be chlamydospores, there is potential for this fungus to be developed for use in feed supplements or controlled release devices for parasitic control.

The extent of infection of sheep and goats from naturally occurring nematode trapping fungi is not known. One study attempted to isolate naturally occurring nematode trapping fungi in fecal samples of sheep and goats in Fiji (Manueli et al., 1999). Out of the 12 pure isolates that were obtained, all of the fungi were from the genus *Arthrobotrys* spp. and no isolates of *D. flagrans* were found. The low level of *D. flagrans* isolates obtained could be explained by the infrequent exposure of the animals to the naturally occurring fungus. They also noted that the nematophagous fungi were isolated only from sheep feces and the majority came from one region. They attributed the lack of isolates found in goats to the difference in feeding behavior between the sheep and goats. At the pasture microenvironment at the soil/forage level the sheep graze is more suitable for the growth of nematophagous fungi, and therefore the sheep have a higher chance of consuming them than the goats that browse trees and shrubs (Manueli et al., 1999).

The method of feeding *D. flagrans* to sheep and its efficacy as a method for decreasing GINP was evaluated in a study by Waller et al. (2001b). In one trial they fed the nematophagous fungi spores in grain at levels of 4, 9, or 13×10^6 spores per day. Within 3–4 days after the feeding of the fungus they reported a decrease in the development of larvae in the fecal cultures obtained from the sheep. They were also able to culture the fungus from feces collected from the treated sheep for 5 days after feeding stopped. This would indicate that the fungus has the potential to have an effect on GINP for some time period after feeding is ended. These results were similar to those of Pena et al. (2002) in which sheep were fed *D. flagrans* at levels of 5, 2.5, and 1.25×10^5 and 5 and 2.5×10^4 spores per day. They reported a reduction in larvae within 2 days of starting the feeding of the fungus. It was determined that daily feeding was necessary to maintain the level of reduction, and there was only a 1 or 2 day limited residual effect after feeding of the fungus stopped.

A second part of the study reported by Waller et al. (2001b) evaluated the effect of feeding the *D. flagrans* fungus incorporated into urea molasses blocks. They were interested in determining if the fungus could survive this type of formulation. If successful this would provide an easier method of administering the fungus to sheep compared with daily feeding of grain treated with spores. The results showed the presence of *D. flagrans* in fecal samples of the sheep, and a reduction of larval development in fecal samples during the time the sheep were consuming the blocks. The proportion of larvae developing in culture stayed low for the first 3 days after the block feeding was discontinued and returned to levels comparable to the pretreatment period. A second aspect of this part of the trial evaluated the shelf life of the blocks with the fungus incorporated. The fungus survived well in blocks with low water content for 18 weeks or more when stored at 4°C. If the blocks contained some moisture then the viability of the fungus declined to low levels after 12 weeks of storage at room temperature. Waller et al. (2001b) hypothesized that this decline in efficacy may be due to the spores germinating in the presence of moisture and this led to a reduction in their ability to survive passage through the digestive tract of the sheep.

Another route of administration that has been evaluated is intraruminal controlled release devices (CRDs; Waller et al., 2001a). *D. flagrans* maintained viability in a tablet form of a CRD for 9 months at 4°C. In addition there was no effect of long-term exposure to room or elevated temperatures (40°C) in air or ruminal gases on the in vitro viability of the spores. When the CRDs were placed in the rumen of sheep, the authors were able to detect viable spores on the erosion surface of the CRD and in the feces of the sheep for 3 weeks after administration (Waller et al., 2001a). Some of the problems associated with the CRDs were what level of spores to incorporate into the device to get long-term efficacy and developing a matrix that will provide a uniform dosage over an extended time period.

Control of the nematode *Ostertagia circumcincta* in sheep by feeding three nematophagous fungi (*D. flagrans*, *Monacrosporium gephyropagum*, and *Harposporium helicoides*) alone or in combination was evaluated by Waghorn et al. (2002). They found that *D. flagrans* and *H. helicoides* alone or in combination reduced the level of infective larvae found in feces. The same study evaluated the presence of earthworms in the soil and the burial of dung as methods to control *Ostertagia circumcincta* in sheep. The burial of dung increased the total number of larvae recovered, and the presence of earthworms decreased the number of larvae. The authors hypothesized that dung burial mimicked the fact that the soil can act as a reservoir for infective larvae that eventually migrate to the herbage where they are re-ingested by the sheep as part of the life cycle of the GINP.

A recent study has evaluated the environmental impact of *D. flagrans* in a pasture environment (Knox et al., 2002). They placed sheep feces that contained or were free of *D. flagrans* spores on pasture plots at various times throughout the year and measured the dispersal of the fungus from the site of deposition. They also evaluated the impact of the presence of *D. flagrans* in the pasture on the populations of nontarget nematodes and microarthropods in the pastures. They reported that *D. flagrans* did not migrate outward from the point of deposition but it did persist for 8–24 weeks in association with the soil under the site of the fecal deposit. There was a negative gradient of

D. flagrans numbers through the soil as depth increased up to 30 cm. There was no impact of the *D. flagrans* on free-living soil nematodes and microarthropods, nor was there any negative effect on the presence of other nematode-trapping fungi. Knox et al. (2002) concluded that there was no negative environmental impact of *D. flagrans* in a pasture. These data add to the attractiveness of the use of nematophagous fungi for GINP control in small ruminants because they demonstrate that nematophageous fungi probably have no impact on the environment, in contrast to many chemical agents used for a variety of purposes in agriculture today.

The use of medicinal plants to control GINP infections in small ruminants has also been evaluated (for a review see Akhtar et al., 2000). In Sweden, Bernes et al. (2000) grazed young sheep on pastures containing *Lotus corniculatus* (birdsfoot trefoil) or *Trifolium repens* (white clover) and measured worm burdens by fecal egg counts collected serially after introduction of sheep into the pasture. At the end of the study the animals were slaughtered and worms were recovered from the digestive tract to identify the species and numbers of GINP. The results showed that there was no effect of either *Lotus corniculatus* or *Trifolium repens* on the number of nematode parasites recovered from the lambs. Bernes et al. (2000) hypothesized that the low level of condensed tannins in the *Lotus corniculatus* variety used and the low intake of the plant by the lambs may have accounted for the lack of parasite control in the study.

Other species of plants that have been evaluated for their ability to control GINP in sheep are *Myrsine africana* and *Rapanea melanophloeos* based on the use of these plants by sheep and goat farmers in Kenya (Githiori et al., 2002). The authors fed either the fruits or the leaves of each plant to lambs that were inoculated with *H. contortus* larvae and collected blood and fecal samples for 2 weeks after feeding to monitor parasite levels and packed cell volume. The fruits and leaves were dried and mixed with water before feeding to the lambs. The authors observed that there was no difference in fecal egg count between control and treated lambs that were fed the plants using the doses and preparation methods used in this study (Githiori et al., 2002). They also indicated that for any plant to be of use to farmers, it needs to have effectiveness in controlling *H. contortus* because this is the most common nematode parasite of sheep, especially in the tropical regions of the world.

Some work has been completed on immunological approach to control of *H. contortus*. Kabagambe et al. (2000) used gut membrane proteins derived from *H. contortus* as antigens to immunize sheep. They found large individual variations in fecal egg counts in both the vaccinated and nonvaccinated sheep that may have masked any treatment effects. Due to what they referred to as varying levels of susceptibility to parasite infection, the authors were unable to make any strong conclusions about the efficacy of the vaccine in the sheep (Kabagambe et al., 2000). They also concluded that more research was needed to fully evaluate the use of gut membrane proteins as antigens for an immunological control of GINP in sheep.

A unique method of controlling *H. contortus* in sheep grazing pasture by the use of copper oxide wire particles was tried by Knox (2002). The copper wire particles were originally used as a method of providing supplemental copper to grazing livestock. The copper oxide particles lodge in the folds of the abomasums and alter the pH, which induces the release of high concentrations of soluble copper. The elevated levels of copper have anthelmintic properties against some species of abomasal nematodes (Knox, 2002). Dosing sheep with 2.5 g of copper oxide wire particles resulted in a 37% decrease in total worm counts. When sheep were treated with either 2.5 or 5.0 g of copper oxide wire particles after 8 weeks of infection, it resulted in an 85% reduction in fecal egg counts. One drawback of this method is the susceptibility of sheep to copper toxicity. More experiments need to be performed to evaluate the effect of feeding the copper oxide wire particles on animal performance. One important procedure that should be performed is the measurement of the copper status of the animals before treatment with copper so the potential for copper toxicity can be evaluated.

Knox (2002) also cautioned about the possibility of copper accumulating in the plants in the pasture from high copper levels in the dung.

Another method of controlling GINP involves selecting for genetic resistance to infection. There are breeds of sheep and lines within breeds that have been identified as having some level of innate resistance to GINP infection. Gauly et al. (2002) compared Rhon and Merinoland sheep for their natural resistance to *H. contortus* infection. They noted that the resistance against *H. contortus* infection was higher and/or developed faster in Merinoland sheep than it was in Rhon sheep, based on higher initial fecal egg counts and a decrease in fecal egg counts in Merinoland sheep over time. Other breeds that have received attention in this area are the breeds of hair sheep found mainly in the Caribbean. One of the desirable traits attributed to this breed is a natural resistance to GINP infection. In many cases parasite resistance evolved in breeds that developed in the tropics, and they are the most productive genotype for that environment. In many cases this genotype is not suited for production in more temperate areas and more productive breeds that were selected and developed in the environment are utilized (Woolaston and Baker, 1996).

Work done by Godfrey et al. (1999) has shown that purebred St. Croix White hair sheep lambs have higher survival rates than wool X hair crossbreds under tropical conditions even though the level of fecal egg counts was similar. It may not be a true case of resistance to parasite infection, because the hair sheep have fecal egg counts and packed cell volumes that are similar to those reported in other breeds, but more a case of tolerance. The term tolerance is used because the hair sheep were able to survive with the elevated fecal egg counts and low packed cell volumes when the wool X hair crossbreds died under the same conditions. In contrast to this Yazwinski et al. (1979) reported that Barbados Blackbelly ewes in North Carolina had lower fecal egg counts and higher packed cell volumes than Dorset (wool) ewes when infected with a mixture of parasites. When the ewes were infected with a pure culture of *H. contortus* there was no significant breed effect, but the fecal egg counts and higher packed cell volumes favored the Barbados Blackbelly ewes. Yazwinski et al. (1979) were not able to detect any breed differences in levels of circulating antibodies that may have been involved in the breed specific resistance.

A method of controlling GINP in small ruminants with the most potential for the livestock industry appears to be the use of nematophagous fungi. The positive aspects of feeding nematophagous fungi as a method of controlling GINP include their ability to control GINP in a manner that will not lead to resistance, they possess a high level of efficacy, and they potentially have little if any negative environmental impact. One of the drawbacks of the method of feeding nematophagous fungi in its current level of development is the fact that it requires daily feeding for maximum effectiveness and there is very little residual effect after feeding stops. Not all sheep and goat producers have the ability to feed their animals on a daily basis, which limits the applicability of the fungi to animals raised on the range. The work of Waller et al. (2001a, 2001b) on the use of CRDs and block formulations may lead to the development of methods that would not require daily treatment of sheep. So far there has not been any move toward commercial production of feed with the nematophagous fungi incorporated into it for general sale to livestock producers. Before this happens it will most likely require testing and approval by federal regulatory agencies in whichever countries decide to pursue this option.

Control of external parasites

In addition to internal parasites there are also external parasites that infest livestock. The current methods of treating cases of external parasites consist of pharmaceuticals that are usually applied topically as a pour-on, spray, or a dip. Similar to the interest in alternative methods, besides pharmaceuticals, for control of internal parasites there is also some interest in alternative methods for controlling external parasites.

An excellent review of immunological control of arthropod ectoparasites of livestock was published by Pruett (1999). He describes the concerns of the agricultural and scientific communities about the dependency of the livestock industry on chemical means of parasite control, which have led to the need for development of environmentally friendly alternative methods for controlling ectoparasites. Unfortunately, the primary area of current research for the control of ectoparasites of cattle evaluates new pesticides and methods primarily using economic criteria. The TickGARD™ vaccine for use in cattle has been evaluated and used in Australia in combination with a reduced use of chemical acaracides (Willadsen, 1997). A product designed specifically for use in sheep and/or goats is not available at the present time.

A protein, vitellin, isolated from the tick *Boophilus microplus* and an 80 kDa glycoprotein isolated from larvae of *B. microplus* were used in efficacy trials in sheep by Tellam et al. (2002). Sheep vaccinated with purified vitellin or the 80 kDa glycoprotein had fewer engorged female ticks with lower weights and a lower level of oviposition. The authors reported that efficacy was eliminated when the protein used was a recombinant form of the 80 kDa glycoprotein, and they attributed this to changes in the folding of the protein or the attached oligosaccharides (Tellam et al., 2002). There is still much research to be done in producing an effective vaccine against ectoparasites in livestock.

Summary

The development of nontraditional methods of controlling gastrointestinal nematode parasites of small ruminants can have a major impact on the industry. By using alternative methods that will be as effective as the chemotherapeutic methods currently in use, but without the negative aspects, producers of small ruminants throughout the world can enhance the growth and productive traits of the animals. Most of the methods that are being developed would not have the problems associated with the development of resistance by the parasites, and would thus have more effectiveness at controlling parasites in sheep and goats in regions where the parasites have developed resistance to the anthelmintics. The immunological methods of controlling parasites have the added benefit of being developed to treat a specific species of parasite and could be used with more precision, and perhaps economic efficiency, than broad spectrum approaches.

References

Akhtar, M.S., Z. Iqbal, M.N. Khan, and M. Lateef. 2000. Anthelmintic activity of medicinal plants with particular reference to their use in animals in the Indo-Pakistan subcontinent. *Small Ruminant Res.* 38:99–107.

Bernes, G., P.J. Waller, and D. Christensson. 2000. The effect of birdfoot trefoil (*Lotus corniculatus*) and white clover (*Trifolium repens*) in mixed pasture swards on incoming and established nematode infections in young lambs. *Acta Vet. Scand.* 41:351–361.

Boersma, J.H. and V.S. Pandey. 1997. Anthelmintic resistance of trichostrongylids in sheep in the highveld of Zimbabwe. *Vet. Parasitol.* 68:383–388.

Bogan, J.A., Q.A. McKellar, E.S. Mitchell, and E.W. Scott. 1988. Efficacy of ivermectin against *Cooperia curticei* infection in sheep. *Am. J. Vet. Res.* 49:99–100.

Chandrawathani, P., M. Adnan, and P.J. Waller. 1999. Anthelmintic resistance in sheep and goat farms on Peninsular Malaysia. *Vet. Parasitol.* 82:305–310.

Coles, G.C., C. Bauer, F.H.M. Borgsteede, S. Greets, T.R. Klei, M.A. Taylor, and P.J. Waller. 1992. Methods for the detection of anthelmintic resistance in nematodes of veterinary importance. *Vet. Parasitol.* 44:35–44.

Echevarria, F.A.M., J. Armour, M.F. Bomba, and J.L. Duncan. 1993. Survival and development of ivermectin resistant or susceptible strains of *Haemonchus contortus* under field and laboratory conditions. *Res. Vet. Sci.* 54:133–139.

Echevarria, F.A.M and G.N.P. Trindade. 1989. Anthelmintic resistance by *Haemonchus contortus* to ivermectin in Brazil: a preliminary report. *Vet. Rec.* 124:147–148.

Egerton, J.R., D. Sudhayda, and C.H. Eary. 1988. Laboratory selection of *Haemonchus contortus* for resistance to Ivermectin. *J. Parasitol.* 74:614–617.

Faedo, M., M. Larsen, and P.J. Waller. 1997. The potential of nematophagous fungi to control the free-living stages of nematode parasites of sheep: comparison between Australian isolates of *Arthrobotrys* spp. and *Duddingtonia flagrans*. *Vet. Parasitol.* 72:145–155.

Farias, M.T., E.L. Bordin, A.B. Forbes, and K. NewComb. 1997. A survey on resistance to anthelmintics in sheep stud farms of southern Brazil. *Vet. Parasitol.* 72:209–215.

Gauly, M., M. Kraus, L. Vervelde, M.A.W. van Leeuwen, and G. Erhardt. 2002. Estimating genetic differences in natural resistance in Rhön and Merinoland sheep following experimental *Haemonchus contortus* infection. *Vet. Parasitol.* 106:55–67.

Githiori, J.B., J. Höglund, P.J. Waller, and R.L. Baker. 2002. Anthelmintic activity of preparations derived from *Myrsine africana* and *Rapanea melanophloeos* against the nematode parasite, *Haemonchus contortus*, of sheep. *J. Ethnopharmacol.* 80:187–191.

Godfrey, R.W., H.A. Buroker, and B.M. Pannagl. 1999. Parasite resistance and physiological responses of hair and wool X hair lambs in a tropical environment. *J. Anim. Sci.* 77(Suppl. 1): 238 (abstract).

Kabagambe, E.K., S.R. Barras, Y. Li, M.T. Pena, W.D. Smith, and J.E. Miller. 2000. Attempts to control haemonchosis in grazing ewes by vaccination with gut membrane proteins of the parasite. *Vet. Parasitol.* 92:15–23.

Knox, M.R. 2002. Effectiveness of copper oxide wire particles for *Haemonchus contortus* control in sheep. *Aust. Vet. J.* 80:224–227.

Knox, M.R. and M. Faedo. 2001. Biological control of field infections of nematode parasites of young sheep with *Duddingtonia flagrans* and effects of spore intake on efficacy. *Vet. Parasitol.* 101:155–160.

Knox, M.R., P.F. Josh, and L.J. Anderson. 2002. Deployment of *Duddingtonia flagrans* in an improved pasture system: dispersal, persistence, and effects on free-living soil nematodes and microarthropods. *Biol. Control* 24:176–182.

LeJambre, L.F., J.H. Gill, I.J. Lenane, and E. Lacey. 1995. Characterization of an avermectin resistant strain of Australian *Haemonchus contortus*. *Int. J. Parasitol.* 25:691–698.

Manueli, P.R., P.J. Waller, M. Faedo, and F. Mahommed. 1999. Biological control of nematode parasites of livestock in Fiji: screening of fresh dung of small ruminants for the presence of nematophagous fungi. *Vet. Parasitol.* 81:39–45.

McKellar, Q.A. and S.E. Mariner. 1987. Comparison of the anthelmintic efficacy of oxfendazole or ivermectin orally administered or ivermectin administered subcutaneously to sheep during the periparturient period. *Vet. Rec.* 120:383–386.

Panitz, E., R.W. Godfrey, and R.E. Dodson. 2002. Resistance to ivermectin and the effect of topical eprinomectin on faecal egg counts in St Croix White hair sheep. *Vet. Res. Commun.* 26:443–446.

Pena, M.T., J.E. Miller, M.E. Fontenot, A. Gillespie, and M. Larsen. 2002. Evaluation of *Duddingtonia flagrans* in reducing infective larvae of *Haemonchus contortus* in feces of sheep. *Vet. Parasitol.* 103:259–265.

Pomroy, W.E. and N.C. Whelan. 1993. Efficacy of mixodectin against an ivermectin resistant strain of *Ostertagia circumcincta* in young sheep. *Vet. Rec.* 132:416.

Pruett, J.H. 1999. Immunological control of arthropod ectoparasites—a review. *Int. J. Parasitol.* 29:25–32.

Rehbein, S, A.F. Batty, D. Barth, M. Vissar, B.J. Timms, R.A. Barrick, and J.S. Eagleson. 1998. Efficacy of an ivermectin controlled release capsule against nematode and arthropod endoparasites in sheep. *Vet. Rec.* 142:331–334.

Sangster, N.C. 1999. Anthelmintic resistance: past, present and future. *Int. J. Parasitol.* 29:115–124.

Santiago, M.A.M., U.C. da Costa, S.F. Bemeninga, E.L. Bordin and J. Grano. 1986. Efficacy of ivermectin against anthelmintic resistant isolates of sheep nematode parasites. *Vet. Rec.* 119: 43–44.

Swan, N., J.L. Gardner, R.B. Besere, and R. Wroth. 1994. A field case of ivermectin resistance to Ostertagia of sheep. *Aust. Vet. J.* 71:302–303.

Swan, G.E., J. Schroder, I.H. Carmichael, J.P. Loud, R.G. Harry, and I. Penderus. 1984. Efficacy of ivermectin against internal parasites of sheep. *J. S. Afr. Vet. Assoc.* 55:165–169.

Taylor, M.A., K.R. Hunt, C.A. Wilson, and D.G. Baggott. 1990. Efficacy of ivermectin against benizimidazole resistant nematodes of sheep. *Vet. Rec.* 127:302–303.

Tellam, R.L., D. Kemp, G. Riding, S. Briscoe, D. Smith, P. Sharp, D. Irving, and P. Willadsen. 2002. Reduced oviposition of *Boophilus microplus* feeding on sheep vaccinated with vitellin. *Vet. Parasitol.* 103:141–156.

Van Wyck, J.A. and F.S. Malan. 1989. Resistance of field strains of *Haemonchus contortus* to ivermectin, closantel, rafoxanide and the benzimidazoles in South Africa. *Vet. Res.* 123:226–228.

Van Wyk, J.A., F.S. Malan, and J.I. Randles. 1997. How long before resistance makes it impossible to control some field starins of *Haemonchus contortus* in South Africa with any of the modern anthelmintics? *Vet. Parasitol.* 70(1–3):111–122.

Vieira, L.S. 1992. *Haemonchus contortus* resistance to ivermectin and netobimin in Brazilian sheep. *Vet. Parasitol.* 45:111–116.

Waghorn, T.S., D.M. Leathwick, L.-Y. Chen, R.A.J. Gray, and R.A. Skipp. 2002. Influence of nematophagous fungi, earthworms and dung burial on development of the free-living stages of *Ostertagia (Teladorsagia) circumcincta* in New Zealand. *Vet. Parasitol.* 104:119–129.

Waller, P.J. 1987. Anthelmintic resistance and the future of roundworm control. *Vet. Parasitol.* 25:177–179.

Waller, P.J. 1997a. Nematode parasite control of livestock in the tropics/subtropics: the need for novel approaches. *Int. J. Parasitol.* 27:1193–1201.

Waller, P.J. 1997b. Anthelmintic resistance. *Vet. Parasitol.* 72:391–341.

Waller, P.J., M. Faedo, and K. Ellis. 2001a. The potential of nematophagous fungi to control the free-living stages of nematode parasites of sheep: towards the development of a fungal controlled release device. *Vet. Parasitol.* 102:299–308.

Waller, P.J., M.R. Knox, and M. Faedo. 2001b. The potential of nematophagous fungi to control the free-living stages of nematode parasites of sheep: feeding and block studies with *Duddingtonia flagrans*. *Vet. Parasitol.* 102:321–330.

Waruiru, R.M. 1997. Efficacy of closantel, albendazole and levamisole on an ivermectin resistant strain of *Haemonchus contortus* in sheep. *Vet. Parasitol.* 73:65–71.

Willadsen, P. 1997. Novel vaccines for ectoparasites. *Vet. Parasitol.* 71:209–222.

Woolaston, R.R. and R.L. Baker. 1996. Prospects of breeding small ruminants for resistance to internal parasites. *Int. J. Parasitol.* 26:845–855.

Yazwinski T.A., L. Goode, D.J. Moncol, G.W. Morgan, and A.C. Linnerud. 1979. Parasite resistance in straightbred and crossbred Barbados Blackbelly sheep. *J. Anim. Sci.* 49:919–926.

Yazwinski, T., A.T. Greenway, S.L. Presson, L.M. Pote, and H. Featherstone. 1983. Antiparasitic efficacy of ivermectin in internally parasitized sheep. *Am. J. Vet. Res.* 44:2186–2187.

Chapter 7
Overview of Research Methods on Medicinal Plants for Livestock: Endo- and Ecto-parasites

Jennifer K. Ketzis

Introduction

The control of endo- and ecto-parasite infections is necessary for the maintenance of healthy, productive livestock. Endo-parasites (e.g., nematodes, cestodes) damage the gastrointestinal (GI) tract, decrease feed intake, decrease nutrient absorption, alter feed utilization, and, in some cases, can lead to livestock death. Ecto-parasites (e.g., mites, lice, flies, and ticks) can distract livestock from grazing, damage hides, cause infections, and transmit diseases (Bowman, 1999; Parkins and Holmes, 1989).

Current endo- and ecto-parasite control methods rely on a combination of management methods and chemotherapeutics (anthelmintics, insecticides, and repellents). Alternatives to the commonly used chemotherapeutics are needed for several reasons. First, many of the available treatments for endo-parasites are becoming less effective. Endo-parasites are becoming resistant to almost every chemical class of available anthelmintics (Prichard, 1994). Second, there are environmental and human health concerns with both types of treatments. For example, ivermectin, which is one of the most commonly used anthelmintics, can potentially kill beneficial soil microorganisms (Pfeiffer et al., 1998). Many of the ecto-parasite treatments are organophosphates, which are cholinesterase inhibitors. Third, there is a growing desire among the general population for more "natural" and environmentally friendly treatments (e.g., the increase in the organic food market). Fourth, in many parts of the world, synthetic endo- and ecto-parasite treatments are either unavailable or are not cost effective (Hammond et al., 1997).

Plants with bioactive compounds are a potential alternative to the chemotherapeutics currently used to control endo- and ecto-parasite infections. Plant treatments for endo-parasites can be given as single oral doses, daily doses mixed with feeds, and planted in pastures. Ecto-parasite treatments can be sprayed on animals and mixed in bedding. Given the wide variety of applications and the need for new treatments, investigation on the use of medicinal plants in veterinary medicine is becoming a fast growing field of research.

In this chapter the basic steps in medicinal plant research for endo- and ecto-parasite treatments are outlined, and some preliminary results are presented by using these steps. In addition, I discuss the efficacy and safety of plant-based treatments and how livestock owners can assist in documenting efficacy.

Basic steps in researching plants as parasite treatments

While there are several approaches to researching medicinal plants, most programs have similar components. These basic components include: (1) identification of potential plant treatments; (2) profiling or identifying the plant compounds; (3) in vitro laboratory screening; (4) preliminary in vivo trials (proof-of-concept); and (5) in vivo efficacy, toxicity, and food residue trials. Differences in the methods and the stress placed on each step depend on the purpose of the research. For example, if the purpose of the research is to validate methods used in ethnoveterinary medicine, stress is placed on in vivo efficacy. If the purpose is to identify active compounds that can be synthesized, stress might be placed on compound identification.

Identifying plants

There are two primary sources of information on plants for endo- and ecto-parasite research: ethnoveterinary and traditional medicine and zoopharmacognosy. Data on the use of plants in ethnoveterinary and traditional medicine can be found in the literature or collected via interviews with people who currently use these treatments. Interviews using participatory techniques have the advantage of providing extensive information on the exact preparation methods and dosing regimes. The literature can indicate how extensively a treatment is used and provide information on the plant (chemistry, other known uses). In zoopharmacognosy, the study of self-treatment, animals are observed to determine if they will eat and/or rub themselves with plants known to contain bioactive compounds or if they will eat and/or rub themselves with plants not normally a part of the diet when they are known to have an endo- or ecto-parasite infection. In addition, animals and birds are observed to determine if they will use unusual plants as bedding or nesting materials (Rodriguez and Wrangham, 1993; Robles et al., 1995).

Participatory techniques were used in the Dominican Republic and Honduras to obtain information on plants used to treat all types of livestock and human ailments (e.g., parasites, stomach pain, diarrhea, skin infections, mastitis, etc.), preparation methods, and doses. Information on over 40 plants was collected. These plants are listed in Table 7.1 along with plants cited in the literature as used in ethnoveterinary treatments.

Voucher specimens of the plants identified were collected and sent to the Jardin Botanico Nacional, Santo Domingo, Dominican Republic or the Bailey Horatorium, Cornell University for identification. Bulk collections of the plants also were made. In all cases, the local informant was asked to verify that the correct plants were collected and labeled with the proper local name.

Preliminary chemical profiles/compound identification

The next step in most research programs is the identification of the chemicals in the plants. The plant material is extracted and concentrated to make a crude extract. This extract can be fractionated several times based on the polarity of the compounds in the plant and the extract solvents used.

To obtain a general idea of the classes of compounds in a plant extract, thin-layer chromatography (TLC) can be used. To obtain more extensive information about the compounds and identify the compounds, many methods can be used including HPLC, GC-MS, and H-NMR. The extent to which the compounds are identified and classified depends on the purpose of the research program. Some secondary plant compounds of special interest and that are known or believed to decrease parasite infections are: ascaridole, eugenol, genistein, methylchavicol, santonin, superoxides, terpineol,

Table 7.1 Plants used to treat endo- and ecto-parasite infections in livestock

Plants used in the Dominican Republic for endo-parasites[a]

Apocynaceae	Chenopodiaceae	Malvaceae	Rubiaceae
Nerium oleander	*Chenopodium*	*Gossypium*	*Coffee arabica*
Arecaceae	*Ambrosioides*	*barbadensis*	*Spermacoce*
Mikania spp.	Combretaceae	Mimosaceae	*assurgen*
Ateraceae	*Laguncularia racemosa*	*Prosopis juliflora*	Rutaceae
Ambrosia	*Conocarpus erectus*	Moraceae	*Citrus aurantifolia*
artemisaefolia	Cucurbitaceae	*Cecropia schreberiana*	*Citrus aurantium*
Bignoniaceae	*Momordica charantia*	Passifloraceae	*Citrus limeta*
Catalpa longissima	Euphorbiaceae	*Passiflora*	Scrophulariaceae
Crescentia cujete	*Jatropha gossypifolia*	*Quadranqularis*	*Capraria biflora*
Cactaceae	Fabaceae	Phytolaccaceae	Smilacaceae
Opuntia ficus indica	*Cajanus cajan*	*Petiveria alliacea*	*Smilax aff.*
Caesalpiniaceae	*Centrosema* spp.	Poaceae	*Rotundifolia*
Cassia grandis	Lamiaceae	*Melinis minutiflora*	Sterculiaceae
Senna alata	*Plectranthus*	Portulacaceae	*Guazuma*
			tomentosa
Senna alexandria	*Ambionicus*	*Portulaca oleraceae*	Vitaceae
Caricaceae	Malphighiaceae	Rhamnaceae	*Cissus verticillata*
Carica papaya	*Bunchosia glandulosa*	*Gouania* spp.	

Plants used elsewhere for endo-parasites

Arecaceae	Burseraceae	Leguminoseae	Palmaceae
Areca catechu	*Boswellia dalzelii*	*Leucaena glauca*	*Cocos nucifera*
Asteraceae	Euphorbiaceae	Menispermaceae	
Senecio lyratipartitus	*Croton macrostachys*	*Cissampelos*	
	Erythrina senegalensis	*Mucromata*	

Plants used in the dominican republic for ecto-parasites[a]

Apocynaceae	Malvaceae	Papaveraceae	Piperaceae
Nerium oleander	*Pavonia fruticosa*	*Argemone mexicana*	*Piper aduncum*
Bixaceae	Melastomataceae	Phytolaccaceae	Rubinaceae
Bixa orellana	*Miconia laevigata*	*Petiveria alliacea*	*Morinda royoc*
Fabaceae	Meliaceae		
Gliricidia sepium	*Azadirachata indica*		

Plants used elsewhere

Annonaceae	Caesalpiniaceae	Leguminosae	Piperaceae
Annona squamosa	*Cassia alata*	*Amorpha fruticosa*	*Piper auritum*
Araceae	Caprifoliaceae	*Baptisia tinctoria*	Polygonaceae
Acorus calamus	*Sambucus canadensis*	Liliaceae	*Polygonum*
			hydropiper
Ascelpiadaceae	Euphorbiaceae	*Aloe ferox*	Solanaceae
Sarcostemma	*Euphorbia bicolor*	*Veratrum album*	*Nicotiana tabacum*
viminale			
Bombacaceae	*Euphorbia marginata*	Meliaceae	Verbenaceae
Adansonia digitata	*Ricinus communis*	*Azadirachta indica*	*Tectona grandis*

[a]Some of the plants listed are used in human medicine and not for animals. Also, some of the endo-parasite plants are used to treat stomach pain and are only used in parasite treatment mixtures.
Sources for plants not used in the Dominican Republic: Hammond et al. (1997), Mateo (1992), Matzigkeit (1990) and Palacpac-Alo (1990).

and thymol (Asha et al., 2001; Bennet-Jenkins and Bryant, 1996; Docampo, 1990; Githiori et al., 2003; Hammond et al., 1997; Kato et al., 2000; Ketzis, 1999; Murillo et al., 2002; Pal and Tandon, 1998; Paula et al., 2003; Pessoa et al., 2002; Reddy et al., 1991; Vasudevan et al., 1999).

If a plant extract is to be developed into a treatment, then at a minimum, marker compounds (primary compounds in the plant) need to be identified and a method for producing an extract with a consistent chemical composition is needed. Plants vary in their composition depending on age (e.g., early bloom versus late bloom) and growing conditions. This variation can directly correlate to levels of efficacy, and hence the need for developing a method of standardizing the extract.

For the plants collected in the Dominican Republic and Honduras, only preliminary chemical profiles were developed using TLC. The bulk collections were air dried and extracted with 95% ethanol, a 50:50 mixture of methanol and chloroform, or hot water (1:5 ratio of plant material to extract solvent). The extracts were filtered and concentrated. Six reagents were used to identify the general class of compounds in the plants. In addition, extensive literature searches were conducted on each plant to collect available information on the chemistry of the plants. Full elucidation of the active compounds is not planned until after it is known that the extract is bioactive. Many of the plants collected contain flavonoids, monoterpenes, phenols, and tannins.

In vitro screens

A variety of in vitro test methods are available to determine if a plant is bioactive. However, the results of in vitro tests cannot be directly related to in vivo activity, especially for endo-parasites. Plants used for endo-parasites can be changed in the gastrointestinal tract. Therefore, the compounds in the extract tested in vitro are not always the same as those that come into contact with the parasites in vivo. In addition, most adult endo-parasites that are the target of plant treatments cannot be cultivated outside of the gastrointestinal tract. Therefore, in vitro tests, substitutes for the adult parasites such as the eggs or larvae of the parasites or adult free-living nematodes (e.g., *Caenorhabditis elegans*) have to be used. Laboratory testing of plants for ecto-parasites can be better correlated to efficacy when used on animals. However, laboratory tests do not take into account how plant compounds are altered when applied to skin/hair, how long they last on an animal, or whether or not they are absorbed into the skin.

Despite these limitations, in vitro and laboratory testing are useful for screening plants and identifying plants for in vivo testing. Some industrial companies use high-throughput screens (largely automated) to quickly test thousands of plant extract fractions. In other cases, small scale, more labor intensive methods are used. In both types of screens, activity against a variety of parasites and life stages can be tested.

Two types of ecto-parasite tests and one type of endo-parasite test were conducted with the crude extracts of the plants collected in the Dominican Republic. In addition, all extracts were screened to determine antibacterial and antifungal properties. Bacteria and fungi used in these tests include: *Escherichia coli, Staphylococcus aureus, Pseudomonas aeruginosa, Bacillus cereus*, and *Candida albicans*.

The Lesser Mealworm (*Alphitobius diaperinus,* a common insect in chicken houses) was used for testing the oral toxicity and repellency of the plant extracts. For the oral toxicity tests, the extracts were mixed with a corn-based feed (1%) and offered as the sole source of food for the mealworms. Total number of dead and live mealworms was counted daily for 10 days. For the repellency tests, filter paper was divided into two halves and one half was treated with 1.5 g of extract/m^2 and the other half left untreated. The number of mealworms on each section of filter paper was counted at 3, 6, and 12 hours postexposure and daily thereafter for 5 days.

Table 7.2 In vitro bioactivity of plants used in endo- and ecto-parasite treatments

Plant	Ovicidal	Larvicidal	Repellent
Bixa orellana (seeds)[a]	X	–	X
Catalpa longissima[a]	X	X	–
Chenopodium ambrosioides[b]	X	X	NT
Cissus verticillata (vinestock)[c]	X	NT	–[d]
Clusia rosea (seeds)[a]	NT	NT	X
Conocarpus erectus[a]	–	X	NT
Crescentia cujete[a]	NT	NT	X
Jatropha gossypifolia[a]	X (leaves) – (roots)	X (leaves) – (roots)	X (root)[d]
Laguncularia racemosa[a]	–	X	NT
Melinis minutiflora (roots)[a]	NT	NT	X
Nerium oleander[d]	NT	NT	X
Passiflora quadranqularis[a]	X	NT	X
Petiveria alliacea(roots)[d]	NT	NT	X
Senna alata[a]	X	NT	–[d]
Senna alexandria[a,c]	X	–	NT

X: exhibited activity; –: did not exhibit activity; NT: not tested
Note: Leaves were used for all extracts, unless otherwise indicated
Ovicidal and larvicidal tests used *H. contortus*
Repellency tests used *Alphitobus diaperinus*
[a] Ethanol extract
[b] Plant oil
[c] Water extract
[d] Methanol/chloroform extract

Egg-hatch tests with *Haemonchus contortus* (a significant parasite of goats and sheep) were used to determine potential endo-parasite activity of the plant extracts (2 ul and higher). Hatched larvae also were categorized as alive or dead to obtain a general idea of activity against larvae. All tests followed general published guidelines (Coles et al., 1992; Hamburger and Hostettmann, 1991; Janssen et al., 1987; Laudani and Swank, 1954; Lorimer et al., 1996).

In the initial tests, relatively high concentrations of the crude extracts were used. Extracts that showed some activity were retested at different concentration levels. A summary of some of the preliminary results from these in vitro tests is presented in Table 7.2. None of the plants exhibited oral toxicity. *Petiveria alliacea* and *Bixa orellana* had the highest indication of repellency properties. The essential oil of *Chenopodium ambrosoides* showed the highest efficacy in the egg-hatch tests. Almost all of the plants showed some level of antimicrobial activity.

In vivo studies

To determine the true efficacy and safety of a plant-based treatment, it must be tested on the target species (e.g., goats, cattle). The first in vivo studies are often referred to as proof-of-concept studies. After proof-of-concept has been confirmed, dose-titration studies and residue studies are conducted. For most proof-of-concept studies, the animals are administered with a challenging infection. For example, with endo-parasites, the animals are given 3,000 or more infective parasite larvae that are allowed to develop into adult worms. Once the adult worms are established in the test animals, the animals are divided into treatment and control groups. After treatment with the test plant, the animals are slaughtered and the adult worms are collected and counted. The number of recovered parasites in the treated animals is compared to the number in the controls.

Once an effective dose is selected, residue studies can be conducted. Animals are slaughtered at different time periods after treatment and tissue samples are collected and analyzed for the plant compounds.

For ecto-parasite treatments two types of "in vivo" tests are conducted. For topical treatments, the plant can be applied to animals and then the animals challenged with a parasite. For facility treatments, identical buildings can be infested with an insect and then one building treated and the other maintained as a control.

Of the plants identified in the Dominican Republic and Honduras, none have been tested on a large scale for ecto-parasite activity. Currently, only one endo-parasite treatment, *C. ambrosioides*, has been tested in vivo. Protocols for the in vivo tests were based on those recommended by the World Association for the Advancement of Veterinary Parasitology (Wood et al., 1995), and included a preliminary efficacy trial, a milk and tissue residue trial, and an efficacy dose-titration trial. Fresh plant material and chenopodium oil were given to kids with *H. contortus* infections, and the number of parasite eggs in the feces and adult parasites in the abomasum were counted and compared to those of untreated kids. Details on the study are found in Ketzis (1999) and Ketzis et al. (2002).

In the in vivo tests, *C. ambrosioides* was found not to be a viable anthelmintic treatment. It did not significantly decrease endo-parasite infection levels. In addition, two of the four kids given the higher doses (0.4 ml oil/kg body weight) died. Kid goats given the lower doses were depressed and rumen activity was decreased for several hours after treatment. In addition, when the oil was given to lactating dose, the active compound (ascaridole) and some of its metabolites could be found in the milk 3–6 hours posttreatment.

Discussion

There is much evidence that plant treatments can be effective. For example, from the 1920s to the 1940s, one of the most commonly used anthelmintics in humans was the oil of chenopodium, derived from *C. ambrosioides*. Also, many of the currently popular ecto-parasite treatments for small animals are synthetic pyrethroids, which are based on the pyrethrins found in *Chrysanthemum cinerariaefolium*. Another common ecto-parasite treatment is rotenone, derived from derris roots (*Derris elliptica*), which is used to treat mite infections in dogs.

There is extensive information available on the use of plants in ethno veterinary medicine, and researchers such as Hammond et al. (1997) and Akhtar et al. (2000) have presented excellent reviews on the potential of plant-based anthelmintics in the tropics and Indo-Pakistan regions, respectively. Many recent conferences, publications, Web sites, and list serves are increasing the dissemination of medicinal plant information. While there is much information available on the historical and current uses of plants in endo- and ecto-parasite treatments, there are few data on efficacy, appropriate doses, safety, and food residues for these alternative methods. These data are essential because many plants can be toxic and because the use of ineffective treatments can lead to a decrease in livestock production.

Traditional use of a plant in ethnoveterinary medicine does not mean that the plant is effective or safe. Also, effectiveness of human traditional medicine does not correspond directly with effectiveness in livestock. In the data presented here, all of the plants tested had activity against either endo- or ecto-parasites in vitro. However, as shown with *C. ambrosioides*, in vitro efficacy does not guarantee in vivo efficacy. In addition, the tests with *C. ambrosioides* showed that natural treatments can be harmful and leave residues in foods (milk, meat).

C. ambrosioides is not the only plant treatment that has been ineffective or raised safety concerns with "natural" treatments. The traditionally used powdered fruits of *Mallotus philippinensis* and *Artemisia cina* were ineffective in vivo (Cabaret, 1996; Jost et al., 1996). Tests with traditionally prepared *Myrsine africana* (leaves at 125 g and fruits at 50 g) and *Rapanea melanophloeos* (fruit at 50 and 125 g) also were ineffective (Githiori et al., 2002). Stem bark of *Zanthoxylum liebmannianum* was effective in vivo, but the active compound (alpha-sanshool) caused seizures in mice (Navarrete and Hong, 1996). Allen et al. (1998) showed that garlic was not effective in treating naturally occurring parasite infections in sheep. While Bromelain (from *Ananas comosus*) and the fruit extract of *Melia azedarach* were effective against various nematode endo-parasites in vitro, neither was effective in vivo (sheep) (Hördegen et al., 2002).

Other in vivo tests with plants have shown more promise. An extract of the whole plant of *Fumaria parviflora* showed activity in vivo (sheep) (Hördegen et al., 2002). Leaves of *Eucalyptus grandis* fed to goats for 7 days significantly lowered *H. contortus* infection levels compared to nontreated goats and did not cause adverse reactions (Bennet-Jenkins and Bryant, 1996). Tests with papaya latex have shown that doses of 4 and 8 g/kg body weight reduce *Ascaris suum* infections in pigs. However, the higher dose did cause transient diarrhea (Satrija et al., 1994). Studies with condensed tannins at various doses and for differing lengths of treatment have shown that they can reduce nematode parasites infections in sheep (Athanasiadou et al., 2000, 2001). Of the plant-based ecto-parasite treatments, one that shows good potential is *Gliricidia sepium*. When applied to cattle, it repelled ticks (*Boophilus microplus*) and warble flies (*Dermatobia hominis*) (Miranda et al., 1999). Studies with *Artemisia verlotorum* also show promise (Perrucci et al., 2001). Many more plant extracts and plant essential oils have been tested for their use as short-lasting repellents for people and treatments for grain in storage. Several leads from these areas of research could be useful to follow-up on for use in livestock ecto-parasite treatments.

Recommendations

Few plants to date have been shown to be effective and safe when used to control endo- or ecto-parasites. However, only a handful of the plants used in ethnoveterinary and traditional medicine have been rigorously tested. Also, much of the current research is focused on plants available in the tropics. These plants are not available to farmers throughout the world. Given the slow process of testing plants and the number of plants to be tested, it might be many years before safe and efficacious treatments are identified.

Many farmers, especially organic and small ruminant livestock producers, use or are experimenting with alternative endo- and ecto-parasite control methods. By following a few experimental guidelines and with better documentation, farmers could contribute significantly to the body of information available on alternatives. This is especially critical since farmers use plants and alternative treatments that are readily available in their area (e.g., easily grown in the climatic zone) or easily purchased. An example protocol to use on-farm for endo-parasite treatments is presented in Table 7.3.

Ecto-parasite research can be more difficult to conduct. For lice research, the number of lice in a defined location and area (e.g., a 2 inch^2 area at the base of the tail) can be counted before and after

Table 7.3   Basic protocol for testing an endo-parasite treatment (given once or for a few days (2–8) consecutively)

1. Determine the average parasite eggs/gram of feces (epg) (e.g., modified McMaster egg count) for all animals to be included in study. To do this, two fecal samples from each animal should be collected on different days. Determining epg is a simple process and many farmers have the equipment and training to do this. Alternatively, the samples can be sent to a laboratory
2. Divide the animals in two groups (of approximately equal age, sex, weight, and epg) with at least six animals in each group. More groups can be used, if more than one treatment is being tested
3. Give one group the alternative treatment. The other group can be given a registered anthelmintic or no treatment
4. Observe the animals at least 1 hour after treatment for any adverse effects (depression, off-feed, etc.). Follow-up observations 12 and 24 hours later also are recommended
5. Approximately 5–7 days after the last treatment, again determine the average epg for each animal by collecting two samples on different days
6. Compare the epg for each group
7. For all steps, record the data for future reference
8. Always save dried samples of the plant material used. If there are any questions from others regarding the material used, chemical composition of the material, etc. having a sample available to distribute is extremely useful
9. Consult with your veterinarian or local cooperative extension agent regarding the design of the study and the results
10. Make use of available resources on study designing methods (e.g., Sooby, 2001) and share results and methods with others (e.g., the EthnoVeterinary Mailing list)

a treatment is used. House fly populations (more of a nuisance than a parasite) can be measured using spot cards.

Whenever alternative plant-based treatments are used, caution should be taken to ensure that unauthorized compounds/drugs do not enter the food chain. Most alternatives are not approved by regulatory authorities (e.g., Food and Drug Administration and AAFCO). Therefore, experimentation should not be done in lactating dairy animals or in animals that are shortly going to market. In cases of farmer conducted research, the farmer is responsible for the safety of the food entering the market.

Conclusions

Documentation on the safety and efficacy of plant treatments for endo- and ecto-parasites is a long process. Much of the current research in this area is in the preliminary stages and few of the results can be transferred into treatments available for on-farm use. Livestock owners who use plant treatments to control endo- and ecto-parasite infections need to be aware of the risks related to these treatments. Uncontrolled parasite infections (due to inefficacious treatments) can lead to decreased livestock productivity and sometimes death. Also, plant treatments can cause some of the same problems as currently used treatments—toxic reactions and food residues. Given the growing interest in these alternative treatments, research into efficacy and safety is essential. Negative and positive results of livestock owner experimentation and laboratory in vivo studies need to be made readily accessible to the general public, and forums for sharing information need to be developed.

Acknowledgments

The assistance of Dr. Manuel Aregullin, Maria Laux and the participants in the Cornell Undergraduate Research Program on Biodiveristy 2000 in this research is appreciated. Also, funding for this research is supported by a National Institutes of Health (NIH) Training grant (#5T32 CA09682) and a NIH Minorities International Research Training grant (#T37 TW00076).

References

Akhtar, M.S., Z. Iqbal, M.N. Khan, and M. Lateef. 2000. Anthelmintic activity of medicinal plants with particular reference to their use in animals in the Indo-Pakistan subcontinent. *Small Rum. Res.* 38:99–107.

Allen, J., M. Boal, and P. Doherty. 1998. *Identifying and Testing Alternative Parasiticides for the Use in the Production of Organic Lamb.* Final Project Report (Grant #98–03). Organic Farming Research Foundation, Santa Cruz, CA.

Asha, M.K., D. Prashanth, B. Murali, R. Padmaja, and A. Amit. 2001. Anthelmintic activity of essential oil of *Ocimum sanctum* and *eugenol. Fitoterapia* 72(6):669–670.

Athanasiadou, S., I. Kyriazakis, F. Jackson, and R.L. Coop. 2000. Effects of short-term exposure to condensed tannins on adult *Trichostrongylus colubriformis. Vet. Rec.* 146:728–732.

Athanasiadou, S., I. Kyriazakis, F. Jackson, and R.L. Coop. 2001. Direct anthelmintic effects of condensed tannins towards different gastrointestinal nematodes of sheep: in vitro and in vivo studies. *Vet. Parasitol.* 99:205–219.

Bennet-Jenkins, E. and C. Bryant. 1996. Novel sources of anthelmintics. *Int. J. Parasitol.* 26(8–9): 937–947.

Bowman, D.D. 1999. *Georgis' Parasitology for Veterinarians.* W.B. Saunders, Philadelphia, PA.

Cabaret, J. 1996. The homeopathic Cina does not reduce the egg output of digestive-tract nematodes in lambs. *Revue de Medecine Veterinaire,* 147(6):445–446.

Coles, G.C., C. Bauer, F.H.M. Borgsteede, S. Geerts, T.R. Klei, M.A. Taylor, and P.J. Waller. 1992. World Association for the Advancement of Veterinary Parasitology methods for the detection of anthelmintic resistance in nematodes of veterinary importance. *Vet. Parasitol.* 44:35–44.

de Paula, J.P., M.R. Gomes-Carneiro, and F.J.R. Paumgartten. 2003. Chemical composition, toxicity and mosquito repellency of Ocimum selloi oil. *J. Ethnopharmacol.* 88(2–3):253–260.

Docampo, R. 1990. Sensitivity of parasites to free radical damage by antiparasitic drugs. *Chemico-Biological Interactions* 73(1):1–27.

Githiori, John B., J. Höglund, P.J. Waller, and R.L. Baker. 2002. Anthelmintic activity of preparations derived from *Myrsine africana* and *Rapanea melanophloeos* against the nematode parasite, *Haemonchus contortus,* of sheep. *J. Ethnopharmacol.* 80:187–191.

Githiori, J.B., J. Höglund, P.J. Waller, and R.L. Baker. 2003. Evaluation of anthelmintic properties of extracts from some plants used as livestock dewormers by pastoralist and smallholder farmers in Kenya against *Heligmosomoides polygyrus* infections in mice. *Vet. Parasitol.* 118(3–4):215–226.

Hamburger, M. and K. Hostettmann. 1991. Bioactivity in plants: the link between phytochemistry and medicine. *Phytochemistry* 30(12):3864–3874.

Hammond, J.A., D. Fielding, and S.C. Bishop. 1997. Prospects for plant anthelmintics in tropical veterinary medicine. *Vet. Res. Commun.* 21(3):213–228.

Hördegen, P., H. Hertzberg, and V. Maurer. 2002. Plants with anthelmintic efficacy against gastrointestinal strongylids: an option for organic agriculture? Abstract and presentation at the 1st *European Symposium: Bioactive Secondary Plant Products in Veterinary Medicine,* Vienna, Austria 4–5 October 2002.

Janssen, A.M., J.J.C. Scheffer, and A. Baerheim Svendsen. 1987. Antimicrobial activity of essential oils: a 1976–1986 literature review. Aspects of the test methods. *Planta Med.* 53:395–398.

Jost, C.C., D.M. Sherman, E.F. Thomson, and R.M. Hesselton. 1996. Kamala (*Mallotus philippinensis*) fruit is ineffective as an anthelmintic against gastrointestinal nematodes in goats indigenous to Balochistan, Pakistan. *Small Ruminant Res.* 20(2):147–153.

Kato S., D.D. Bowman, and D.L. Brown. 2000. Efficacy of *Chenopodium ambrosioides* as an antihelmintic for treatment of gastrointestinal nematodes in lambs. *J. Herbs, Spices, Med. Plants* 7(2):11–25.

Ketzis, J.K. 1999. The anthelmintic potential of *Chenopodium ambrosioides* in goats. Dissertation, Ithaca, New York.

Ketzis, J.K., A. Taylor, D.D. Bowman, D.L. Brown, L.D. Warnick and H.N. Erb. 2002. *Chenopodium ambrosioides* and its essential oil as treatments for *Haemonchus contortus* and mixed adult-nematode infections in goats. *Small Ruminant Res.* 44(3):193–200.

Laudani, H. and G.R. Swank. 1954. A laboratory apparatus for determining repellency of pyrethrum when applied to grain. *J. Econ. Entomol.* 47:1104–1107.

Lorimer, S.D., N.B. Perry, L.M. Foster, E.J. Burgess, P.G.C. Douch, M.C. Hamilton, M.J. Donaghy, and R.A. McGregor. 1996. A nematode larval motility inhibition assay for screening plant extracts and natural products. *J. Agric. Food Chem.* 44(9):2842–2845.

Mateo, C. 1992. Herbal medicine in livestock and poultry production. In *Proceedings 8th Congress of the Federation of Asian Veterinary Associations*, 21–25 November 1992, Philippines, pp. 783–792.

Matzigkeit, U. 1990. Natural Veterinary Medicine: Ectoparasites in the Tropics. AGRECOL. Weikersheim, Margraf.

Miranda, Y., S. Lozano, J. Vaquedano, W. Romero, J.D. Vellojín, and D. Suárez. 1999 (unpublished). Comparacíon de productos químicos y extractos naturales (*Gliricidia sepium y Lippia alba*) para el control de ecto y endoparásitos. Escuela de Agricultura de la Región Tropical Húmeda, Guácimo, Costa Rica.

Murillo, E., A. Viña, and M. Linares. 2002. Chemical composition, insecticidal and antifungal activity of Ocimum micranthum Willd. *Revista Colombiana de Entomología* 28(1):109–113.

Navarrete, A. and E. Hong. 1996. Anthelmintic properties of alpha-sanshool from *Zanthoxylum liebmannianum. Planta Med.* 62(3):250–251.

Pal, P. and V. Tandon. 1998. Anthelmintic efficacy of Flemingia vestita (Fabaceae): Genistein-induced alterations in the esterase activity in the cestode, *Raillietina echinobothrida. J. Biosci.* 23(1):25–31.

Palacpac-Alo, A.M. 1990. Save your animals! Try medicinal herbs. *PCARRD Monitor.* 18(2):3, 8–9.

Parkins, J.J. and P.H. Holmes. 1989. Effects of gastrointestinal helminth parasites on ruminant nutrition. *Nutr. Res. Rev.* 2:227–246.

Perrucci, S., G. Flamini, P.L. Cioni, I. Morelli, F. Macchioni, and G. Macchioni. 2001. In vitro and in vivo efficacy of extracts of *Artemisia verlotorum* against *Psoroptes cuniculi. Vet. Rec.* 148:814–815.

Pessoa, L.M., S.M. Morais, C.M.L. Bevilaqua, and J.H.S. Luciano. 2002. Anthelmintic activity of essential oil of *Ocimum gratissimum* Linn. and eugenol against *Haemonchus contortus. Vet. Parasitol.* 109:59–63.

Pfeiffer, C., C. Emmerling, D. Schroder, and J. Niemeyer. 1998. Antibiotics (ivermectin, monensin) and endocrine environmental chemicals (nonylphenol, ethinylestradiol) in soils. *Umweltwissenschaften und Schadstoff-Forschung.* 10 (3):147–153.

Prichard, R. 1994. Anthelmintic resistance. *Vet. Parasitol.* 54(1–3):259–268.

Reddy, G.B.S., A.B. Melkhani, G.A. Kalyani, J.V. Rao, A. Shirwaikar, M. Kotian, R. Ramani, K.S. Aithal, A.L. Udupa, G. Bhat, and K.K. Srinivasan. 1991. Chemical and pharmacological investigations of *Limnophila conferta* and *Limnophila heterophylla. Int. J. Pharmacognosy* 29(2):145–153.

Robles, M., M. Aregullin, J. West, and E. Rodriguez. 1995. Recent studies on the zoopharmacognosy, pharmacology and neurotoxicology of sesquiterpene lactones. *Planta Med.* 61(3):199–203.

Rodriguez, E. and R. Wrangham. 1993. Zoopharmacognosy: the use of medicinal plants by animals. In *Recent Advances in Phytochemistry* (eds K.P. Downumend and H.A. Stafford), pp. 89–105. Phenam Press, New York.

Satrija, F., P. Nansen, H. Bjorn, S. Murtini, and S. He. 1994. Effect of papaya latex against *Ascaris suum* in naturally infected pigs. *J. Helminthol.* 68(4):343–346.

Sooby, J. 2001. *On-Farm Research Guide*. Organic Farming Research Foundation, Santa Cruz, CA.

Vasudevan P., S. Kashyap, and S. Sharma. 1999. Bioactive botanicals from basil (*Ocimum* sp.). *J. Sci. & Ind. Res.* 58(5):332–338.

Wood, I.B., N.K. Amaral, K. Bairden, J.L. Duncan, T. Kassai, J.B. Malone, J.A. Pankavich, R.K. Reinecke, O. Slocombe, S.M. Taylor, and J. Vercruysse. 1995. World Association for the Advancement of Veterinary Parasitology 2nd edn of guidelines for evaluating the efficacy of anthelmintics in ruminants (bovine, ovine, caprine). *Vet. Parasitol.* 58(3):181–213.

BISHOP BURTON COLLEGE
LIBRARY

Section II
Historical Review of Alternative Methods

Chapter 8
Forage Quality and Livestock Health: A Nutritionist's View

Jerry Brunetti

Introduction

The resurrection of interest amongst graziers in medicinal plants seems to parallel the burgeoning movement of livestock operators into organic (and ecological) meat, milk and egg production, rotational managed grazing, and the stockman's increasing interest to be less dependent upon pharmaceutical drugs, due to their costs, side effects, and concerns of residues in meat, milk, and egg products. There are numerous books available as to the medicinal properties of various plants, many of which are considered to be "weeds" as they occur in pastures and meadows on farms.

Sadly, the trend in crop management, even on organic farms, is oriented toward high yielding domesticated grasses and legumes. This is due to the ability of these forages to efficiently and economically contribute to yields of milk and/or gain of body weight.

Evidence points to the profitability of managing warm and cool season cultivars in one's meadow or paddock, but it is very important to recognize that indigenous herbs, many of which are deep rooted perennials, provide a number of other attributes. These attributes include their medicinal properties, nutrient density (i.e. forage quality), drought resistance, palatability, perennial persistence, soil conditioning characteristics, abilities to accumulate minerals, and even indicators of certain soil conditions. Agricultural authors such as Newman Turner (*Fertility Pastures and Cover Crops*, and *Fertility Farming*), Hugh Corley (*Organic Small Farming*), Robert H. Elliot (*The Clifton Park System of Farming and Laying Down Land to Grass. A Guide to Landlords, Tenants, and Land-Legislators*), Julliette de Bairacli Levy (*The Complete Herbal Handbook for Farm and Stable*), and J. Russell Smith (*Tree Crops a Permanent Agriculture*) make strong cases for incorporating various herbs and other plants in the seed mixtures and hedgerows for their paddocks.

Turner, who discusses the importance of sub-soiling "every 7 or 8 years" states "…once deep rooted herbal leys have been all round the farm, and are continued in the rotation, even sub-soiling should not be necessary. There is no better means of aerating the subsoil than by roots of herbs like chicory, burnet, lucerne, and dandelion, all of which penetrate to a depth of three or four feet and more in as many years." (Turner, 1951, pp. 52–53). Turner continues: "I have seen my Jersey cattle going around patches of nettles, or docks, eating off the flowering tops and relishing something that they have been unable to obtain from the simple shallow rooting ley mixture. So the thing we must do is to get back into our dairy pastures as many herbs as possible to assist the health of the cattle grazing the leys and to benefit the topsoil in a way any amount of chemical dressing can never do. All my leys contain a high proportion of these weeds deliberately sown-burnet, chicory, plantain, wild vetch, sheep's parsley, dandelion, sweet clover, chickweed- and when the leys have been down four years and developed roots to a depth of several feet they are then most relished by cattle. The cattle did anything to get from the younger shallower-rooting leys, when I still had some, to those herbal leys that had penetrated the valuable untapped resources of the deeper subsoil." He adds that, "bloat has become a thing of the past since such leys were used, whereas before I lost cattle every year when I practiced the method of sowing leys with three or four ingredients only." (Turner, 1951, p. 54)

I do not have the luxury of disclosing all the enlightened methods Newman Turner incorporated on Goosegreen Farm in Somerset, UK in the 1940s and 1950s, including composting, mineralizing, crop rotation, green manuring, silage making, paddock management, pig and poultry inputs, and so on. As elucidated in his two farm journal books, Turner was quite the naturalist, quite the generalist, and an astute observer of his farm from a whole phenomena perspective. That being said, he was an unprecedented enthusiast for plant diversity for reasons that are more revealing today than when he was farming over a half a century ago.

The number of plant species Turner recommended for seeding a paddock after harvesting oats is many and varied. His list included two varieties of perennial ryegrass, cocksfoot, timothy, rough-stalked meadow grass, red clover, white clover, chicory, burnet, yarrow, sheep's parsley, alsike clover, sweet clover, vetch, alfalfa, plantain, dandelion, and fennel (Turner, 1951, p. 58). He stressed that adequate organic matter and calcium are prerequisites for this mixture to become adequately established and emphasizes "a mixture containing deep-rooting herbs is essential to soil, crop and animal health, assisting in the aeration of the topsoil and to cycle important minerals and trace elements." He adds "Hedgerows should contain comfrey, garlic, raspberry, hazelnut, docks and cleavers, etc."

Turner was amazed that soil samples taken from fields that didn't receive lime for 10 years indicated no need for lime. "He (Castle Hill Quarry analyst) said that he had never before sampled the soil of a dairy farm without having got an order for some lime. It is now evident that organic methods, which include subsoiling and deep-rooting herbs over a period of years, maintain a correct soil balance even on farms which are sending away large quantities of milk." (Turner, 1951, pp. 112–113). He adds ". . . subsoiling will be unnecessary once deep-rooting herbs have been included in a ley on each field." (Turner, 1951, p. 131).

In his subsequent book, *Fertility Pastures*, Turner conducts a test to determine which forages were most and least preferred by his Jersey cattle. In 1952, Turner put out 35 individual plots, each sown with a single plant species of the herbal ley, using 1/2 lb of seed of each of the herbs, clovers, or grasses. The plant species seeded in the individual plots were: five varieties of ryegrass, three varieties of fescue, three varieties of cocksfoot, two varieties of meadow grass, eight types of clover, three varieties of alfalfa, yarrow, burnet, sheep's parsley, kidney vetch, plantain, sainfoin, and chicory (Turner, 1974).

Plots most relished by Turner's Jersey cattle were single stand of sheep's parsley, plantain, and chicory (in that order); least preferred were ryegrasses, meadow fescue, and hard fescue. Second in preference were burnet, kidney vetch, sainfoin, and alsike. Interestingly, lucerne (alfalfa) and American sweet clover went untouched in the presence of other options. The grasses most preferred were short rotation ryegrass and meadow fescue; all other grasses appeared to be desired equally, except hard fescue, which was not liked at all.

Turner points out a significant issue. He states, "It would be interesting to know whether soil conditions . . . deficiencies and varying availability of the different minerals and trace elements, organic content and moisture, and even breed of cow had any bearing on the choice for the cow. The only way that this information could be provided, and I think it is vital that it should be, would be for my experiment to be repeated on all classes of soil in different parts of the country and with different breeds of cattle." (Turner, 1974, p. 137).

Looking at yields was another matter, except in the case of chicory, which produced the heaviest bulk, followed by Lucerne and American Sweet Clover. Research conducted in the late 1890s and reported by Robert Elliot in his 1898 classic *The Clifton Park System of Farming and Laying Down Land to Grass. A Guide to Landlords, Tenants, and Land-Legislators* features the remarkable properties of chicory, as well as other unconventional forages. During a severe drought in 1895 in Scotland, Elliot noted chicory, burnet, kidney vetch, and yarrow withstood the drought almost intact. Apparently, chicory was first introduced and cultivated in England in 1787 by Arthur Young, who brought it from Italy, where it was ubiquitous forage. The English farmers found that chicory was much more prolific than lucerne, producing 11 tons of hay per acre (compared to lucerne at $4^1/_2$ tons), with six cuttings yielding 30 green tons in northern Scotland in 1788. Elliot had actually observed the roots of chicory traveling 22 inches in 5 months and 30 inches in 15 months.

It didn't take Thomas Jefferson very long to hear of this remarkable plant that grew in a wide range of soils and provided unrivaled nutrient density for cattle, sheep, horses, and hogs. It was the basis of an American political scandal as Jefferson was attempting to import chicory into America when British-American relations were strained. Based upon bulk yield as the sole criterion, Newman Turner proposed a mixture in order of preference (without suggesting proportions) as follows: chicory, lucerne, New Zealand ryegrass, cocksfoot, timothy, meadow fescue, perennial ryegrass, late flowering red clover, S.100 white clover, sheep's parsley, yarrow, tall fescue.

Turner's field and grazing experiments resulted in his various formulas for "Herbal Ley Mixtures." These included: (1) Early "Grazing Herbal Ley Mixture" that circumvents "forcing" growth with nitrogen fertilizers with their attendant impact of reducing energy and increasing nonprotein nitrogen; (2) Midsummer Grazing Herbal Ley, to withstand drought damage; (3) Herbal Ley Mixture for Autumn and Winter Grazing chosen from herbs and grasses growing later into autumn and winter; (4) Herbal Ley Mixture for Very Thin, Dry Soils, consisting of species predominantly of the deepest-rooting varieties; (5) All Purpose Herbal Ley Mixtures providing maximum grazing yield for most of the year; and (6) Herbal Hedgerow Mixture, to supplement existing pastures, particularly for goats, and to be sown in or near the hedgerows. There are then mixtures for Light Land, Heavy Land both direct seed and undersown with a nurse crop; Pig and Poultry Leys with a strong emphasis on chicory, plantain and a lesser amount of burnet, sheep's parsley, yarrow, and kidney vetch.

Turner credits much of his inspiration of Herbal Ley Mixtures to Robert Elliot's detailed experiences, as documented in *Clifton Park System of Farming*, and suggests, as one of Turner's chapters is entitled, to "Consult the Cow." Indeed, Turner demonstrated in a trial that lasted 4–5 years and compared two fields of similar soils but seeded to mixtures: field 1—a simple mixture consisting of cocksfoot, perennial ryegrass, late flowering red clover, S.100 white clover and 1 lb per acre of chicory, a total of 25 lb of seed being sown per acre; and field 2—containing the same legumes and grasses as field 1, but in addition the following were added: 3 lb/acre chicory, 4 lb of burnet, 2 lb sheep's parsley, 2 lb of kidney vetch, 1 lb yarrow, 2 lb lucerne, and 2 lb of American sweet clover for a total of 45 lb of seed per acre.

Both fields achieved equal results, yet no matter what the variation of growth was, which was deliberately varied for test purposes, whenever cows were led from field 1 to field 2 (the Herbal Ley) milk yields always increased. This was so even when cattle were removed from field 1 (with ample grazing available) and moved to field 2 where grazing might have been even less than adequate. This makes the case that there is more to nutrition than the usual nutritional parameters surrounding protein, energy, TDN, NDF, ADF, and so on. Perhaps the diversity of such a mixture in a paddock provides critical trace elements, or various plant hormones, enzymes, aromatic oils, tannins, amino acids, fatty acids, alkaloids, pigments, vitamins and their co-factors, unidentified rumen flora stimulants, etc. The point is that there is no substitute for diversity; there is no way to quantify all the possible and synergistic interactions amongst these identifiable and unidentifiable components.

Livestock producers must have faith (and many professionals in animal husbandry do not) that livestock are the best judges for their diet (when not in confinement); that such livestock are able to make dietary choices that reflect the fertility of the soil; and that livestock health is a primary, not secondary consideration with regard to farm profitability. Only then will the attributes of diversity be more closely investigated and researched to determine in many ways how it can contribute so readily to a stockman's bottomline.

The foremost concerns or questions by stockman in regard to the grazing of unconventional forages are probably their palatability and toxicity. Researchers such as Fred Provenza have compiled a vast amount of data in cooperation with Utah State University, the USDA Natural Resources Conservation Service Grazing Lands Technology Institute, and the Utah Agricultural Experiment Station, which has been made available in a publication entitled *Forage Behavior: Managing to Survive in a World of Change* (Provenza, 2003). Provenza suggests that livestock develop a "nutritional wisdom" that results from interactions between flavors, nutrients, and toxins. Decreases in palatability occur due to foods containing excessive levels of either nutrients or toxins, and foods causing nutrient imbalances and deficits. Animals are able to discriminate between foods based upon feedback from nutrients, including protein, energy, and mineral levels. Grazing animals typically eat a variety of plants because no single food contains all the necessary nutrients and all plants contain various amounts of toxins. Livestock "learn" that eating a variety of plants not only helps them obtain their nutrient requirements and regulate their intake of toxins, but also provides compounds that can either neutralize toxins or activate metabolic pathways to eliminate toxins. This is a healthier model than constraining livestock to a single food even if that food is nutritionally "balanced." Since animals prefer familiar foods to novel foods, rotational grazing methods that incorporate low stock densities may have actually detrimentally modified the behavior of generations of livestock to "eat the best and leave the rest," thus accelerating a decline in biodiversity. According to Provenza heavy stocking for short periods encourages diet mixing. Mothers then "teach" their young, beginning as early as an embryo in the womb and later through the mother's milk as well as grazing examples, which plants are suitable and desirable for consumption.

Recognizing the fact that rhizospheres of plants are actual ecosystems in and of themselves, it's agronomically critical to take into consideration that a diverse number of species, consisting of perennial deep rooted herbs, legumes, perennial grasses, annual grasses, biennial legumes, and herbs, provide an indescribable substrate upon which a very complex food web can be established. The food web includes multiple species of bacteria, protozoa, fungi, arthropods, earthworms, nematodes, and so on. This diversity in the soil creates the same opportunities for the higher life forms that are dependent upon the "plankton of the earth," whether these ecosystems are grasslands, rain forest, coral reef, bayou, or the savannah.

Life begets life continually because predation, digestion, and recycling occur effectively when there is this diversity. An example of the monoculture myth was a tale of two plots on the same field on a farm in Ohio where I had the privilege of visiting. Plot A consisted of only perennial ryegrass seeded to glyphosate treated soils. The soils were generously fortified with lime, phosphate, potash, boron, gypsum (for sulfur), and, of course, nitrogen. Plot B consisted of the same soil fertility (without nitrogen) program but white clover (Alice variety), Festulolium, red clover, and orchard grass were included in the seeding. The short version of this story is that the ryegrass-only plot took off running and clearly was in the lead for producing more dry matter per acre. By mid-summer, and during hot and humid conditions, the ryegrass-only plot exploded with a devastating outbreak of rust. The diverse plot next to it was completely unscathed. Clearly, the only difference in these two plots was forage diversity and clearly, the diversity in this instance made a strong case for plant immunity against disease. Who can specifically determine what mode of action was at work in this protection? How many identifiable, as well as unidentifiable variables were involved in this phenomenon?

Note Elliot's observations in *Clifton Park System* in the late 1800s: "I have now to observe that if the conclusions I have arrived at are correct, that is, a grass mixture should consist of the seeds of plants, some of which are of deep-rooting and drought resisting character, so as at once to draw support from the lower strata of the soil, supply food when other plants should, besides, be of a kind especially calculated to promote the health of the stock, and also act as a preventive against disease." (Elliot, 1943, chap. 6, p. 2).

The miracles of roots

A remarkable experiment Elliot conducted on a "deep, strong soil on a low-lying alluvial flat" for the purpose of breaking up hardpan was described as

the following mixture, on the 25th April 1895, was sown with a thin seeding of oats: 5 lb each of cocksfoot, meadow foxtail, and tall fescue; 7 lb of meadow fescue; 4 lb of timothy and 1 lb each of wood meadow grass and rough-stalked meadow grass; 2 lb each of white clover, alsike, and perennial red clover, kidney vetch, and lucerne; 3 lb chicory, 8 lb burnet, 1 lb of sheep's parley, and $1/2$ lb of yarrow. The field of fifteen acres was in 1896, cut for hay, which amounted to 36 tons, 14 cwt, or nearly $2^{1}/_{2}$ tons per acre, and the aftermath grazed with lambs, was an excellent crop. Two trenches were cut in the field to a depth of about three feet, and on 11th September 1896 . . . I carefully inspected the land in order to estimate the depth to which some of the plants had penetrated. The results were particularly interesting as regards chicory, which seemed to have a profound contempt for the very hard pan, which we found at about fourteen inches below the surface, and which was about ten inches to a foot in thickness and was so hard that a powerful man with a sharp spade had to use great force to break it open when we were tracing the descent of the chicory roots, which had passed straight downwards without any deflections . . . in passing through the pan, the strong roots of these plants, notably the chicory, had succeeded in disintegrating the apparently impenetrable pan. This pan was composed of very small particles of soil washed down from the soil above. This pan evidently was not formed solely from ploughs and horses, but owed much of its hardness and compactness to the smallness of the washed down particles, which may be so small as to arrest capillary attraction. Altogether, we estimated that the roots had gone down about thirty inches. The burnet and vetch roots had gone down about twenty inches, and the Lucerne from eight to ten inches. . . . Altogether we came to the conclusion that the roots of these plants are capable of doing all the work of a subsoiler."

All this occurred in only 1 year!

It's interesting to see that lucerne (alfalfa) only penetrated this soil 8–10 inches, compared to the "unconventional" forages. Elliot aptly states, "Of all the cultivating agencies, then, roots stand by far at the head, and it is by applying this principle to our arable lands that we shall at once manure, aerate, and cultivate them in the cheapest manner. . . ." Hugh Corley's British classic *Organic Small Farming: The Exciting Story of Scientifically Controlled Methods used on Pucketty Farm* (Corley, 1975), first published in 1957, gives praise to the same deep-rooting champions as his other English compatriots and stockman did. He points out that it is necessary to sow deep rooting and tap-rooting plants, so that the greatest possible depth of soil is permeated by their roots. And it is sensible to sow a variety of herbs to ensure the health of the grazing animals, and the palatability of the herbage. These herbs probably benefit the soil too, toning up the soil organisms and making better humus when ploughed in. Bacteriological work by the Soil Association at Haughley suggests that phosphate-dissolving bacteria thrive best in compost made from a big variety of different wastes. Similarly, the humus made from a mixture of herbs and grasses may well be much more beneficial than that made from one grass and one clover. (Corley, 1975, p. 61)

The soil connection

It is my responsibility to alert the reader of this chapter that this discussion endorsing forage diversity that includes herbs does not address forage quality and pasturing success as it pertains to sound pasture management. This of course includes managed intensive rotational grazing, with adequate rest periods in between for recovery, etc. Nor does this chapter suitably address soil fertility and agronomic practices that my experience has proven to be necessary for optimum forage quality. There are soil fertility parameters that have a direct correlation to the nutrient density of forages, which in turn are necessary for livestock to be productive and healthy. On soils that tend to be imbalanced and/or poor in fertility, species diversity including deep rooted herbs can assist in bringing up fertility from below and hastening the decay process in order to recycle nutrient residues associated with urine, manure, and forage, both foliage and roots. This can especially be helpful when the soils in question are natively deficient, or depleted from abuse or neglect, and the economics of having to purchase fertility from off farm sources becomes a prohibitive option.

Forage quality requires a quality soil and most nutritionists use a wide range of lab determinants to gauge the quality of forage. My first inclination is to look at the mineral levels to see if I'm "on target." What I mean by that is certain mineral levels and mineral ratios give clues as to the quality of protein, the presence of energy, the ability of that forage to supplement an animal's needs for immunity and reproduction and so forth. If the mineral levels are lower than those shown in Table 8.1, I am doubtful as to whether this forage can supply the necessary essentials for productivity and health, regardless of what the crude protein, or relative feed value is. Of course, the "proof of the pudding lies in the eating," and ultimately the livestock will prove the quality of their forage based upon

Table 8.1   Target concentrations of various minerals for productive forage

Nitrogen	3.50%
Calcium	1.60+% ⎫ Ideally at
Potassium	2–3% ⎭ 1:1 ratio
Magnesium	0.50%
Phosphorus	0.50%
Sulfur	At least 10% of nitrogen level
Chloride	0.40%
Iron	<200 ppm
Manganese	35+ ppm
Copper	15+ ppm
Boron	40+ ppm
Zinc	30+ ppm
Aluminum	<200 ppm

production, reproduction, immunity to disease, healthy offspring, milk and meat quality, including flavor, keeping and cooking characteristics, and so forth. Keep in mind that typical soil and forage analyses often do not test for all the critical trace elements required by livestock, including selenium, chromium, cobalt, iodine, silica, vanadium, etc. This fact makes a strong case for diversity, especially of deep rooted plants, which then lessens the vulnerability of a farm in relying on a few species, that although may be efficient in accumulating certain minerals would be inefficient in accumulating others.

Forage mineral importance

For domesticated forages, having calcium levels approaching 2.0% provides a superior quality of protein than for forages with less than 1.5% calcium levels. Additionally, high calcium levels indicate forages rich in energy, synthesized as calcium pectate. Although crude protein levels are preferred in the 20–22% range (or 3.3–3.5% nitrogen), sulfur levels should comprise at least 10% of the nitrogen. That is because a 10:1, or less, nitrogen to sulfur ratio indicates there is less nonprotein nitrogen (NPN), and therefore a protein that has a more complete amino acid profile. Sulfur is also a vital component of the essential amino acid methionine, as well as cysteine, precursors to glutathione, a tripeptide antioxidant which also happens to be a building block of glutathione s-transferase, an important liver detoxifier, and glutathione peroxidase, a critical immune activator. Phosphorus is a necessary element of ATP and ADP, energy molecules associated with the Krebs cycle. Magnesium is associated with over 300 enzymatic reactions, including energy production in animals.

Trace element deficiencies, quite common in today's conventionally grown crops, are associated with soil depletion, soil erosion, and hybridization (Bergner, 1997). Volumes have been written on the multiple catalytic properties of trace elements, so necessary for immunity, reproduction, growth, and performance. Zinc, for example, is associated with at least 200 enzyme processes in the body; copper is a component of healthy red blood cells; manganese is absolutely necessary for conception; and boron is associated with the parathyroid gland. These comments address just a few of the many elements necessary for optimum health and production, and I haven't even provided a scintilla of their numerous functions and benefits, as they relate to profitable livestock production.

Unconventional forages

During the Pennsylvania summer of 2000, which also happened to be a year of severe drought and record heat, I conducted a small research project to determine how various indigenous herbs, brambles, and woody plants fared against a good sample of alfalfa. A typical analysis was conducted on random samplings from plants growing in noncultivated, nonfertilized soils and is illustrated in Tables 8.2 and 8.3.

The only comparison I could find to such a study was one that compared the mineral analysis of 16 "weeds" to those of timothy and red clover (Klingman et al., 1982) as shown in Table 8.4.

The data in Table 8.4 are from a study originally published in 1953 (Vengris et al., 1953) and re-published in 1982 by Klingman et al. Curiously, some of the plants that were enthusiastically recommended by Turner, Corley, and Elliot, namely dandelion, plantain, and narrow leaf plantain (ribgrass) scored higher on this limited analysis than other competitors, with the exception of wild carrot and milkweed. In the report I conducted on 24 plants (Tables 8.2 and 8.3), I also found some

Table 8.2 Analysis of herbs, brambles, and woody plants compared to alfalfa

	Alfalfa	Dandelion	Lamb's quarter	Chicory	Comfrey	Plantain	Nettle leaf	Burdock	Cleavers	Curly dock	Yarrow (in bloom)	Purslane	Jewelweed
Protein (%)	20.97	25.00	31.70	19.5	23.7	19.6	25.7	29.0	11.7	32.7	15.2	18.6	24.9
Digestable protein (%)		24.40		14.7	18.5	14.7	20.4	23.5	7.3	26.9	10.7	13.8	19.6
Soluble protein (%)				4.7	2.7	2.9	4.3	3.9	1.2	1.6	1.3	5.2	2
Protein solubility (%)	50.07	18.10	18.10	24.2	11.4	15.0	16.8	13.4	9.9	4.9	8.8	27.7	0.08
Nitrogen/sulfur ratio	11:1	10:1	12:1	8:1	14:1	6:1	4:1	5:1	7:1	15:1	14:1	12:1	14:1
Acid detergent fiber (%)	32.10	19.20	15.00	32.8	29.8	34.1	22.6	25.1	40.6	19.5	34.6	26.4	12.9
Neutral detergent fiber (%)	43.61	30.00	21.90	46.8	42.2	45.8	34.4	36.5	49.1	44.7	43	38.5	22.2
Relative feed value (%)	136.20	229.00	329.00	126	145	127	193	177	108	153	134	165	330
TDN (est.) total digestible nutrients	63.89	80.90	85.60	63.5	66.8	64.4	74.5	71.8	57.1	77.8	61.7	72.9	87.9
ME (mcal/lb)		1.33	1.41	1.04	1.10	1.06	1.22	1.18	0.94	1.28	1.01	1.2	1.44
Est. net energy (therms/cwt)		69.9	74.3	54.0	57.0	54.7	64	61.6	48	67.1	52.2	62.6	76.4
NE/lact (mcal/lb)	0.65	0.85	0.9	0.65	0.69	0.66	0.77	0.75	0.58	0.81	0.63	0.76	0.92
NE/maint (mcal/lb)		0.895	0.959	0.648	0.697	0.661	0.806	0.768	0.551	0.853	0.62	0.784	0.989
NE/gain (mcal/lb)		0.6	0.655	0.383	0.426	0.394	0.523	0.490	0.295	0.564	0.358	0.504	0.681
Calcium (%)	1.58	1.04	1.10	0.89	2.73	1.84	4.38	2.10	1.3	0.83	0.99	1.3	1.21
Phosphorus (%)	0.37	0.33	0.39	0.31	0.20	0.26	0.41	0.34	0.39	0.37	0.43	0.38	0.32
Potassium (%)	2.05	4.46	7.66	3.59	3.94	2.97	3.01	3.28	2.46	3.53	3.25	3.17	2.05
Magnesium (%)	0.46	0.26	0.55	0.26	0.39	0.17	0.39	0.43	0.25	0.64	0.29	0.8	0.29
Sodium (ppm)	759			0.04	0.04	0.011	0.005	0.028	0.014	0.020	0.034		
Sulfur—total (%)	0.31	0.41	0.43	0.37	0.27	0.53	0.94	0.90	0.26	0.35	0.17	0.24	0.29
Iron (ppm)	171	657	91	195	176	83	349	149	70	111	100	4419	180
Copper (ppm)	15	15	8	14	29	12	11	26	13	13	17	37	12
Zinc (ppm)	30	34	46	43	46	44	40	32	127	38	40	265	52
Manganese (ppm)	23	35	138	36	192	30	36	47	66	36	71	163	48
Boron (ppm)	50	30	44	28	42	29	67	32	15	31	26	29	26

Rankings for alfalfa
(a) Protein: 14
(b) Protein solubility: 3
(c) N:S ratio: 9
(d) TDN: 20
(e) Energy: 22
(f) Calcium: 10
(g) Phosphorus: 8
(h) Potassium: 16
(i) Magnesium: 6
(j) Sulfur: 9 (tie)
(k) Copper: 11 (tie)
(l) Zinc: 21
(m) Manganese: 25
(n) Boron: 5

Table 8.3 Analysis of herbs, brambles and woody plants compared to alfalfa

	Alfalfa	Day lily leaf	Day lily blossom	Echinacea leaf	Wild grape leaf	Wild rasp leaf	Willow leaf	Hazlenut leaf	Mulberry leaf	Chinese chestnut leaf	Linden leaf	Elder leaf	Honey locust leaf
Protein (%)	20.97	20.6	23.4	15.7	22.1	15.2	19.8	14.1	26.2	21.8	16.5	24.2	17
Digestable protein (%)		15.7	18.3	11.1	17.1	10.6	14.9	9.6	20.9	16.7	11.9	19.0	12.3
Soluble protein (%)		5.4	14.8	1.8	1.2	0.4	1.5	0.7	3.6	14.7	0.06	2.5	1.3
Protein solubility (%)	50.07	26.4	63.0	11.4	5.6	2.8	7.5	4.9	13.7	67.7	3.4	10.4	7.4
Nitrogen/sulfur ratio	11:1	19:1	20:1	12:1	14:1	16:1	7:1	14:1	17:1	11:1	14:1	12:1	14:1
Acid detergent fiber (%)	32.10	28.2	17.0	20	19.5	22.6	24.9	20.2	21.5	41.2	19.8	18.0	34.6
Neutral detergent fiber (%)	43.01	35.7	23.5	29.3	34.6	43.1	37.6	42.3	34.2	70.9	35.3	27.4	48.2
Relative feed value (%)	136.20	175	299	233	198	154	172	161	197	75	194	255	120
TDN (est.)	63.89	70.9	83.4	77.3	77.8	74.5	72	77.1	75.7	54.6	77.5	79.4	61.7
ME (mcal/lb)		1.16	1.37	1.27	1.28	1.22	1.18	1.27	1.24	0.9	1.27	1.30	1.01
Est. net energy (therms/cwt)		60.7	72.2	66.6	67.1	64	61.8	66.4	65.1	45.7	66.8	68.6	52.2
NE/lact (mcal/lb)	0.65	0.74	0.87	0.81	0.81	0.77	0.75	0.8	0.79	0.55	0.081	0.83	0.63
NE/maint (mcal/lb)		0.756	0.929	0.845	0.853	0.806	0.771	0.842	0.823	0.513	0.848	0.875	0.620
NE dain (mcal/lb)		0.479	0.629	0.557	0.564	0.523	0.493	0.555	0.538	0.259	0.560	0.583	0.358
Calcium (%)	1.58	0.81	0.39	2.57	1.91	0.85	1.45	1.44	3.09	1.37	2.79	1.72	1.33
Phosphorus (%)	0.37	0.25	0.43	0.25	0.32	0.16	0.23	0.12	0.26	0.2	0.20	0.25	0.24
Potassium (%)	2.05	2.24	2.17	2.22	0.95	1.6	1.71	0.75	1.85	0.84	0.88	1.87	1.17
Magnesium (%)	0.46	0.20	0.17	0.02	0.25	0.29	0.27	0.31	0.34	0.37	0.53	0.23	0.16
Sodium (ppm)	759	0.025	0.05	0.02	0.02	0.01	0.011	0.04	0.016	0.015	0.02	0.03	0.02
Sulfur—total (%)	0.31	0.17	0.19	0.21	0.25	0.15	0.44	0.16	0.24	0.31	0.19	0.31	0.19
Iron (ppm)	171	203	86	131	502	100	117	118	154	120	196	274	82
Copper (ppm)	15	10	22	21	16	18	13	19	12	15	19	14	11
Zinc (ppm)	30	25	66	32	32	35	105	27	36	61	26	21	33
Manganese (ppm)	23	54	40	132	89	210	101	373	63	160	65	48	52
Boron (ppm)	50	49	16	66	31	23	34	28	36	72	52	38	20

Rankings for alfalfa
(a) Protein: 14
(b) Protein soluability: 3
(c) N:S ratio: 9
(d) TDN: 20

(e) Energy: 22
(f) Calcium: 10
(g) Phosphorus: 8
(h) Potassium: 16
(i) Magnesium: 6

(j) Sulfur: 9 (tie)
(k) Copper: 11 (tie)
(l) Zinc: 21
(m) Manganese: 25
(n) Boron: 5

Table 8.4 Chemical composition of grassland weeds compared to timothy and red clover (sampling date June 5–10) (Vengris et al., 1953)

Plant	Growth stage	Number of samples	Mean percentage composition (air-dry basis)				
			N	P	K	Ca	Mg
Timothy	Early heading	19	1.55	0.26	2.17	0.34	0.10
Red clover	In buds, before bloom	19	2.84	0.25	1.09	1.88	0.42
Tufted vetch	Early bloom	3	3.58	0.30	1.52	1.52	0.30
Yarrow	In buds, before bloom	8	1.56	0.31	2.35	0.82	0.18
Oxeye daisy	50% heads in bloom	7	1.63	0.34	2.48	0.94	0.21
Daisy fleabane	In buds, before bloom	11	1.47	0.38	2.12	1.12	0.20
Common dandelion	Mostly leaves	14	2.25	0.44	3.39	1.21	0.43
Yellow rocket	After bloom	7	1.44	0.24	1.55	1.23	0.17
Plantain	Mostly leaves	11	1.48	0.30	2.10	2.55	0.46
Narrowleaf plantain	Mostly leaves	5	1.85	0.37	1.90	1.90	0.33
Yellow dock	50% heads in bloom	13	1.84	0.30	2.29	1.11	0.42
Tall buttercup	In bloom	7	1.45	0.31	1.98	0.94	0.25
Wild carrot	Vegetative growth leaves	5	2.52	0.54	2.37	1.92	0.44
Mouseear chickweed	In bloom	11	1.73	0.41	3.14	0.70	0.26
Cinquefoil	Early bud stage	2	1.49	0.28	1.31	2.08	0.33
Common milkweed	Vegetative growth	2	3.02	0.47	3.08	0.80	0.45
Sensitive fern	Vegetative growth	6	2.27	0.48	2.50	0.65	0.39
Quackgrass	Before heading	11	1.82	0.28	2.14	0.36	0.10

Source: Weed Science.

correlations to the British experiment with certain plants, namely dandelion, chicory, and yarrow. In addition, other plants (which amounted to a small sampling of what should be analyzed) demonstrated some surprising values with regard to their nutritional functionality.

Curiously, all the samples of these unconventional forages submitted for analysis, with the exception of day lily blossom and chestnut leaf, indicated very low protein solubility, indicating that most of the protein doesn't degrade in the rumen to produce rumen ammonia. Alfalfa contains highly soluble, rumen degradable protein, so much so that rations that are predominantly alfalfa or other highly soluble protein forages require that a portion of this protein be replaced by commercial, less soluble protein supplements, such as corn distillers. The reason is that too much rumen degradable protein yields excessive amounts of blood urea nitrogen (BUN) or milk urea nitrogen (MUN), which may contribute to immunosuppression, reproductive failure, and metabolic energy deficits.

Dandelion (*Taraxacum officinale*) proved to be quite high in protein as well as in sulfur. As expected it was rich in potassium, appropriate for an effective diuretic herb to possess. It especially concentrates the trace minerals copper, iron, zinc, and manganese; is moderately rich in phosphorus; and slightly low in calcium and boron. Corley's praise of dandelion is such that he states, "Probably no other herb has such a well deserved reputation for putting bloom on a horse's coat. And probably dandelion, as much as anything is responsible for the healthy dapplings that appears in my red cows' coats in summer time." (Corley, 1975, p. 64)

Profuse populations of dandelion usually are an indication of calcium deficiency (Walters, 1999) and so getting the calcium/magnesium/potassium ratios corrected is called for. Julliette de Bairacli Levy, in *The Complete Herbal Handbook for Farm and Stable*, says this plant is one of the most valuable known to the herbalist. It has an important effect upon the hepatic system, is blood cleansing, and a tonic. Steve Brill's excellent volume *Identifying and Harvesting Edible and Medicinal Plants (And Not So Wild Places)* describes the plant as especially endowed with vitamins B-1, B-2, B-3, B-6, B-12, C, E, P, beta carotene, biotin, inositol, as well as the sugar inulin.

Lamb's quarter (*Chenopodium album*), also called "fat hen" or "goose's foot" and also referred to as wild spinach, since it's a cousin, is very high in protein, high in total digestible nutrients (TDN), as well as potassium, phosphorus, and magnesium and sulfur, and quite rich in trace elements boron, manganese, and zinc. Lamb's quarter is an encouraging indicator plant suggesting good soil fertility where it readily finds a home. Also called "muck weed" and "dung weed" for those reasons, it's rich in B-vitamins, vitamin C, along with beta-carotene.

Chicory (*Cichorium intybus*), one of the more heroic fodder herbs and a favorite of grazing champions, weighs in as a forage rich in protein, has high TDN, and good acid detergent fiber (ADF) and neutral detergent fiber (NDF) levels. It is also rich in sulfur and potassium, the trace minerals copper, zinc, and manganese and has an excellent nitrogen to sulfur ratio.

Medicinally, chicory is related to milk thistle and has the same notoriety of protecting the liver as its more popular cousin has, with lab animal research to back it up (Duke, 1998). Turner credits chicory for being able to feed his cows on pasture through the worst British droughts of 1949 and 1955, while his neighbor's parched leys caused them to tap their winter hay inventory.

Comfrey (*Symphytum officinale*), a prolific producer of fodder, is very rich in protein, calcium, potassium, magnesium, and trace minerals including copper, zinc, manganese, and boron. It contains moderate levels of sulfur and phosphorus and has impressive TDN, ADF, and NDF values. In his first book, *Fertility Farming*, Turner claims that comfrey is capable of producing 20–30 tons of green fodder the first year and 120 tons per acre by the fourth year! Its downside is that it is a persistent plant lasting up to 40 years, so it's suggested to "try" this plant in waste places, or along hedgerows and tree lines. Medicinally, comfrey is also known as knitbone and bruise wort because of its abundance of an amazing alkaloid called allantoin, a powerful cell proliferant. The word "comfrey" is a corruption of "con firma," and the botanical name "symphytum" comes from the Greek term "symphyo." Both words are defined as "to unite." Rich in vitamins B-complex, C, E, and beta-carotene, this plant is especially attractive as forage in its early growth stages.

An entire volume is dedicated to comfrey research, entitled *Comfrey: Fodder, Food and Remedy* by Lawrence D. Hills. He was the director of the Henry Doubleday Research Association, which was involved in extensive research on comfrey production. The one caveat associated with comfrey consumption pertains to concerns of a hepatotoxic group of alkaloids known as pyrrolizidines. Research coordinated in the UK between the Chemistry Department of the University of Exeter, the Toxicology Unit of the Medical Research Council at Carsholton, and the Michaelis Nutritional Research Laboratory at Harpenden strongly suggests that comfrey employed as a fodder to livestock does not present a danger to the stock or humans consuming animal products.

Plantain (*Plantago major* and *Plantago lanceolata*) is highly relished by domestic stock for many reasons. It's high in protein, very high in calcium, sulfur, potassium, and zinc as well as indicates very good TDN, ADF, NDF values. Like comfrey, plantain produces a healing mucilage containing astringent and soothing, cooling properties for inflammation/irritation. The seed heads contain a soluble fiber that is found in abundance in a larger cultivated variety, which is called Psyllium and is used in natural laxatives such as "Metamucil." It was referred to in medieval times as "waybread" inferring that it was a traveler's botanical resource.

Common Nettle (*Urtica urens*), also called stinging nettle, is avoided by most livestock for the same reasons humans avoid them—the stinging hairs covering the plant contain formic acid (some say ammonium bicarbonate) which causes skin irritation upon contact. However, when common nettle is cut and allowed to wilt and dry, there is no better fodder for livestock. A long tradition of cultivating nettles as a fodder plant for hay exists in Scandinavia, Russia, Germany, Holland, and Egypt. (During World War I, the Germans ambitiously employed this tradition to provide nourishment for their military draft animals.) Victor Hugo in his famous "Les Miserables" writes

> One day he (Monsieur Madeleine) saw some peasants busy plucking out nettles; he looked at the heap of plants uprooted and already withered and said- 'They are dead. Yet it would be well if people knew how to make use of them. When the nettle is young, its leaf forms an excellent vegetable, when it matures it has filaments and fibres like hemp and flax. Nettle fabric is as good as canvas. Chopped, the nettle is good for poultry; pounded it is good for cattle. The seed of the nettle mingled with fodder imparts a gloss to the coats of animals; its root mixed with salt produces a beautiful yellow color. It is excellent hay, and can be cut twice. . . .'

In looking at the forage analysis it appears to have some exceptional numbers. It's very high in protein, TDN, calcium, phosphorus, potassium, magnesium, sulfur, zinc, and boron. Medicinally, nettle is not only reputed to be one of the best tonics, but also a diuretic, an expectorant, and a restorative for liver, gallbladder, and kidneys.

Burdock (*Arctium lappa*), although not to be considered as paddock forage, is an incredible botanical food and medicinal wonder and should be considered at least as a hedgerow resident. Burdock is one of the best blood purifiers and diuretics and is wonderful for the liver. Livestock will often medicate themselves with this plant when they are recovering from a bout of illness. Nutritionally, burdock commands a good dose of respect. It's very high in protein, TDN, calcium, phosphorus, potassium, magnesium, sulfur, copper, zinc, and manganese. Burdock exhibits an excellent nitrogen to sulfur ratio.

Cleavers (*Gallium aparine*), also known as "bedstraw" and "goosegrass," is perhaps best known as forage suited for poultry. Nutritionally it is rich in phosphorus, potassium, and trace minerals such as zinc and manganese and is reputed to be high in iodine. Cleavers has the reputation of providing tonifying properties to the blood and lymphatic systems as well as being a benign diuretic.

Curly Dock (*Rumex crispus*), also known as yellow dock, is another herb that should be allowed in the paddock in limited quantities due to its both prolific and lack of palatability qualities. Since it is a deep-rooted plant it has the ability to bring up generous levels (as demonstrated in these analyses) of phosphorus, potassium, copper, zinc, and manganese. Its foliage proved to contain the highest level of protein of all forages tested in this sampling. Medicinally, yellow dock has a long tradition in addressing liver ailments and blood and lymph purification and is known for having mild laxative properties. Docks in profusion are usually an indication of wet, poor draining, and often lime deficient fields.

Yarrow (*Achillea millefolium*) is a herb of choice for the British stockman Turner, Coley and Elliot. In my analysis, yarrow was an impressive accumulator of phosphorus, potassium, zinc, and manganese. ADF and NDF were in good ranges, as were TDN. It abhors "wet feet," so its presence is an indication of land that freely drains. The other indication, however, is that a profusion of this plant indicates a need for calcium. Yarrow, the medicinal, is famed by its botanical name because the Greek warrior Achilles used this plant to heal the wounds of his soldiers. Thus, yarrow is effective for all kinds of hemorrhages, including uterine, gastrointestinal as well as topical. Grieve, in her *Modern Herbal*, Volume II, states it is especially useful as a " . . . diaphoretic, astringent, tonic, stimulant and mild aromatic . . . is a good remedy . . . in the commencement of fevers . . . ."

Purslane (*Portulaca oleracea*) is a low growing succulent and is known to be the terrestrial plant with the richest concentration of linolenic acid (alpha-omega-3 fatty acid). Purslane was cultivated for thousands of years, first in its native India and Persia, and then later by early Europeans. Although succulent, it survives hot weather effectively as long as there is some moisture in the topsoil. Julliette de Bairacli Levy calls it "an important fodder herb and should be grown for its blood-cooling properties.... And as a blood cleanser and to refresh the digestive system...." Purslane is an exceptional accumulator of magnesium, potassium, copper, zinc, and manganese and displays a very good TDN analysis and good phosphorus levels.

Jewelweed (*Impatiens* species) is also called "touch-me-not" and grows profusely in moist soils, especially along stream banks, flood plains, and swamps. It favors partial shade. As a curious aside, this plant's stem juice is the antidote to poison ivy. It contains 2 methoxy-1, 4 naphthoquinone, an anti-inflammatory and antifungal compound, which happens to be an active ingredient in Preparation H. I chose to analyze this herb because by mid-July 2000, at the height of the drought, it was one of the few plants around to sample. The plants either produce orange or yellow flowers and supposedly, orange flowers indicate soils low in calcium and yellow flowers suggest lime is present. Jewelweed is very high in protein but most of the protein is highly insoluble or by-pass protein. It's exceptionally high in TDN and has good reserves of phosphorus and potassium. My chickens, which had very little free-range grass or clover available to them due to the drought, readily devoured jewelweed leaves, which also happen to be effective accumulators of selenium.

Day Lily (*Hemerocallis fulva*) is another plant, like jewelweed, which prefers to inhabit moist flood plain areas. It's quite high in protein, TDN, potassium, manganese, and boron and has a palatable advantage for most stock. The blossoms are equally nutritious and are additional reservoirs of phosphorus, copper, zinc, and potassium. Day Lily is a urinary tract tonic and cleanser and a mild diuretic.

Purple Coneflower (*Echinacea purpurea*) is currently ranked as the most widely used herb amongst people in the United States. A native of the prairies, it was one of the most popular plants used by Native Americans. Dr. H. C. F. Myer introduced this plant into mainstream medicine in the 1870s as a "blood purifier" and it subsequently became one of the most widely used herbs in the United States, especially in the treatment of infection. It was added to the National Formulary in 1916. Echinacea seems to enhance nonspecific type of immunity, increasing the number of white blood cells and spleen cells, increasing macrophage phagocytosis, improving levels of properdin (associated with complement activity), reduces inflammation, enhances the production of hyaluronic acid, etc.

Evidently, the nutrient density of Echinacea is worth a second look. It has very good levels of TDN, exceptional levels of calcium, magnesium, copper, manganese and boron, and very good levels of zinc and potassium.

Wild grape (*Vitis species*) isn't mentioned as a medicinal by most herbalists. However, some of the most powerful "nutraceuticals" are found in grapes. Resveratrol, being one of them, is the premier antioxidant and is also found in Japanese knotweed, a wetland invasive. Grapes also provide potassium, tartaric acid, quercitrin (the most powerful bioflavonoid), tannins, malic acid, potassium bitartrate, niacin, beta-carotene, etc. The leaves act as a mild astringent and it's a mild liver tonic. Wild grape is an outstanding nutritive and all stock love it. Domesticated grape varieties could easily be incorporated into a silvapasture system of two-tiered grazing, especially for browsing animals such as goats. Grape leaf is a very good source of protein, very rich in calcium, copper, zinc, and manganese and has good levels of phosphorus and potassium.

Wild raspberry (*Rubus strigosus*), like other members of the bramble family (blackberries, wineberries, dewberries), is best described as hedgerow specimens. The berries themselves are rich in carotenoids, vitamins B-complex, C and K as well as calcium, phosphorus, sugars, citric and malic acids, pectin, silica, and iron. Medicinally, the leaves are one of the most reputable botanicals for the female reproductive system. They strengthen the uterine wall, balance female hormones, and hasten recovery from birth. They also act as an astringent. All stocks relish this family of plants and nutritionally they have demonstrated reasons for this. They have a high TDN and are rich in potassium, copper, zinc, and especially manganese, the fertility element.

Clearly, I have submitted a small sampling of plants for forage consideration. Scores of other plants exist in any locale that could and should be analyzed for their nutritionally functional benefits.

Nicolaus Remer in writing his biodynamic work *Laws of Life in Agriculture* suggests that high yielding bulk fodder plants (15 tons of dry matter per hectare; or 6.7 tons per acre) could consist of the following forages: sorghum (fodder millet); Jerusalem artichokes; timothy at 2–3 cuts/year; *Phalaris tuberosa* (reed grass); meadow fescue and tall fescue; comfrey (for silage); and lucerne. All these examples provide a much better amino acid profile than corn.

Remer emphasizes that representatives from three plant families should be encouraged to be either grown as a medicinal supplement or seeded in the pastures where appropriate. From an anthroposophical perspective, these plants are capable of incorporating the light forces to activate the different organs systems of livestock. The *Umbellifarae* (or Carrot family) activates the nerve-sense system, which fosters alertness, quick reactions, and well-formed growth. Good bone formation and mobility are also benefits. The following are edible roots of this family: carrots, parsnips, angelica, masterwort, loveage, parsley, and celeriac. It's important to supplement silage with the following foliage of these plants since they are associated with lactic acid fermentation: caraway, dill, loveage, celeriac, angelica, parsley, and chervil. Finally, the seeds of this plant family have a profound effect on digestion, being rich in essential oils, thus quite aromatic.

The *Labiatae* (mint family) support the rhythmic system (upper and lower) of animals. These plants, also rich in essential oils, are activators of the sense of taste and glandular activity. Remer includes the following as his choice list: Sweet basil, marjoram, hyssop, summer and winter savory, thyme, lemon balm, bergamot, peppermint, and sage.

The *Compositae* (daisy family) are all perennials. In this family the light filled flower forces accumulate to produce bitter substances in the leaf capable of combating inflammation and sepsis in the digestion system, cleansing the organs and discouraging parasites. They would include southernwood, rue, mugwort, wormwood, tarragon, goldenrod, tansy, and blessed thistle. The dried flowers, receptacles of the sulfurous element, are highly medicinal and utilized for internal ulcers, inflammation, and to enliven the metabolism. Chamomile, yarrow, calendula (marigold), dandelion, arnica, common daisy, cornflower, sunflower petals, birdsfoot trefoil, cowslips, and St. John's wort are all plants associated with producing these valuable blooms.

The trees and woody plants

I found Newman Turner's praise for trees in *Fertility Farming* to be nothing less than eloquent, poetic reverent, scientific, and wonderfully pragmatic. He writes

> We farmers have almost forgotten about trees and our only thoughts about them nowadays are to decide how best we can cut them down, to make way for larger and more powerful machines. But the slow disappearance of trees from our farmlands has resulted in serious flood and drought problems, and in declining fertility. Trees take up moisture and hold it as required, and it is now common knowledge that the serious drought areas are those with few trees. Further, the roots of trees penetrate to a great depth,

bringing up minerals and trace elements to the leaves.... Leaf fall may seem to be a small contribution to fertility, but it is an extremely valuable one, which cannot be satisfactorily substituted artificially. Optimum fertility is therefore as dependent on a proportion of the farm being devoted to trees as on the application of manures. At least one-twentieth of the farm acreage should be occupied by trees, most of which will of course be in hedges." (Turner, 1951, p. 54–55)

In my opinion the best book ever written on this subject is *Tree Crops, A Permanent Agriculture* by J. Russell Smith. It was first published in 1929; Smith believed that "farming should fit the land" and that to know how to properly farm a local region requires one to observe how nature does so. That modern agriculture assumes that flatland, mechanized farming should apply to all but the most adverse circumstances of topography has led to a "Forest-Field-Plow-Desert" rotation. Tree crops offer a way out of the dilemma of using the land while not ruining the land, i.e. highly erodible soils, the majority of which the world has to contend with. Smith's vision was to put together a Mountain Institute to develop parent trees and to implement long-range experimental plots, testing newer cultivars of these trees as crops for humans and for livestock. Smith's suggestions for fodder trees included oak (acorns), honey locust, chestnuts, persimmons, mulberries, and "many, many others." In addition to trees being the obvious choice for erodible land, Smith points out that economically they are also the best choice for level land as a form of two-story agriculture. An example of success he noted was the Spanish island Majorca where the tree crop might be figs, almonds, olives, or acorn bearing oaks. The understory consisted of a rotation of wheat, clover, and chickpeas. Sheep grazed the 2-year clover during the second year. It was noted that one might get about 75% of the possible yield of each crop; but that makes a yield of 150%, while minimizing risks with frost, drought, and so on. He provides an excellent metaphor for the economic justification of this by comparing this kind of agriculture to a ship which fills three-fourths of her tonnage capacity with pig iron and five-sixths of her cubic capacity with light wood manufactures.

New Zealanders John and Bunny Mortimer published a very useful, farmer-friendly publication entitled *Shelter and Shade—Creating a Healthy and Profitable Environment for Your Livestock with Trees*. I would have added "and Sustenance" since it provides a fair amount of information on trees as fodder. They point out that browse feed values remain high for most of the year, especially for protein and sugars (and compared to grasses). Browse is clearly better suited to goats and sheep than cattle, but cattle are amazingly adaptable to at least supplement their grazing ration with browse. Goats make excellent companion graziers to beef stocker cattle in humid environments. Sheep and goats, however, should never be the centerpiece in humid regions, due to parasite susceptibility. Rather, cattle as the centerpiece, with goats and sheep, is the rule. In arid environments sheep and/or goats should be the dominant choice due to their superior browsing ability where there's more browse resources on the range.

The Mortimers concluded from studies conducted in New Zealand that 3-year pasture growth on land previously eroded still produced 80% less growth than on uneroded land. Even after 50 years, the pasture growth on previously eroded land was down 23% from uneroded ground. Smith observed similar conditions worldwide, but especially in the Appalachian United States where agroforestry would have been a profitable and ecologically sound alternative to soil destructive row cropping.

Some of the fodder trees acclaimed by the Mortimers include poplars, willow, chestnuts, pecans, persimmons, honey locust, honey mesquite, and acorn oaks. One poplar tree's "testament" concerns Tinai, New Zealander, Jim Pottinger, who during a severe drought in July 1978 fed his nearly 200 mixed age in-calf beef cows nothing but a diet of poplar leaves, twigs, and branches for 2 months and nothing else! This was on a total acreage of 111 acres.

Willow (*Scalix* sp.) is discussed by the Mortimers with a great deal of encouragement and for very good reasons. Willows are capable of producing 15 tons of edible dry matter per hectare (or 6 tons per acre) on 48 trees per acre. Now add in the yields from the forages and you begin to realize that two-tiered pasturing isn't merely a nice idea for naturalists. The analysis of willow (Table 8.3) speaks highly of its quality with very good protein levels, excellent TDN, sulfur, zinc and manganese, and good calcium and potassium concentrations. Willow, according to Levy, is a refrigerant herb, valuable for fevers and inflammation. This is associated with its salicin content, a precursor to salicylic aid (aspirin). It is also a tonic, astringent, and antiseptic. Willow is good for the respiratory tract, colic, and enteritis. I also like it because it's very early forage for bees following wintertime. Willow is easily propagated by cuttings and grows rapidly. Farms that are burdened with marshy areas that won't support conventional grasses (reed canary being an exception) might seriously look to willow as their browse fodder of choice. Their fibrous root systems oxygenate and purify the water table and they are adaptable and able to grow on dry land as well. A better fodder is hard to come by!

Honey locust (*Gladitsia triacanthos*) is another remarkable specimen lauded by the Mortimers and Smith for its productivity, fast growth, forage production (leaves and especially pods), bird habitat, and fence posts. A cousin to the pod producing carob and algarroba (keawe) trees, honey locust is adaptable from Canada to the deep south and can also grow in semiarid conditions since it is a specimen with a great deal of drought hardiness. Research conducted at the Alabama Agricultural Experiment Station in Auburn, Alabama from 1942 to 1945 demonstrated 48 trees per acre produced an average of 60 lb of pods per tree (dry wt.) or 2,923/lb/acre, while also producing 2.5 tons of lespedeza sericea hay per acre as an understory crop. Although the leaf analysis I obtained suggested honey locust to be a not-so-spectacular forage with medium levels of calcium and potassium as well as very good levels of zinc and manganese, the real prize of this fodder tree is the grain concentrate equivalent of its pods. The above yields would be comparable to 100 bushels of oats or 50 bushels of corn. Sugar content ranged from 29% to 39% providing a nonstarch source of energy, rivaling sugar concentrations in sugar beets and sugar cane! Protein levels tested at 13%.

Mulberry (*Morus* sp.) is referred by Smith as the "king of crops," no doubt due to its proven track record of fattening hogs in the deep, south early in the 20th century. These trees are such prolific producers of spring fruit that reports from farmers and researchers at that time suggested one tree could totally support two or more hogs for 3 months. USDA analysis of dried mulberries showed that they contain 70% invert sugar. Dr. George Washington Carver of the Tuskegee Institute and the man who made peanuts a U.S. staple found that mulberries were higher in total carbohydrates than pumpkins. Smith provides a multitude of reasons why every livestock farm should have such an orchard: it grows rapidly, sets fruit earlier than any other tree, tolerates shade, has a long fruiting season, rebounds from killing frosts, is very resistant to diseases and insects, propagates easily, and the trunks make good fence posts.

Mulberries have been propagated for centuries in the Orient and Middle East as a food source for man and livestock. The one "livestock" developed to feed exclusively on the fodder of this tree is unique to the Orient, the silkworm. The leaves I sampled were analyzed and found to be very rich in protein, high in TDN, outstanding in calcium levels, and have very high numbers for zinc, manganese, and potassium. The consequence of the Asians developing this tree for silkworm production was that a number of Mediterranean countries incorporated mulberry trees into silvopasturing systems in yet another example of two-tiered agriculture.

Medicinally, Levy considers the berries to be a refrigerant and antagonist to internal parasites. Both the berries and young shoots have good blood purifying, lymphatic cleansing, and laxative properties.

Linden (*Tilia* sp.), also known as lime tree or basswood, produces very fragrant, yellow-white flowers in late spring and is quite attractive to livestock and pollinators. The test results from my laboratory analysis indicated foliage with excellent TDN values, as well as exceptional levels of calcium, copper, manganese, and boron. The leaves are very palatable to herbivores. Medicinally, leaves and blossoms have the reputed notoriety, as reported by Levy, Grieve, and other herbalists, of addressing concerns of nervous ailments and spasmodic conditions such as asthma and epilepsy. It's helpful for colds, flu, and mucous congestion and is a diaphoretic and a mild diuretic.

Elder (*Sambucus* sp.) is a ubiquitous shrub that naturally inhabits lowlands, flood plains, and stream banks. Nutritionally, this plant ranks high on the limited analysis returned from the forage lab. It's highly endowed with protein and exhibits a high TDN value, good levels of calcium, potassium, copper, manganese and boron, and excellent sulfur levels. Medicinally, elder is a renowned member of the botanical elite. The flowers and berries both have expectorant, diaphoretic, and astringent properties. The berries contain compounds that are uniquely antiviral. The leaves are edible, although livestock seem to graze upon them preferentially. The leaves apparently repel flies. According to Levy, the entire plant has benefits for gastric, hepatic, and pulmonary ailments.

Persimmon (*Diospyros virginiana*), although not analyzed by me due to lack of availability, is a native American tree revered by J.R. Smith and has enviable cultivars in Asia and is persuasive as a fodder tree. Persimmon has some unique characteristics. First, since animals don't like the foliage, persimmons are ideal candidates for planting without protection in pastures. They don't bloom until very late in the spring which avoids late frosts. Persimmons are a long season producer, dropping fruit from August through January or February. Consequently, it is a wonderful companion tree to mulberries when feeding hogs on pasture over an extended feeding interval. Persimmons can grow virtually in any soil. Its deep taproot obtains nutrients even in the most impoverished substrates. The fruit is extremely nutritious, containing a whopping 35% solids (apples contain 13%) and 32% sugars (apples contain 10%). This relative of the ebony tree provides fruit rich in calories, potassium, calcium, vitamin C, phosphorus, beta-carotene, and the proteolytic enzymes found in papaya and pineapple, namely papain and bromelain respectively.

Chinese chestnut (*Castanes* sp.). Following the demise of the native American chestnut from blight introduced in the late 1800s, there have been breeding attempts to produce Asian cultivars that provide flavor, nutrition, and yield. Today, thanks to breeding experiments primarily in the Upper Midwest, the chestnut can rightfully proclaim its title as the "corn tree." Chestnuts are capable of producing as much, or more calories as maize, while also providing an understory crop of hay and pasture. Chestnut orchards established in Corsica by the Romans in the 2nd century A.D. were found to be very established and productive when Smith toured Corsican farms around 1925. Chestnut-fed pigs produce hams of exceptional flavor. Chestnuts test out on a dry basis with approximately 11% protein, 8% fat, and 70% carbohydrates. The forage sample I had analyzed was 22% protein, 67.7% of it being soluble, the highest value of all samples submitted, even more than the typically highly soluble protein of alfalfa. Although moderately high in the macronutrients, chestnut demonstrated outstanding levels for sulfur, copper, zinc, manganese, and boron. As a two-tiered tree crop, considering nuts, foliage and understory pasture, this crop packs a nutritious wallop.

Hazelnuts (*Corylus* sp.). Just as chestnuts pose to be a permaculture replacement for corn, hazelnuts offer the same possibility as an alternative to soybeans. However, this tree offers an additional advantage of being a North American substitute tree for the olive since it produces very large quantities of oleic fatty acid oil (also known as omega-9), thanks to innovative and ambitious plant breeders who crossed European filberts with hazels (such as Turkish hazels). Laboratory analysis of filberts indicates the nuts contain 16% protein, 64% fat, and 12% carbohydrates. Leaf analysis demonstrates a high value for TDN and exceptional trace mineral levels, especially for copper and manganese.

The symbiosis of trees, forbes and livestock

Clearly, tree crops have a proven track record of providing agricultural, ecological, and economic prosperity throughout the world for thousands of years. Not only are there numerous kinds of trees and companion crops, but livestock also effectively and naturally dovetail into this system. Intensive tree crop practices that incorporate livestock actually increase tree growth and productivity. Economic risk is minimized, since animal products (meat, milk products, eggs, and livestock) are not challenged by the same pests (insects, disease, and parasites) and weather phenomena (frosts, temperature, etc.), as are tree crops. They sell into different markets and require different inputs. Shade is a huge economic consideration for livestock production. Studies conducted on the Southern Plains Experimental Range in Woodward, Oklahoma found that shade increased summertime gain of yearlings Hereford steers by 19 lb/8.6 kg per head in a 4-year study (Mortimer and Mortimer, 1996). Humidity that exceeded 45% when temperatures exceeded 85°F/29°C became detrimental factors that reduced gains by 1 lb/0.45 kg per day.

Grazing positively impacts tree growth if done properly. Grasses have fibrous root systems that compete for soil moisture and nutrients. Grazing, by removing adequate leaf area and thereby causing roots to self-prune, can dramatically reduce unfair competition by grasses prior to dry weather making an appearance. This reduces or eliminates stress from summer moisture deprivation. Additionally, since herbivores can only utilize a fraction of the nutrients they ingest, the majority of those nutrients are excreted in the form of urine and manure, as highly available plant foods for fast growing or fast producing trees. Manure and urine also provide biological inputs in the form of enzymes, auxins, hormones, and microbes (cow manure consists of 25% bacteria by weight), stimulating the soil food web ecosystem.

Summary and conclusions

Incorporating biodiversity of plants on a livestock farm in turn increases the diversity of animal-required nutrients, including minerals, vitamins, pigments, enzymes, amino acids, fatty acids, sugars and other carbohydrates, sterols, hormones and the numerous myriad of phytochemicals, known and unknown, that are able to provide countless medicinal and metabolic properties. Increasing the farm's plant biodiversity provides weatherproofing from heat, drought, frost, and excessive moisture. It minimizes the vulnerability that monocultures have with the vagaries of weather, because different plants have different strengths and weaknesses with regard to climatic influences. Additionally complex plant polycultures create numerous microclimates on the farm, which are able to buffer the extremes of temperature and moisture. Shade from trees and hedgerows can offset production losses associated with heat and humidity impacting live weight gain and milk production. Windbreaks can reduce winter feed requirements by effectively reducing, and even eliminating the "wind-chill" quotient.

An extended food supply can be more readily realized with a biodiverse livestock operation starting with early growing grasses, legumes, and herbs and then later arriving browse as leaves, and finally berries, fruits, and nuts late in the season. Woody plants have the advantage of actually having a year-round growing season, thus being more efficient than grasses and certainly row crops in producing biomass. Winter browse on terminal buds provides exceptional medicinal components and a high level of nutrient density.

Plant diversity increases the diversity and numbers of other wildlife including songbirds and bats, which consume insect pests affecting plants and animals. These in turn attract raptors which then prey upon rodents. Pollinators and predatory insects are able to find habitats and in turn help increase yields of crops bearing seeds, fruits, and nuts. The soil food web, or soil ecosystem is enhanced due to a permanent polyculture of plants growing on undisturbed soils. This means more efficient nutrient recycling and healthier root systems for all plants, again contributing to farm productivity. A healthy polyculture also means improved water percolation and purification, translating into cleaner groundwater and surface water, devoid of silt and excessive nutrients, ultimately affecting the ecosystems of invertebrates and fish in streams and lakes.

Plant diversity with livestock can very readily provide the opportunity for two or three cash flow income streams for the farm, while improving the health of the farm. Animal products as livestock, meat, eggs, and dairy products and timber as lumber or fence posts, along with fruits, nuts and berries (to offset purchased feed and/or sold directly to the human marketplace) all offer multiple economic rewards that don't necessitate additional (net) human labor investments. This is especially true when factoring in the reduction or elimination of conventional agricultural practices and/or equipment.

References

Bergner, P. 1997. *The Healing Power of Minerals, Special Nutrients and Trace Elements*. Prima Lifestyles, Prima Publishing, Rocklin, CA.

Brill, S. 1994. *Identifying and Harvesting Edible and Medicinal Plants (And not so Wild Places)*. William Morrow and Co., New York, NY.

Corley, H. 1975. *Organic Small Farming: The Exciting Story of Scientifically Controlled Methods Used on Pucketty Farm*, 2nd edn. Bargyla and Gylver Rateaver, Pauma Valley, CA.

De Bairacli Levey, J. 1991. *The Complete Herbal Handbook for Farm and Stable*, 4th edn. Faber and Faber, London.

Duke, J. 1998. The Green Pharmacy: the ultimate compendium of natural remedies from the world's foremost authority on healing herbs. *The Green Pharmacy*. St. Martin's Paperbacks, New York, NY.

Elliot, R.H. 1943. *The Clifton Park System of Farming and Laying Down Land to Grass. A Guide to Landlords, Tenants, and Land-Legislators*. Faber and Faber, Ltd., London.

Grieve, M. 1971. *A Modern Herbal*, vol. 2. Dover Publications, Mineola, NY. Available on the Web at www.Botanical.com

Hills, L.D. 1976. *Comfrey: Fodder, Food and Remedy*. Universe Books, New York, NY.

Klingman, G.C., F.M. Ashton, and L.J. Noordhoff. 1982. *Weed Science: Principles and Practices*. John Wiley and Sons, New York, NY.

Mortimer, J. and B. Mortimer. 1996. *Shelter and Shade: Creating a Healthy and Profitable Environment for your Livestock with Trees*. Green Park Press, Jackson , MS.

Provenza, F.D. 2003. *Foraging Behavior: Managing to Survive in a World of Change*. Utah State University Press, Logan, UT.

Remer, N. 1995. *Laws of Life in Agriculture*. Steiner Books, Anthroposophic Press, Herndon, VA.

Smith, J.R. 1929. *Tree Crops a Permanent Agriculture*. Harcourt, Brace and Co., New York, NY.

Turner, N. 1951. *Fertility Farming*. Faber and Faber Ltd., London.

Turner, N. 1974. *Fertility Pastures and Cover Crops: Based On Nature's Own Balanced Organic Pasture Feeds*. Bargyla and Gylver Rateaver, Pauma Valley, CA.

Vengris, J., M. Drake, W.G. Colby, and J. Bart. 1953. Chemical composition of weeds and accompanying plants. *Agron. J*. 45:213–218.

Walters, C. 1999. *Weeds: Control without Poisons*. Acres, USA.

Chapter 9
Livestock Treatments Links from the Past to Holistic Alternatives of the Present

Hubert J. Karreman

Animals have been treated for illnesses since man began to keep livestock. Many treatments were barbaric and had virtually no basis in science. Blood-letting was commonplace for many conditions (Varlo, 1785; Richardson, 1828). Bleeding would often leave an animal dead due to lack of blood volume. Mercury, arsenic, and lead salts were often used, even up to the early 20th century. Reading various manuscripts of the 18th and 19th centuries proves quite revealing as to the common treatments of the day, which of course centered on beasts of burden. Many common diseases for which we now have a highly developed nosology (nomenclature) were basically called by their descriptions, for example, grease, scab, red water, blackleg, the rot, etc. Intellectual reasoning was at times offered but was usually based solely on loose associations and observable signs.

The actual description of the course of a disease in anatomic terms could be fairly accurate in the late 1700s to early 1800s, but there commonly lacked any sort of correct pathophysiology or etiology (bacteriology was still 100 years away). In blackleg as it was called (and still is), it was pointed out that "the best lambs and calves are most generally subject to it" (true, because usually the fastest growing grain-fed young stock succumb to clostridial disease). However, the belief was that blackleg was essentially a blood disorder, owing to "over-rankness of blood, that is, the whole body is overloaded with blood." Old time descriptions of blackleg continue in some detail about how the veins cannot discharge the blood quickly enough so that the blood spills out of "its latitude" (the vessels) and that it "corrupts or rots all the flesh near it." It was known that the disease may be prevented but is not treatable. Perhaps the prevention worked to some degree, but it is quite different than that of today (which is vaccination, based on Pasteur's discoveries). The prevention of blackleg based on advice Varlo provided greater than 200 years ago is given below:

> On the 1st of May or thereabouts, make 2 quarts of very strong rue tea, for every calf you have, and to every 2 qts. of tea, put 2 qts. of salt, bottle it up for use. Drive up your calves every Monday morning, or once a week, and give each calf a half pint, and bleed them in the neck-vein once every fortnight, give your lambs each half the quantity every week, and bleed them in the tail every fortnight, by this precaution, you in all probability, will loose neither lamb nor calf; though I call them lambs or calves, they are generally a year old before they take this disorder. (Varlo, 1785, pp. 293–295).

Another treatment from the same manuscript for treatment of "red water" in bullocks, which could have been leptospirosis, bacillary hemoglobinuria, or cystitis, stated:

> to cure the red water in a bullock take a piece of lean hung beef, dry and bruise it to powder, do the like to a red herring, mix these powders together, then add to them an ounce of bole armoniac(?), and a handful of shepherd's purse, stamped very small, mix all these together in a quart of the strongest, oldest ale you can get, this will make two doses, give it two mornings together lukewarm (Varlo, 1785, p. 291)

A concoction such as this never made it into the modern world of veterinary medicine. However, some treatments did persist well into the 1900s and even some of the individual ingredients would still have merit today, albeit as an alternative or natural treatment (without the mercury), such as the following for ectoparasites which incorporates tobacco (with its poisonous active ingredient nicotine): "In every 2 qts. of water, boil a quarter pound of tobacco, in this dissolve $^1/_2$ oz. of corrosive sublimate (mercury), add a gill of the spirit of turpentine and a gill of train-oil, bottle it up for use." (Varlo, 1785, p. 295)

Nearly 50 years later in the 1830s there was not much change in the treatments. There was more variety in terms of plants used, but some very crude treatments persisted. There were also some diseases for which a modern trained veterinarian would have no idea as to the actual disease. For instance, in suspected "Horn Ail":

> this disease is seated in the horns of cattle, the inside becomes carious, putrefies and is discharged from the nose. The beast that is taken with this disorder will frequently shake its head, and appear to be dizzy. Take a nail gimblet and perforate the horn, if it is hollow and no blood follows, it is the horn ail. Bore each horn into the hollow part, then inject into it strong vinegar and camphorated spirits; this will cleanse the horn, and generally effect a cure. (Richardson, 1828, pp. 31–32)

Granted, modern cattle are dehorned at an early age and we would not see this, but there are farms (such as biodynamic farms) which keep horns on for the entire life of the cow and yet "Horn Ail" is an unknown disease. Perhaps it was a nutritional deficiency, or perhaps a migrating parasite.

Another interesting disease was the so-called worm in the tail.

> For the worm, you may presently perceive it by the tail, for sometimes the hair will go off where the worm lieth, and most commonly the joints of some of them is eaten asunder, which you may feel, knock one beside the other. Cure-You must be sure that you slit the skin of the under side, above the decayed joint, just against the vein, and prick the vein, and it will bleed very well; then take garlick, butter, and salt, and bind it on, and it will mend. (Richardson, 1828, p. 240)

As for "inflammation of the eyes" (pinkeye?),

> you must first cord them in the neck, and bleed them in the temples under the eyes: let them bleed very well, and put in some burnt alum and live honey mixt together every day, and they will mend for certain.

An alternative to the bleeding treatment for sore eyes is:

> Take six egg shells and put the meat clean forth, then lay the shell betwixt two tile-stones, & lay the stones and shells in the hot glowing fire, and burn them well, and cover the edge of the tiles with clay for to keep the ashes from the shells; and when they are burnt, pound them to powder and sift them finely, and with a

quill blow the powder into the beast's eye, and it will mend presently; but blow it in three times a day. Also take white sugar-candy, pound it small and blend it with the aforesaid powder of the shells and Maybutter (without salt) and work it into a salve, so anoint the eyes morning, noon and night, and it will help them. (Richardson, 1828, p. 234).

Maybe the bleeding would have been easier. These are examples of veterinary medicine as it was practiced before about 1850.

Veterinary medicine reached a turning point by about the middle of 19th century. Individuals began to rebel against frequent use of blood-letting and other absurd, baseless methods. Some practitioners began to think about their approaches to their patients and how better to care for them, taking into account a different view of "the brutes" (beasts) under their care. It seemed as though a sense of compassion began to dawn upon parts of the medical community. This was the time of the beginning of the Eclectic medical school of thought that strongly promoted botanical therapeutics with Dr. John Scudder as one of its leaders. Not too long before, Samuel Hahnemann laid down the principles for his homeopathic school of thought. Both of these schools were vehemently opposed to the barbaric methods of the conventional school, and their early adherents were respectful of each other's approaches to patients. The philosophical underpinnings of both the Eclectic and homeopathic schools were to work with nature instead of forcibly controlling it. The issue of rearing of animals in their natural surroundings versus the artificial confinement rearing of animals is still a main divide among modern farmers, who either allow cattle to graze and fulfill their ecological niche or continuously confine their animals to live inside barns and force maximal production. In *The American Eclectic Practice of Medicine, as Applied to the Diseases of Domestic Animals*, written in 1865, the practitioner Nelson N. Titus was clearly ahead of his time as a forerunner of the holistic veterinary movement. His introduction is thus:

I have found by experience and observation that the diseases of horned cattle are few and simple. When animals live in their wild and natural state, they are seldom or never sick; but when deprived of all natural and healthy conditions, by shutting them up and depriving them of pure air, water, exercise, and their proper food, they get sick, the same as we do; and we have veterinary surgeons, cow-doctors, etc. to cure them. As cattle live under more natural conditions, and are not compelled to transgress the laws of nature so frequently as the horse, they are not so subject to disease. All the cattle-doctors have treated on a variety of diseases, – diseases, that exist nowhere except in the imaginations of the authors. But their books must be filled up; they must be scientifically written, having the appearance of wisdom at least. But a practical work is what people want; a work based upon observation and experience – a practice that will apply in the diseases of their animals. My experience teaches me that there are but few diseases among cattle; which diseases will be treated in a plain and comprehensive manner. In doing so, I shall lay down general principles upon which all diseases must be treated. I care nothing about names of diseases, if I only understand their nature and cause. By understanding the laws that govern in life and health, disease and death, we can treat disease successfully without going into the minutiae of diagnosis or discrimination of disease. (Titus, 1865, p. 180)

Nowhere in his book is there a mention of the nearly incessant need for blood-letting as was prevalent in the earlier veterinary literature. His entire book is essentially a plant based materia medica with mention of inorganic mineral compounds—a breath of fresh air compared to the practices which were very crude. The medical conditions described would be easily understood by any trained veterinarian today. But one old condition "Horn Distemper" is addressed (also called "Horn Ail"), but notice his position in contrast to the previously described treatment:

> Cause-From the circumstance that we never knew cattle in good condition affected with this complaint, we attribute it, generally, to poor keeping and hard work. Symptoms-The animal appears dull, weak, and languid; taking it by the horn, you will find it cold quite down to the head. Treatment-The horn is generally bored with a gimlet, and found to be entirely hollow and empty; pepper and vinegar is then introduced. This treatment is both cruel and absurd, and originated in ignorance of the disease. What nature has so guarded as to enclose in a tight case of horn, ought not to be laid open to the action of the atmosphere; but to introduce such foreign and acrid or pungent matter into the horn, is still more revolting. It should be treated on more philosophical principles. As the disease originates from a depraved condition, the first thing that should be looked to is to give the animal a liberal allowance of nutritious food, and give alteratives to operate on the secretions and excretions. For this purpose, give 4 oz. powdered mandrake root, 2 oz. powdered bloodroot, 1 oz. powdered ginger root and 1 oz. powdered goldenseal root. Mix and divide into 10 powders; give one each morning for 10 mornings, and rasp the horn thin next to the head, and apply spirits of turpentine. Wait 10 days after the application of the medicine, and then, if the condition of the animal is not much improved, repeat the medicine as before. This treatment is effectual, if given in time. (Titus, 1865, p. 201–202)

Whether or not this treatment was truly efficacious against so-called Horn Ail is not as important as the difference of approach. For if neither the older conventional nor the Eclectic approach worked, at least Titus' treatment seemed to be more caring toward the animal and based on a little more thought as to treating the whole animal. Near the end of a section in which he detailed (correctly) various obstetrical procedures, Titus shows his understanding of how a veterinarian must approach work that is summed up herewith:

> When you are called upon to assist a cow in calving, be cool and deliberate in your proceedings, and never attempt to force nature; let nature do her own work in her own way, and when she fails, assist her. Remember that nature is the only true midwife. Use no force or violence, and never attempt to do anything that you do not understand; if you cannot do any good, do no hurt. (Titus, 1865, p. 199)

During the same era, modern chemistry was coming of age and plants, which for long had been part of the medical armamentarium, were being investigated as to their constituents. Whereas the homeopathic and Eclectic approaches to case taking differ in their focus upon patient symptoms, with the Eclectics being more attuned to an exhaustive physical examination while the homeopaths honed in on more uniquely peculiar symptoms, both schools strived to diagnose a *specific remedy* for the symptoms presented. John Scudder from the Eclectic approach states their ideas this way:

> We propose studying the expressions or symptoms of disease with reference to the administration of remedies. It is a matter of interest to know the exact character of a lesion, but it is much more important to know the exact relationship of drug action to disease expression, and how the one will oppose the other, and restore health. If I can point out an expression of disease which will be almost invariably met by one drug, and health restored, I have made one step in a rational practice of medicine.
>
> I have no hesitation in affirming that if we have once determined such relationship, we have determined it in all diseases alike, in all persons, and for all time to come. If, with this symptom or group of symptoms, my Aconite, Nux or Podophyllin cures today, it will cure tomorrow, next year, and so long as medicine is practiced. (Scudder, 1874, pp. 14–15)

This differs completely from conventional medicine for those doctors made their diagnosis according to the received nosology, and then prescribed the name (Scudder, 1874, p. 14). Although the homeopaths and Eclectics each knew their own materia medicas in detail, their approaches to actual treatments were definitely not of the same philosophy. The homeopathic method aims primarily to stimulate the body's own defense mechanisms to cure itself on an energetic level. This is thought to work by using an extremely dilute, succussed (which is defined as forcefully shaking usually by hitting on a hard surface) material for a set of symptoms which a low dose of the same crude material itself would have induced in a healthy person. This is what the homeopaths call the simillimum and is arrived at by repertorizing the case: taking detailed notes about the symptoms (common and peculiar) and then matching them with a remedy having gone through its own provings. Homeopathic provings were the detailed accounts of healthy persons who had taken the remedy in low dose and recorded their symptoms in detail, from a physical, behavioral, and mental level. The information from these provings was pooled together and this formed the basis of the homeopathic materia medica. By taking a case and by repertorizing it, a remedy was diagnosed and was administered in its highly dilute and energized form to stimulate the body's vitality. This is contrasted by the Eclectics whose primary goal was also to diagnose a correct remedy—but the thrust of Eclectic treatment was to directly antagonize and subdue a given condition with small yet chemically quantifiable amounts of a remedy. Again, Scudder states:

> The first lesson in therapeutics is, that all remedies are uniform in their action; the conditions being the same, the action is always the same ... Then we study the action of drugs upon the sick, and when we find them exerting an influence opposed to disease and in favor of health, we want to know the relation between the drug and the disease – between disease expression and drug action.
>
> I do not say that we should not study a drug action in health – indeed I think it is a very important study. You may, on your own person, study a wholly unknown drug, and determine its proximate medicinal action. How? Easy enough. You will feel *where* it acts; that points out the local action of the drug, and as a matter of common sense, you would use it in disease of that part, and not of a part on which it had no action. You will feel *how* it acts – stimulant, depressing, altering the innervation, circulation, nutrition and function. If now you want to use it in disease, use it to do the very things it did in health, and not as our Homeopathic brethren would say, to do the very opposite things. (Scudder, 1874, p. 16)

During the late 1800s and into the early 1900s, it was evident that a given remedy as used by an Eclectic practitioner was not altogether different from the one used by a homeopath, at least in its strength/potency. One of the great homeopaths, Boericke, for instance, says the remedy Nux vomica is one of the greatest of polychrests, because the bulk of its symptoms correspond in similarity with those of the commonest and most frequent of diseases and finishes by saying to use it in the 1st to 30th potency and higher (Boericke, 1927, p. 475). In Boericke's book, *Materia Medica and Repertory*, an overwhelming number of entries explicitly state to use the specified remedy in a concentration ranging anywhere from the tincture to the homeopathic 30th potency, with an obvious majority being in low homeopathic potency (i.e., 3X, 6X, etc.). The French homeopath Jousset under the heading of Tetanus in his *Practice of Medicine* proclaims:

> *Nux vomica*, Brucine and especially Strychnine are entirely homeopathic to tetanus since poisoning with these substances produces a perfect picture of tetanus. The renewal of paroxysms by the least motion and even by the simple touch is the characteristic sign of the indications for these drugs. Several cures have resulted from the administration of Nux Vomica even in the hands of our adversaries (conventional school), who explain this favorable action of the drug by *substitutive medicine*. Dr. Stille, cited by Richard Hughes,

records eight cases of traumatic tetanus cured by Strychnine, at a dose of 1/16 to 1/8 of a grain. Jahr affirms having cured with the 3rd dilution (3X). Doses: from the crude drug up to the 30th dilution. I preferably advise the use of Strychnine sulphas, 1st trituration. (Jousset, 1901, p. 445)

Another passage of Jousset, regarding the treatment of endocarditis, is as follows:

Aconitum – A majority of authors recognize, like ourselves, that Aconitum is the principal remedy in acute endocarditis. Aconitum is the remedy for the early stage; it is indicated when there is intense fever, pulse hard and quick, energetic cardiac palpitations, with cutting pains, sensation of a violent blow at the precordial region or at the epigastrum, heat and redness of the face, thirst, tendency to syncope, breathing short, urine dark. The intermittent pulse is not a contra-indication. Dose: From 20–30 drops of the mother tincture in 200 grams of water, a tablespoon every two hours. *Cactus* is similar to Aconitum…Dose: the low dilutions and the mother tincture should be preferred in very acute cases. We usually prescribe 3 drops of the mother tincture in 200 grams of water, a tablespoonful every 2 hours. (Jousset, 1901, p. 848)

These doses are nearly the same as Eclectic doses to treat the exact conditions, but homeopathic mother tinctures are 1:10 dilute whereas Eclectic tinctures varied anywhere from 1:2 to 1:10. The Eclectics widely used tinctures but they used fluid extracts even more, especially "specific medicines" that were potent in very low concentrations. They also used some inorganic minerals such as mercury, arsenic, and antimony but only to a small extent (especially when compared to the conventional school). By definition, a USP fluid extract is a plant derivative with a concentration of 1:1 (plant:solvent). Tinctures, on the other hand, are not as strictly defined but generally are thought of as dilution up to 1:10 as the weakest (usually in alcohol or as a glycerite). Homeopathic "mother tinctures" are, by the HPUS definition, a 1:10 dilution, usually in an alcohol solvent. A mother tincture is the beginning point from which a multitude of further homeopathic dilutions are derived. Thus, if a homeopath would prescribe a 2X potency of a remedy, this would be roughly equivalent to using one part of an Eclectic 1:10 plant tincture placed into ten parts of water to be given orally. The difference being that a homeopathic remedy is diluted and *succussed* (to release the starting material's energy) while the Eclectic tincture, if put into water, is simply diluted. Dr. Humphrey, a medical doctor who later learned to be a veterinarian, used "homeopathic veterinary specifics," an abbreviated form of homeopathy which used a combination of low potency homeopathic preparations (mainly of plants). Some of Humphrey's recipes for various ailments are shown in Table 9.1. Usually 5–10 drops of the solutions shown in Table 9.1 would be placed on the back of the tongue (Humphrey, 1881).

Low potency homeopathic remedies (like Humphrey's) had true pharmacologic activity owing to there being actual material still present. But they were "energized" due to one or a few succession of steps. These succussed, low dilutions were small enough not to wreak havoc with the animal's system as a highly concentrated version of the same remedy most likely would (as given by the conventional school). The term "specific" seems to have been a term used in the late 1800s and mainly in the province of the Eclectic tradition but also by homeopaths who used low dose potencies (such as Humphrey). A "specific" remedy appears to have denoted the *exact* correct remedy for a given condition—the correct diagnosis, especially in reference to Eclectic diagnostics.

Conventional veterinary medicine in the early 20th century certainly used plant medicines, but in full strength. A Scottish veterinarian, Finlay Dun, in writing *Veterinary Medicines*, provided a materia medica which gives in-depth pharmacologic and physiologic descriptions of medicines used at the time, a great multitude of which are plants. Plants such as belladonna, bryonia, cinchona, digitalis, ergot, gelsemuim, gentian, ginger, ipecachuahana, lobelia, nux vomica, sabina (and a multitude more)

Table 9.1   Humphrey's homeopathic veterinary specifics[a]

AA = Acon 2X, Verat Vir 3X, Bell 3X
  Fever, inflammation, congestion
BB = Rhus tox 2X, Ruta 2X, Arnica 2X, Calc F 3X
  Strains, injuries, lameness (tendons, ligaments, joints)
CC = Phytolacca 2X, Merc Iod F 13X, Kali Bich 13X
  Influenza, quinsy, nasal gleet, catarrh
DD = Acon 2X, Ars Alb 4X, Ferr Sulph 12X
  Worms, bots, grubs
EE = Ars Iod 12X, Bell 2X, Phos 2X
  Coughs, bronchitis, inflamed lungs
FF = Colocynth 2X, Colch 2X, Bell 2X, Nux 2X, Dioscorea 3X
  Colic, belly-ache, wind-blown, diarrhea
GG[b] = Cimicfuga 2X, Caulophyllum 2X, Secale 10X
  Miscarriage, imperfect cleansing or hemorrhage
HH = Apis 2X, Chim Umb 2X, Canth 2X
  Urinary and kidney diseases, and dropsy (increase urine output)
II = Rhus 2X, Ars Iod 4X, Hepar 4X
  Eruptions, ulcers, mange, grease, farcy, abscesses, fistulas, unhealthy skin, eczema
JJ = Nux 2X, Ant crud 12X, Sulph 5X, Lycopod 4X
  Indigestion, over-feed, bad condition, paralysis, stomach staggers, loss of appetite

[a] Thanks to Jack Bornemann, R.Ph for deciphering these patent medicine formulas.
[b] Theorized by author, but not verified.

were all used full strength; some had a very narrow range of safety (i.e. aconite) while others had a wide range of safety (peppermint). Most of the time prescriptions were written by the tending veterinarian to be filled at an apothecary. These prescriptions were commonly mixtures of both plant and inorganic mineral materials. The veterinary textbook *Veterinary Materia Medica and Therapeutics* by Kenelm Winslow of Washington State University is divided equally into "inorganic agents" and "vegetable drugs." Books such as these are a wealth of information on the known active compounds of medically useful plants and inorganic mineral medicines. They were essentially working with crude drugs, usually given orally, and based their use on direct observations and the known actions of the plant constituents. Accounts of the actions of a medicine as observed in small numbers of animals (usually horses and dogs) seem to have been the standard from which clinical use of a substance was made. (This was the scientific method prior to the post-World War II double blind random controlled trials that pharmaceutical companies and the FDA adopted as the only standard from which to validate single active compounds.) Veterinary students back then were taught a standard materia medica based on inorganic and plant substances; in addition, they were taught how to correctly combine ingredients and how to write an apothecary prescription using Latin terminology. In *Veterinary Doses and Prescription Writing*, Pierre Fish of Cornell University describes in detail the pharmacy side of veterinary practice. By the time the 6th edition of his book came out in 1930, botanical therapeutics in the veterinary profession were at its zenith. After that time, organic chemistry developed to such an extent that many of the known isolated, active principles of the crude drugs could be synthesized in the laboratory much more cheaply than actual extraction of the active ingredients from plants. With time, more and more synthetic compounds, especially those derived from "coal-tar" (petroleum), came into use with advances in hydrocarbon chemistry.

Plant material was then, and still is today, studied for potential pharmaceutical use. The one time predominance of plant medicine in the therapeutic arena, however, is usually belittled today by mainstream veterinary medicine. The only time students hear about plants is in the toxicology section of their pharmacology course. Plants should not only be looked upon merely for their toxic potential, for they contain a vast source of therapeutic compounds as well. The main difference between historical conventional veterinary use of plant medicines and the Eclectic use is that when conventional medicine was able to obtain the purified, synthetic active principles of plants, they immediately began to use them, to further the inherent reductionist quest of science—trying to elucidate exact mechanisms of action. The Eclectic approach never aimed to only use isolated active ingredients but rather the whole juice of the plant, with all its biologically complex constituents still together (holistic approach). Thus conventional medicine was ripe for acceptance of synthetic versions of active ingredients while the Eclectic method never was.

For Eclectics, their custom line of "specific medicines" were a special class of remedies, not of the official USP of the time, but manufactured by John Uri Lloyd, who founded Lloyd Brothers Pharmacy in Cincinnati, Ohio. He was responsible for the formulation of this body of plant extracts, which were based on the philosophy and recommendations of John Scudder. These specific medicines were colloids, which seemed to have a more potent biological activity than their USP fluid extract counterparts and were administered in much smaller doses. Lloyd was concerned with the difference between the quality of a medicine and the strength of a medicine. Pharmacognosy expert Lloyd states:

> An error common to a superficial, as well as to a one-sided or fragmentary conception of pharmacy, is that of considering *strength* and *quality* as synonymous terms. As we have said, it is a common error, but it is established by very high authority. The truth is that, although more or less related, the constituent that gives the factor *strength* is often less important than are the attributes that go to make up *quality*, which, perhaps more than does strength, leads to high excellence. Let us define *strength* as a dominating something that stands out boldly, and which, in toxic drugs, produces a violent or energetic action, as does the poisonous something that produces death when an overdose of a toxic drug is administered. Let us define *quality* as a balanced combination of other something, with just enough of the toxic agent to make a complex product that, as a whole, has wider functions than are possible if the single death-dealing substance dominates. But we need not confine ourselves to toxic drugs, for, from all time, in many familiar directions, such as tea, coffee, spices, tobacco, etc. standards of strength have been differentiated from those of quality.
>
> The dominating, poisoning agent in nux vomica is a strychnine compound, and on this substance rests the official (U.S.P.) strength of the drug. But nux vomica contains other alkaloidal structures and essential oils, as well as other organic complexities, which, balanced in Eclectic pharmacy and then used in Eclectic therapy, are necessary to the quality of the Eclectic nux vomica. In the standardizing of nux vomica, the U.S. Pharmacopoeia recognizes strychnine only, whilst the Eclectic physician considers strychnine, in undue proportion, objectionable in that it dangerously overbalances *quality*. (Lloyd, 1914)

Although current veterinary medicine does not deny that plants have active constituents, there appears little need to study such things anymore since synthetic compounds abound. This is unfortunate for veterinary practitioners who have clients with USDA Certified Organic livestock, for the USDA National Organic Program (NOP) prohibits all synthetic substances while all natural substances are allowed for animal treatments. Although there are a few synthetic drugs allowed for relieving pain and suffering, there are none allowed for the vast majority of common ailments of animals for which a practitioner may be called to examine. For instance, there are no synthetic antibiotics allowed. Thus, it would seem prudent to know what natural products may be useful in order to help treat an infectious process. Only by going back to the old veterinary books that are stocked with plant and inorganic mineral treatments (which also describe their known pharmacologic properties) will a practitioner gain insight as to how a certified organic animal could potentially be treated. If for no other reason, practitioners might enjoy seeing what their colleagues of yesteryear were required to learn. In addition, this was the best scientific knowledge available at the time. Although medicine continually sifts out worthless treatments, the treatments prior to the onslaught of synthetic medicines generally fell into disuse only because they were replaced by the cheaper, mass produced synthetics, not necessarily because they themselves were useless.

Western herbal medicine has much of its roots in the Eclectic tradition, and the Eclectics' own use of plants may have originated from what natives (in many countries) were found using when settlers came into contact with them (as well as rebelling against the barbaric methods of the time). They used scientific discoveries of plant constituents to bolster their view of the medicines, distancing themselves from traditional herbalists' use of folklore and oral tradition. With a sound basis in 21st century veterinary science and medicine, it might be possible for a knowledgeable and open-minded practitioner to extrapolate from early 20th century medical textbooks and integrate modern knowledge to come up with what may be of value for a given clinical case on an organic farm. Clinical experience will help shape the course of action, as it always does.

When addressing conditions affecting certified organic livestock, it is good to know when a given condition is life threatening or when the condition will allow some leeway as far as trying natural medicines. This is *not* to say that natural medicines cannot be used for life-threatening situations, it is just that intense emergency situations may require really strong measures. Certainly, modern medicine's crowning achievements are in the realms of surgery and emergency/critical care needs. Indeed, livestock practice has its share of emergencies and critical care needs, but they are dealt with to a much lesser extent than is practiced in small animal medicine and not at all to the extent that occurs in human emergency rooms. In other words, heroic medicine and surgery is generally not the mainstay of daily livestock practice. It may be safe to say that in livestock practice, specifically dairy practice, there are many more situations that would be considered "acute" but not life threatening. General dairy practice often entails regularly scheduled herd fertility exams, diagnostic testing as done for parasites and mastitis causes, lameness diagnosis and treatment, obstetrics, surgery, and acute medical problems. Typical acute medical conditions would include (but not limited to) milk fever, ketosis, off-feed, fever, mastitis, pneumonia, and youngstock parasitism. Although the conditions of milk fever (hypocalcemia) and ketosis were not fully understood as far as etiology and definitive treatment prior to World War II were concerned, many treatments were tried on cows being off-feed due to fever, respiratory problems, parasites, and mastitis. Prior to the advent of antibiotics for infectious diseases, the best techniques included treatments such as antitoxins, antisera/passive antibodies, and vaccination. Active treatments (antitoxins), metaphylaxis (antisera), and prophylaxis (vaccination) are still in use today, especially vaccination.

It is interesting to note that even though a century divides modern from historical veterinary medicine, the same time honored husbandry principles of clean, dry housing and good ventilation are still echoed today by veterinary practitioners. One aspect of farm management, that of nutrition, has made gigantic leaps as far as the metabolic and production needs of livestock species are concerned. However, the traditional use of pasture (and textbook information regarding it) has all fallen to the wayside in favor of high-tech ration formulation, very much paralleling the decline of botanical therapeutics in favor of high-tech pharmaceuticals.

The rest of this chapter will focus on treatment plans for common, acute conditions. They are mainly for dairy cows, but some other species will be mentioned as well. To those readers already applying natural treatments to livestock, many of the ingredients should sound familiar. For veterinarians reading these prescriptions, try to picture what it must have been like before antibiotics were discovered and perhaps piece together professional training with basic pharmacology to arrive at an understanding of why these prescriptions were used. These prescriptions are from old veterinary texts as well as books written by veterinarians for the livestock owner. In reading some of the books for livestock owners it is rather amazing to think that farmers generally had some very potent crude drugs on hand. When reading the following nonsynthetic ("natural") treatments it should be noted how a combination of ingredients was usually formulated, whereas modern synthetic drugs tend to rely on one single active ingredient (dexamethasone, flunixin, prostaglandin, gonadorelin, ampicillin, etc.). Concerning being in agreement with evidence-based medicine (or proven by its dictates), these recipes may not be, if only because they pre-date the concept of double-blind random controlled trials. But it should be remembered that although items such as dexamethasone, flunixin, and ampicillin may have been individually proven in double-blind studies, the common cocktail mixtures that practitioners put together and administer to animals in clinical situations have *not* themselves been proven by evidence-based medicine. So, at least in view of the lack of double-blind studies on these plant based formulas, it suffices to say that the modern veterinarian equipped with "shotgun" treatments practices in a manner not unknown to previous generations of practitioners. If these treatments are taken in earnest and tried out today, keep in mind that a multiprong approach may be needed (e.g., supplemental fluids, stomach tube feeding, etc.) especially when thinking of how much more milk dairy cows produce in modern times and how important it is to get a cow back into production as quickly as possible due to strong economic pressures. It may be possible for a person to go ahead and use the information presented in the rest of the chapter so as to treat livestock without reverting to antibiotics and hormones. Of course, antibiotics have their therapeutic place (as in bacterial pneumonia) and professional veterinary involvement is critical in many situations. The following compilation of information is at best just one half of the medicine box and the concurrent prudent use of modern veterinary science will provide the other half of the box. In trying to bridge the "old" with the "new" to help farmers who are trying to farm "naturally/organically," no stone should be left unturned.

Since the formulas are drawn mainly with dairy cattle in mind, it is appropriate to begin with the presentation of known information about potential residues (Table 9.2). Even before the era of antibiotics, tainted milk was a consideration for marketable milk. Just because only antibiotics are checked for regularly in modern times doesn't mean that other substances which are not regularly checked for can be dismissed out of hand.

Current regulatory status for herbal medicine is a "gray area." Probably the best source of information for maximum residue limits on *some* plant medicines can be found at www.emea.eu.int/htms/vet/mrls/a-zmrl.htm. This is the Web site of The European Agency for the Evaluation of Medicinal Products. It is mainly for injectable pharmaceutical compounds but has many popular plant based remedies as well.

The general action of drugs is shown in Table 9.3. The classification of medicines according to their physiologic actions is shown in Table 9.4, and doses of medicines are shown in Table 9.5. Most of these treatments have never been rigorously tested, but many veterinaries and stockman relied on them for treating livestock before modern treatments replaced most of the treatments.

Table 9.2 Drugs excreted by the mammary gland

Acid, boric; acid, carbolic; acid, salicylic; aloes; antipyrin; arsenic and its salts; atropine; bromine and its compounds; chloroform; copper and its salt; croton; ether; iodine and its compounds; lead and its salts; mercury and its salts; potassium and antimonium tartrate; rhubarb; sodii sulph.; turpentine
(Fish, 1930, p. 176)

Opium; all volatile oils; purgative salts; rhubarb; senna: castor oil; scammony; jalap; iodine; potassium iodide; antimony; arsenic; mercury; lead; zinc; iron; bismuth; neutral salts; ammonia; acids; sulfur; atropine; copper; carbolic acid; colchicum; euphorbium; ergot; salicylic acid; veratrine; strychnine; croton oil; aloes; turpentine
(Winslow, 1919, p. 49)

BISHOP BURTON COLLEGE
LIBRARY

Table 9.3 General actions of drugs. (Winslow, 1919, pp. 19–58)

Drugs acting on the digestive organs:
Stomachics:
  Bitters-Gentian, calumba, quassia, hydrastis, taraxacum
  Aromatic bitters-Cascarilla, chamomile, serpentaria
  Aromatics-Coriander, capsicum, pepper, ginger, cardamom, fennel, fenugreek, anise, calamus,
    mustard, spearmint, peppermint, alcohol, ether, chloroform, alkalis
Antacids:
  Sodium carbonate, sodium bicarbonate, potassium carbonate, potassium bicarbonate, solution of
    potash, ammonia, ammonium carbonate, magnesia, magnesium carbonate, calcium carbonate
    (chalk), solution of lime (lime water)
Antiseptics:
  Carbolic acid (phenol), creosote, creolin, napthol, naphtalin, bismuth subnitrite, bismuth
    subcarbonate, bismuth subsalicylate, sodium sulfite, bisulfate and hydrosulfite, hydrogen dioxide
    (hydrogen peroxide)
Emetics:
  Specific-apomorphine, lobeline, morphine, senega, squills
  Mixed-tartar emetic, ipecac, copper sulfate, zinc sulfate
  Local-tepid water, mustard, salt, alum, ammonium carbonate
Gastric sedatives and antiemetics:
  Ice, hot water, bismuth subcarbonate, bismuth subnitrate, carbon dioxide, hydrocyanic acid,
    morphine, menthol, carbolic acid, creosote, aconite, belladonna, hyoscyamus, cocaine, cerium
    oxalate, lime water, minute doses of: arsenic, ipecac, alcohol, iodine, silver nitrate; chloroform,
    chloral, bromides, nitrites, brandy and champagne
Laxatives:
  Olive oil, cottonseed oil, magnesia, sulfur, nux vomica, small dose: linseed oil, castor oil; liquid
    petrolatum and other mineral oils (mechanical lubricant, not absorbed)
Simple purgatives:
  Aloes, calomel (mercury), linseed oil, castor oil, rhubarb, senna, cascara sagrada, phenolphthalein,
    frangula, bryonia
Drastic purgatives:
  Croton oil, colocynth, gamboges, scammony, jalap, elaterium
Saline purgatives:
  Magnesium sulfate, sodium sulfate, sodium phosphate, potassium bitartrate
Direct cholagogues:
  Sodium salicylate*, podophyllum*, aloes, rhubarb, colchicum, sodium sulfate, sodium phosphate*,
    ipecac, euonymus, nitro-hydrochloric acid*, corrosive sublimate (mercury)
  *Have been found by clinical evidence to be most active

Drugs acting on the circulation
Drugs acting upon the blood
  Hematinics-iron and its salts, copper salts, potassium permanganate, manganese dioxide

Drugs acting on the heart:
Increase the force of the heart beat:
  Digitalis, adrenalin (epinephrine), squill, physostigmine, strophanthus, sparteine
Increase the rate of the heart beats:
  Belladonna, atropine, hyosctamus, stramonium, cocaine
Increase the force and rate of heart beats:
  Alcohol, chloroform, ether, ammonia, ammonium carbonate, strychnine, caffeine, quinine, arsenic
Decrease the force and rate of the heart beats:
  Aconite, veratrum viride, ergot, antimony salts, prussic acid

Drugs acting on the blood vessels:
Systemically to contract vessels:
  Cocaine, ergot, atropine, digitalis, strophanthus, squill, sparteine, strychnine, hamamelis, hydrastis,
    physostigmine, adrenalin (epinephrine), pituitary extract

Table 9.3 *Continued*

Systemically to dilate vessels:
  Amyl nitrate, nitroglycerin, spirit of nitrous ether, alcohol, salicylates, ether, chloroform, thyroid
    secretion, chloral, aconite, opium, secondary action of belladonna, hyoscyamus and stramonium

Drugs influencing the brain:
Cerebral excitants:
  Campor, caffeine, quinine, cocaine
Cerebral depressants:
  Anodynes, by reason of their action on the brain: Codeine, morphine, opium, alcohol, anesthetics,
    chloral, cannabis indica, gelsemium, bromides
  Narcotics: opium and its derivatives, alcohol, anesthetics, chloral, cannabis indica, belladonna,
    stramonium, hyscyamus
  Hypnotics: opium, morphine, chloral, bromides, cannabis indica
  General anesthetics: ether, chloroform, nitrous oxide, methylene bochloride
Stimulate the motor centers:
  Strychnine, atropine, physostigmine
Depress the motor centers:
  The bromides, chloral, alcohol, anesthetics
Drugs acting on the spinal cord:
Stimulate motor cells of inferior cornua:
  strychnine, brucine, thebaine, ammonia, anesthetics, opium, ergot
Depress the motor cells of inferior cornua:
  physostigmine, bromides, ergot, nitrites, gelsemium, emetine, turpentine, saponin, chloral, morphine,
    apomorphine, alcohol, ether, chloroform, camphor, carbolic acid, nicotine, veratrine, mercury,
    arsenic, salts of magnesium, sodium, potassium, lithium, antimony, zinc, silver
Drugs acting on the nerves:
Influence peripheral sensory nerve endings:
  Stimulate: counter-irritants
  Depress local anodynes: aconite, menthol, carbolic acid, atropine, morphine, chloral, prussic acid,
    sodium bicarbonate, veratrine, heat, cold
  Depress local anesthetic: cocaine, eucaine, stovaine, novocaine, holocaine, cold, ether spray, methyl
    chloride spray
Influence motor nerve-terminations:
  Stimulate: strychnine, pilocarpine, aconite, nicotine, pyridine
  Depress: curare, conium, atropine, amyl nitrate, cocaine, camphor, prussic acid, lobeline, nicotine
    (and many others)

Drugs acting on the nerves of special sense:
Act on the eye:
  Mydriatics-paralyze third nerve endings: atropine, homatropine, hyoscyamine, hyoscine,
    scopolamine, gelsemine. Cocaine stimulates sympathetic endings.
  Myotics-acting locally-stimulate third nerve endings: physostigmine, pilocarpine-*acting centrally*:
    anesthetics, opium

Drugs acting on the respiratory organs:
Expectorants:
  Increase secretion: apomorphine, potassium iodide, ipecac, pilocarpine, ammonium chloride, squill,
    camphor, balsams, sulfur, tar, turpentine, terpin hydrate, terebene, volatile oils
  Decrease secretion: belladonna, hyoscyamus, stramonium, opium, volatile oils (first increase, then
    decrease secretions)
  Altering the nutrition of bronchial mucous membrane: cod-liver oil, sulfur, potassium iodide,
    ammonium chloride
  Exerting an antiseptic action: turpentine, terebene, terpine hydrate, balsam of Peru, Balsam of Tolu,
    Cubebs, Copaiba, tar, ammoniacum
  Locally stimulating and antiseptic to mucous membranes: eucalyptol, guiacol, creosote

(continued)

115

Table 9.3 *Continued*

Drugs stimulating the respiratory centers:
  Strychnine, atropine, caffeine, cocaine, belladonna, hyoscyamus, stramonium, ammonium carbonate, strong ammonia

Drugs depressing the respiratory centers:
  Morphine, codeine, heroin, chloral, bromides

Drugs relaxing spasm of the bronchial muscular tunic and relieving cough:
  Locally: white of egg, linseed tea, syrups, mucilage, external counter-irritation and heat
  Systemically: opium, codeine, heroin, hyoscyamus, stramonium, cannabis indica, nitrites, chloral, bromides, chloroform, phenacetin, adrenalin (epinephrine)

Drugs allaying spasm and cough:
  Opium with belladonna

Drugs acting on the urinary organs:
Diuretics:
  Increase the glomerular fluid: water, potassium acetate, citrate, bitartrate; ammonium acetate; digitalis, squill and strophanthus (when the circulation is poor); caffeine, nitrites
  Stimulating renal cells or lessening absorption from tubular cells, or both: caffeine, theobromine; volatile oils, resins, or aromatics such as buchu, juniper, turpentine, cantharides; glucosides such as scoparin and asparagin; all salts, glucose and alkalies
Urinary antiseptics:
  Benzoic acid, boric acid, methylene blue, salicylic acid, salol, buchu, copaiba, cubebs, volatile oils
Urinary sedatives:
  Hyoscyamus, belladonna, opium, alkalies (with an acid urine)

Drugs acting on the sexual organs:
Influencing chiefly the male generative organs:
Aphrodisiacs:
  Direct aphrodisiacs: strychnine, phosphorus, alcohol (act on centers); cantharides (local irritant); yohimbine (causes congestion of the sexual organs)
  Indirect aphrodisiacs: iron, strychnine, arsenic, full diet
Anaphrodisiacs:
  Opium, bromides, purgatives, nauseants, bleeding (venesection), spare diet
Influencing the female sexual organs:
Emmenagogues:
  Direct: savin, rue, cantharides (irritants); ergot
  Indirect: aloes (purgative); iron, arsenic, strychnine, full diet (in debility)
Ecbolics (oxytocics):
  Ergot, quinine, hydrastis, savin, corn smut, cotton root bark, pituitrin
Restraining uterine contractions:
  Cannabis indica, bromides, chloral, anesthetics
Influencing milk secretion, increase flow of milk (galactogoues):
  Pilocarpine, leaves of the castor oil plant, alcohol, extracts of the pituitary, and mammary glands, full diet
Drugs influencing metabolism:

Alteratives (vague, indefinable word used to describe the action of certain drugs modifying tissue change and improving nutrition in some disorders):
  Iodine and its salts, cod liver oil, colchicum, sarsaparilla, sulfur

Tonics (a word even more vague then "alterative"—impossible to define precisely. Tonics improve the general nutrition and health, and generally understood to refer to drugs promoting appetite and digestion (gentian); the state of the blood (hematinics, as iron); the condition of some organs (heart, as digitalis; nervines, strychnine). Tonics are indicated in the treatment of debility (general or special) and anemia.

Table 9.3 *Continued*

Drugs influencing body heat:
Diminish metabolism:
  quinine
Dilate superficial vessels:
  Salicylic acid, alcohol, ammonium acetate, nitrous ether, opium and ipecac
Depress circulation:
  Aconite, veratrum, digitalis, antimony, and venesection (bleeding)
Antipyretics (synthetics which act directly on the heat-regulating centers):
  Acetanilid, antipyrin, phenacetin

Drugs influencing the skin:
Dilate superficial vessels:
  Cantharides, iodine, mustard, capsicum, croton oil, oil of turpentine, and other volatile oils, camphor,
    heat (and mineral caustics, not mentioned)
Contract superficial vessels:
  Hamamelis, ergot, hydrastis, cocaine, tannic acid and drugs containing it, cold (and mineral salts, not
    mentioned)
Styptics (hemostatics):
  Ferric alum, ferric chloride, and subsulfate; adrenaline
Emollients:
  Lard, petrolatum, cacao butter, olive oil, cottonseed oil, lanolin
Demulcents (soothing, protecting and softening influence on the mucous membrane of the alimentary
    canal when given internally):
  Acacia, linseed infusion or tea, licorice, syrup, molasses, honey, glycerin, white of egg, milk, starch,
    sweet oil
Diaphoretics (stimulate sweat):
  Pilocarpine, alcohol, opium, ipecac, aconite, camphor, external heat, blankets
Anhidrotics:
  Atropine, belladonna, hyoscyamus, stramonium, nux vomica, quinine, salicylic acid (locally), cold
    externally

Drugs which destroy microorganisms and parasites:
Disinfectants or germicides:
  Carbolic acid, lime, chlorinated lime, chlorine, heat
Antiseptics (external/surgery):
  Tincture of iodine, alcohol, carbolic acid, hydrogen peroxide, potassium permanganate, zinc
    chloride, zinc sulfate, iodoform, salicylic acid, boric acid, thymol, Balsam of Peru
Antiseptics (internal):
  Salol, carbolic acid, bismuth salicylate, bismuth subnitrite, quinine, volatile oils
Anthelmintics removing tapeworms:
  Aspidium (horse and dog), oil of turpentine, kousso, areca nut (sheep), pumpkin seed, aloe,
    linseed/cottonseed/or castor oil
Anthelmintics removing ascarids:
  Horses: oil of turpentine, copper sulfate, carbon bisulfide
  Dogs: santonin, spigelia, oil of chenopodium
Anthelmintics removing pinworms:
  Oil of chenopodium, thymol, and cathartics (orally)
  Salt, lime solution, quassia, iron salts, phenol, tannic acid, oil of turpentine (enema)
Anthelmintics removing strongyles:
  Thymol, oil of chenopodium, turpentine, copper sulfate, chloroform
Anthelmintics removing bots (gastrophilus spp.):
  Carbon disulfide

(continued)

Table 9.3 *Continued*

Anthelmintics against lungworms:
  Carbolic acid (intratracheal injections)
  Turpentine
  Chloroform (injections in nostrils)
Vermifuges (to expel dead parasites from bowels after anthelmintics):
  Aloe and oil
Antiparasitics (skin):
  Against fungi of ringworm (Trichophyton spp.): tincture of iodine, glycerite of phenol, creosote, chrysarobin ointment, cantharides, croton oil, formalin, salicylic acid, boric acid, thymol
  Against ray fungi of lumpyjaw (Actinomyces): tincture of iodine, potassium iodide, glycerite of carbolic acid, iodoform, copper sulfate
  Against fungi of thrush or aptha, sporadic aphthous stomatitis: boric acid, potassium chlorate, potassium permanganate, alum, salicylic acid
  Against mites of scab, itch or mange: sulfur, lime-sulfur dips, tar, crude petroleum, Peruvian balsam, phenol, salicylic acid, cantharides
  Against lice: staphisagria, oil of tar, Peruvian balsam, oil of anise, phenol, tobacco, pyrethrum, creosote preparations
  Against fleas: pyrethrum, carbolic soap, oil of anise, creosote preparations (for dosages, see dosage Table 9.5 from Fish (1930))

Table 9.4 Classification of medicines according to their physiologic actions (Fish, 1930, p. 156–172, abridged)

Anthelmintics:
Aloes (enema), aspidium, chenopodium, koussein, naphtalin, oil turpentine, extract male fern, pelletierine tannate, pumpkin seed, quassia infusion, santonin wth calomel (mercury), sodium chloride, sodium santoninate, spigelia, thymol

Antipyretics:
Acetanilid, benzoic acid, carbolic acid, salicylic acid, aconite tincture, ammonium acetate solution, ammonium benzoate, aspirin, phenacetin, quinine and salts, resorcin, veratrum viride tincture

Carminitives:
Anise, calumba, capsicum, cardamom, caraway, cascarilla, chamomile, cinchona, cinnamon, cloves, gentian, ginger, nutmeg, nux vomica, oil cajeput, oil mustard, orange peel, pepper, pimenta, quassia, sassafras, serpentaria

Galactogogues:
Lactic acid, alcohol, ammonium chloride, castor oil (topically), extract malt, jaborandi, pilocarpine hydrochloride

Gastric tonics:
Alkalies: before meals, aromatics, berberine carbonate, bismuth salts, bitters, carminitives, hydrastis, ichthalbin, nux vomica, quassin

Oxytocics (ecbolics):
Cotton root bark, ergot, hydrastine, hydrastine hydrochloride, pennyroyal, quinine, rue, savine

Tonics, general:
Vegetable: Bitters, berberine carbonate, cinchona alkaloids and salts, cod-liver oil, eucalyptus, hydrastis, quassin, salicin

Table 9.5 Veterinary doses (Fish, 1930, pp. 8–41—abridged)

	H&C[a]	Sh&Sw[b]		H&C	Sh&Sw
Aconite T[c].	2–6	0.25–1	Glycerin	30–60	8–15
Aloe	8–40	4–15	Glycyrrhiza	15–60	4–15
Areca nut	15–30	2–6	Gossypium F.E.	8–30	2–8
Arnica .T	15–30	4–8	Granatum F.E.	15–30	4–12
Asafetida T.	60–120	8–15	Guarana F.E.	8–30	2–4
Balsam Copaiba	15–60	2–8	Gum Tragacanth	60–90	15–30
Balsam Peru	15–60	4–8	Hamamelis F.E.	30–60	8–15
Balsam Tolu	15–60	2–4	Helleborus Niger F.E.	4–15	0.6–2
Belladonna leaves T.	15–30	4–8	Hematoxylin F.E.	15–45	6–12
Brandy	60–120	30–60	Humulus T.	30–120	4–15
Bryonia T.	15–30	2–4	Hydrastis F.E.	8–30	4–8
Buchu leaves F.E.	30–60	2–4	Hydrastis glycerite	8–30	4–15
Calendula T.	15–30	4–8	Hydrastis T.	30–60	4–15
Calumba T.	60–120	12–24	Hydrogen peroxide 3%	15–60	4–15
Cannabis Indica T.	15–45	2–4	Hyoscamus T.	30–90	8–15
Cantharides	1–2	0.3–1	Ignatia F.E.	2–4	1.3–2.6
Capsicum	4–8	0.6–2	Iodine T.	8–15	1.3–2.6
Cardamom T.	60–90	12–24	Ipecac F.E.	4–8	1–2
Cascara sagrada F.E.	8–45	0.6–4	Jaborandi F.E.	8–15	2–4
Cascarilla bark F.E.	15–30	4–8	Juniper oil	4–8	0.6–2
Castanea F.E.	30–60	8–15	Kamala F.E.	15–30	4–12
Castor oil 500	60–120		Kava kava F.E.	15–30	4–12
Catechu C/T.	30–60	8–15	Kino F.E.	30–60	4–12
Chamomile	30–60	4–8	Kousso F.E.	15–60	4–12
Chaulmoogra Oil	2–12	0.3–2	Krameria F.E.	15–30	4–8
Chenopodium Oil	6–12	0.6–1.3	Lactucarium F.E.	8–30	1–4
Chimaphila F.E.	30–60	4–15	Laudanum	15–60	4–15
Cimicifuga T.	30–90	8–15	Lobelia T.	30–60	4–12
Cinchona bark C/T.	60–120	15–30	Male fern F.E.	12–24	4–8
Cinnamon oil	2–6	0.3–0.6	Matico T.	30–60	8–15
Coca F.E.	30–120	15–30	Mentha piperitae oi	1–2	0.3–0.6
Cod liver oil	60–120	15–30	Myrrh T.	8–15	4–8
Colchicum root T.	15–45	4–6	Nux vomica T.	4–24	1.3–2.6
Conium F.E.	4–8	0.6–1.3	Opium T. (paregoric)	60–120	15–30
Convallaria	4–8	0.6–1.3	Pareira F.E.	15–30	4–8
Cotton root bark	15–60	4–8	Physostigma F.E.	1–2	0.13–0.25
Creolin, as anthelmintic	15–30	2–4	Phytolacca F.E.	4–8	1.3–3
Digitalis T.	12–24	3–10	Pichi F.E	8–24	2–4
Dioscorea F.E.	8–24	2–4	Pilocarpus F.E.	8–15	2–4
Echinacea F.E.	4–15	2–4	Pipsissewa F.E.	30–60	4–15
Epsom salts	60–120	15–30	Pomegranate	30–60	4–12
Ergot T.	15–60	4–15	Polygonum F.E.	15–30	4–8
Eriodictyon F.E.	15–60	2–8	Prunus Virginian F.E.	15–60	4–8
Eucalyptus oil	8–15	1.3–3.3	Pulsatilla F.E.	2–8	0.3–0.6
Fennel	30–60	8–12	Pyrethrum	15–30	2–6
Fenugreek	30–60	8–12	Quassia F.E.	30–60	8–15
Gamboge	15–30	1.3–4	Quercus Alba F.E.	15–30	4–8
Gaultheria oil	8–30	2–8	Quinine (antipyretic)	8–15	1.3–2.6
Gelsemium T.	15–60	4–12	Rhamnus F.E.	30–60	4–8
Gentian F.E.	15–30	4–8	Rhubarb F.E.	30–60	4
Geranium F.E.	8–30	2–4	Rhus glab. F.E.	15–30	4–8
Glauber's salts	600	45	Rumex F.E.	30–60	4–8

(*continued*)

Table 9.5   *Continued*

	H&C[a]	Sh&Sw[b]		H&C	Sh&Sw
Ruta F.E.	15–30	15–30	Tanacetum oil	1.3–4	0.13–0.4
Ruta oil	2–4	0.13–0.6	Taraxacum F.E.	30–60	8–15
Sabina F.E.	30–60	2–4	Terebene	8–24	2–4
Sabina oil	8–15	0.5–1	Thiosimanin	2–4	0.5–1
Sanguinaria F.E.	4–24	0.6–2	Thymol	2–8	0.3–2
Santal F.E.	15–60	8–12	Tiglii oil	1–2	0.3–0.6
Santal oil	4–12	0.6–3	Tonga F.E.	8–30	2–4
Santonin	15–30	4–8	Triticum F.E.	30–60	8–24
Sarsaparilla F.E.	30–60	4–8	Turpentine oil		
Sassafrass F.E.	30–60	4–8	(carminative)	30–60	4–15
Sassafrass oil	2–8	0.3–0.6	(anthelmintic)	60–120	15–30
Scoparius F.E	15–30	4–8	Ustilago F.E.	15–60	2–4
Scutellaria F.E.	15–30	4–12	Uva ursi F.E.	60–120	8–15
Senega F.E.	4–15	1–2	Valerian F.E.	30–60	4–8
Senna F.E.	120–150	30–60	Valerian oil	2–4	0.6–1.3
Serpentaria F.E.	15–30	2–4	Veratrum viride F.E.	2–4	1.3–2
Spigelia F.E.	4–30	2–4	Veratrum viride T.	8–12	2.6–4
Squill F.E.	4–8	0.3–1.3	Viburnum Prunus F.E.	30–120	8–15
Squill T.	24–48	6–12	Vinegar	30–120	2–8
Stillingia F.E.	4–30	2–8	Whiskey	60–120	30–60
Stillingia T.	15–45	4–8	Wintergreen oil	8–30	2–8
Stramonium F.E.	1.3–4	0.3–0.6	Xanthoxylum F.E.	15–60	4–12
Stramonium T.	4–8	0.6–2	Zea F.E.	30–60	8–15
Strophanthus T.	4–15	0.3–1.3	Zingiber F.E.	8–30	4–8
Sumbul F.E.	8–24	1–4	Zingiber T.	30–60	8–15
Sumbul T.	15–30	2–8			

[a] H = horse, C = cattle.
[b] Sh = sheep, Sw = swine.
[c] T. = Tincture (1:10), C/T. = compound tincture (mixture), F.E. = fluid extract (1:1). Doses are "full strength"; all doses are in cc (ml) and to be given orally.

References

Boericke, W. 1927. *Materia Medica & Repertory*, 9th edn. Reprint edition: B. Jain Publishers Pvt. Ltd. 1994.

Dun, F. 1910. *Veterinary Medicines*, 12th edn. David Douglas, Edinburgh, UK.

Fish, P.A. 1930. *Veterinary Doses and Prescription Writing*, 6th edn. The Slingerland-Comstock Publ. Co. Ithaca, NY.

Humphrey, F. 1881. *Manual of Veterinary Specific Homeopathy*. Humphreys' Specific Homeopathic Medicine Co., New York, NY, USA.

Jousset, P. 1901. *Practice of Medicine, Containing the Homeopathic Treatment of Diseases*. A.L. Catterton & Co., New York, NY.

Lloyd, J.U. 1914. *The Eclectic Medical Journal*. Cincinnati, OH.

Richardson, J. 1828. *The New-England Farrier, and Family Physician*. Published by Josiah Richardson. Exeter, MA.

Scudder, J. 1874. *Specific Diagnosis*. Wilstach, Baldwin & Co., Printers, Cincinnati, OH.

Titus, N.N. 1865. *The American Eclectic Practice of Medicine as Applied to the Diseases of Domestic Animals*. N.N. Titus. Union, NY.

Varlo, C. 1785. *A New System of Husbandry*, Vol. 1. Philadelphia, PA.

Winslow, K. 1919. *Veterinary Materia Medica and Therapeutics*, 8th edn. American Vet. Publishing Co., Chicago, IL.

Chapter 10
Herbs and Alternatives in Equine Practice
Joyce C. Harman

Introduction

Complementary and alternative veterinary medicine (CAVM) in equine practice is a broad subject encompassing acupuncture, chiropractic, homeopathy, herbal medicine, and nutrition. This chapter will discuss alternative medicine in equine practice and its relationship to soil health. Intestinal health is directly related to soil health in that both function optimally when the beneficial bacteria are in balance. As feed becomes more processed, less nutrition is available for the horse. A brief introduction to the treatment of disease in equine practice covers homeopathy, herbs, and nutrition related to the intestinal tract.

What is health?

When looking at medicine holistically, the first question to ask is what is health? Health is defined as freedom from disease. In conventional medicine "normal" chronic conditions are accepted as healthy, as long as the animal is considered free from devastating illness. In other words, many signs of chronic disease, when not life threatening, are accepted as normal health. According to this definition many domesticated horses are not truly healthy. Many horses have low-grade problems that few people regard as signs of ill health; the practitioner simply treats each symptom as it appears.

True health in holistic terms is freedom from any signs of disease. It includes the ability to acquire common, self-limiting diseases, such as the flu, and have adequate immunity such that the illness is short-lived and requires little medication to recover. A healthy individual should mount a strong reaction to an infectious disease, often running a high fever (up to 105°F or more) for a short period of time, followed by a quick recovery.

A horse, by nature, is a prey animal. It lives in areas with scrubtype vegetation and moves 20 hours a day eating, with about 4 hours spent resting and sleeping. We expect horses to adapt to our ways of living, eating, and exercise, and, for the most part, horses do this very well. However, the levels of stress brought on by the unnatural living conditions create chronic disease and weakened immune systems.

Signs of chronic disease

Signs of disease manifest as mental or physical symptoms that range from mild to severe. Any deviation from health can be considered a sign of disease, but may only indicate an imbalance in feed. It is important for humans as guardians of animals to become more observant of the signs of disease.

Mental signs that chronic disease may be present include excessive fears, nervousness, and inability to adapt to change. Horses with repetitive behaviors such as weaving, stall-walking, self-mutilation, or cribbing that appear addicted to these behaviors are probably not dealing well with the stresses of confinement. If a horse is having a difficult time adapting to the stress of confinement, the immune system is probably compromised and the horse's health may deteriorate.

Typically horses that are either consistently underweight or overweight have a problem with chronic disease. Underweight horses may have trouble digesting or utilizing food, or they may have low-grade liver disease or cancer. Horses chronically overweight, especially those with fat deposits and "cresty" necks, may have metabolic problems but may simply be overfed and underexercised.

The respiratory system is commonly affected in the chronically ill horse. Allergies usually manifest as heaves and allergic coughs (although allergies with itchy skin are commonly seen in the warm climates). Allergies are a sign of immune system imbalance and overreactivity. Many high-speed horses (racing, eventing, steeplechasing) bleed from the lungs, showing signs of weakness in the respiratory tract. Foals with upper respiratory "snots" of several months duration may be considered normal by conventionally trained individuals. However, from a holistic perspective, protracted infections are an indicator of disease.

Skin is the largest organ in the body, and internal health and nutritional state are reflected in the skin and hooves. The dry, dull, bleached coats on which people spend fortunes can be best treated from the inside using a complete holistic approach. One of the primary signs of a healthy horse is a deep rich color to the hair. Truly healthy horses have a glow to their coat and they do not bleach out in the sun.

Allergies, especially itching eruptions, are signs of chronic immune system problems (Dodds, 1993), and though skin allergies are difficult to cure with any form of medicine, the holistic approach is often successful. Often, seemingly simple conditions like dermatophilis ("rain rot," etc.) are signs of subtle disease. All horses on a given property may be exposed to a causative agent, yet only a subset of the horses succumb to the infection. As horses are cured from chronic disease, skin conditions including warts, sarcoids, oily or sticky sweat, discharges from the sheath, poor wound healing, and excessive scar tissue production tend to resolve.

Feet are an adaptation of the skin structures, and the old adage, "no foot, no horse," is as true today as when it originated. Poor nutrition, chronic disease, and weather conditions play important roles in the health of the foot, as does the quality of the farrier work. Cracked, brittle, or dry feet as well as soft or crumbly feet can be signs of chronic disease. Thrush, white line disease, abscesses, and seedy toe need to addressed from a holistic standpoint and be considered as subtle signs of disease.

Gastrointestinal disorders are an important disease entity, as colic causes the maximum number of horse deaths. However, most facilities where colic is common have identifiable management problems, especially when taking into account horses' natural grazing and exercising habits. Lack of correct roughage is one of the primary causes of colic, since the equine gut is designed for long stem roughage and not concentrates. The stress of confinement contributes to colic, as does the overuse of antibiotics and dewormers. Horses with chronic digestive tract problems including dry feces, soft feces, ulcers, sensitivity to change in diet or weather, odiferous stools, failure to digest completely, cravings for dirt, salt or wood, fussy eaters and various mouth problems probably suffer from chronic disease.

The reproductive system is affected by nutrition, management, heredity, and chronic disease. Horses are selected for desirable performance and are not selected for reproductive health as they are in the wild. Mares have many problems, both physical and behavioral, associated with their heat cycles. Infertility of the male and female, including lack of libido, sterility, ovulation problems, and chronic uterine infections of all types, can often be corrected holistically.

Equine musculoskeletal problems, which usually manifest as lameness, are a common reason for horse owners to seek veterinary services. Lameness is yet another sign that can be an indication of disease in the horse. Muscle stiffness and tying up, as well as weak tendons and ligaments, may have a nutritional or chronic disease origin. Arthritic changes in the joints, including navicular syndrome, can result from an ill-fitting saddle, shoeing, nutrition, or chronic disease. From a Chinese perspective, constant swelling or stocking up of the legs indicates poor digestion (Xie, 1994).

The signs discussed above are merely an introduction to the signs of chronic disease and are presented to stimulate thought about the current state of health in our horses. Typically disease symptoms are resolved best by treating the chronic disease with the appropriate therapy (homeopathy, acupuncture, chiropractic, herbal medicine, and others), nutrition, and management changes.

Intestinal health as the foundation of all healing

Horses are designed by nature as foraging animals; they are made to graze on whatever scrub, grass, and weeds were available for the greater part of each day. During this time they move continually, except for relatively short periods spent sleeping. If they become ill, a wide selection of herbs (weeds) are available, in many pastures, to help remedy their health problems. Today, commercialization of nutrition into bags of feed and supplements along with rich cultivated pastures have changed equine nutrition habits from rough forage to processed feeds and rich grass. The lack of biodiversity in the pastures plus the modern feeding practices contribute to poor intestinal health.

Physiology of equine digestion

The equine digestive tract is a unique system that allows the animal to obtain nutrients and energy from a variety of feedstuffs. Horses use acid digestion in the stomach and fermentation in the cecum in the digestive process. The stomach absorbs water and begins protein digestion primarily through the action of pepsin. The stomach's acidic environment allows for ionization and subsequent absorption of some minerals such as calcium, magnesium, manganese, and iron (Kimbrough et al., 1995). The small intestine then hydrolyses the protein, fat, and carbohydrates into the final form for absorption. The fermentation vat, the cecum, is perhaps the most important part of the equine digestive tract since it is here that the fiber portion of the diet is digested. The cecum is designed to break down and ferment long stem fiber and through bacterial metabolism produce vitamins and fatty acids. Horses evolved to graze continually in the wild to keep the digestive tract full and moving. The common practice of feeding twice a day does not keep the food moving continually through the cecum and can lead to poor digestion or colic (Clarke, 1990; White et al., 1993).

The intestinal environment is a miniature ecosystem where each player has a place and a job, just as a symphony, and if any piece is out of place, the whole is affected. The intestinal tract contains bacteria and protozoa designed to digest food, manufacture vitamins and fatty acids, and make minerals available. Bacteria inhabiting the intestinal tract are pH specific in their requirements for growth, so they are found where the correct pH is for each bacterial species. The bacteria use dietary fiber in the digestive tract as an energy source. They live on the fiber, not in the intestinal wall. Consequently when fiber is deficient, the bacterial population is not healthy (Folino et al., 1995). When the horse is fed mostly concentrates in the form of grain and very little long stem fiber such as hay, the incidence of colic is higher.

Bacteria and the pH of the digestive tract are intimately related. The normal pH of the intestinal tract changes from acidic in the stomach and upper small intestine, moves toward neutral in the lower small intestine, and becomes close to neutral in the large intestine. With incomplete digestion and poor quality feeds, the pH and motility can become altered, allowing pathogenic bacteria to move up from the alkaline large intestine, into the acidic small intestine potentially causing diarrhea. Alternatively, if the pH of the large intestine becomes more acidic, and the acidophilic bacteria move down, the large intestine can become irritated.

Natural, raw food has all the bacteria and enzymes needed to aid digestion; however, processing often destroys them. The healthy digestive tract can still digest good quality cooked or processed food because the healthy bacteria and the enzymes already present in the digestive tract will continue to function even though new bacteria are not introduced in processed food. The unhealthy digestive tract has difficulty functioning with poorer quality feed. Live foods also appear to have a "life force" that cannot be put into a package or processed into a ration.

Anything that occurs in the animal's life to upset the natural balance of the intestinal tract flora will affect digestion and direct utilization of the food. A course of oral antibiotics upsets the digestive flora balance and should only be used in specific appropriate situations (Schmidt et al., 1993). Overuse of antibiotics and nonsteroidal anti-inflammatory drugs has been shown to increase intestinal permeability, allowing improperly digested or foreign material to enter the bloodstream. One of the side effects of antibiotics is suppression of the immune system.

Other factors that appear to disturb the normal digestive flora are frequent use of dewormers, illness, confinement, the stress of being worked while in pain (a common happening in today's horse world), and changes of diet. The latter are very common since most feed manufacturers use least-cost programs to formulate feed. The more horses are confined, stressed, and managed by humans, the more nutritional deficiencies and imbalances the veterinarian will find.

Minerals

Mineral availability and balance is probably the most important aspect of nutrition and healing in equine practice. Most modern farms consist of chemically fertilized soils planted repeatedly with the same crops. This can lead to depletion of trace soil minerals and subsequent mineral depletion of harvested grains used as feed. There is a complex interaction between many minerals; even a slight excess of one mineral in a diet can mean another mineral may not be properly processed. In nature each "weed" has a trace mineral associated with it, so if a particular mineral is needed the horse will eat the weed. Also, if the soil needs a particular mineral a certain weed will grow there to provide that mineral (McCaman, 1994).

A new branch of science called zoopharmacognosy involves the study of animals and their natural ability to select plants and herbs according to their needs and particular illnesses (Lipske, 1993; DeMaar, 1993). Horses will naturally select from free-choice minerals as long as they are not too sick to sense their needs through instinct and odor recognition. Conventional nutrition research reports that no species can accurately select free-choice minerals. However, upon observation it becomes apparent that seasonal variations in mineral and vitamin consumption are significant.

Free-choice minerals need to be fed with salt provided separately. If both are fed together with salt in a mineralized salt block, the salt will limit the mineral intake due to the high salt content (about 95%). When horses are given plain free-choice minerals the quantity they eat is often astounding. Most horses will eat two to three times the normal intake for a few months or until they have balanced their minerals, then will taper off to a maintenance level. Artificial flavorings, salt and molasses should not be used in combination with free-choice minerals as they may affect the natural selection of the nutrient.

In the author's opinion, the best way to approach mineral nutrition is through a free-choice system, with the salt and mineral separated. Very few companies provide a plain mineral supplement; usually salt will be in the top half of the ingredient list. Avoid unbalanced single minerals or combinations of just a few minerals unless they are given free-choice (and are palatable for that purpose). Many products are formulated based on human requirements, which may not be appropriate for the nutritional needs of the horse. Racehorses are constantly given iron tonics to "build their blood," but most horses this author has tested had normal levels of iron.

Soil and plant health

Horses are often not considered as having a role in sustainable agriculture. However, the ownership of horses is vitally important to maintaining open land in rapidly developing areas. In fact, horses are a primary source of agribusiness in many states.

Since feedstuffs are grown in soil it is important to understand soil health as much as it is to understand animal nutrition. Knowledge of soil health is almost nonexistent in the equine world, as horse owners and veterinarians do not consider themselves farmers or caretakers of the land. Very little organic grain is used in the equine world, even by people who are heavily into natural healing. This is due in part to the lack of availability.

Achieving soil health parallels achieving intestinal health in many ways. Soil minerals become available to the plants through bacterial action. Soil organic matter provides the substrate for healthy bacterial growth just as soluble fiber does in the intestinal tract (Ridzone and Walters, 1994). A lack of a healthy bacterial balance in the soil can lead to poor mineral absorption, soil compaction, and poor plant health (Walters and Fenzau, 1996). Poor plant mineral content can lead to poor animal nutrition, even though the grain or hay produced may look big, green, and healthy after adding nitrogen.

The soil in which most of our grains are grown is heavily fertilized with conventional fertilizers, replacing only three of the nutrients needed to make the plants look healthy. Many horse owners religiously fertilize their soils with high levels of nitrogen, leading to grass that is too rich for the digestive system of the horse. Some use herbicides to improve the aesthetic appearance of the pasture, which they equate with their lawn. Many do not realize that the weeds (herbs) have a place in the ecosystem of the pasture, nor do they understand the toxic load placed on their horses' liver and kidneys by the use of herbicides.

Most herbicides contain estrogenic compounds. The estrogenic nature of these chemicals can alter the balance of hormones in the body (Krimsky, 2000). In the world, mares are supposed to go into a winter anestrus (no heat cycles); however, in recent years most of the mares in this author's practice cycle through the winter routinely. This indicates an imbalance in the hormonal system.

Genetically modified grains are used in increasing amounts. Most bags containing corn have at least some genetically modified grain present. The implications of genetic alterations of food are unknown at this time.

Once the feed is harvested, it is heavily processed in most cases. Horse feed is frequently ground, cooked at high temperatures, and extruded or pelleted in a process similar to dog food manufacturing. It is impossible to determine the exact quality of ingredients going into the processed feed. Preservatives are being used increasingly, which can add to the liver's toxic load. The ideal way to provide better nutrition is to select precleaned (dust-free) plain whole grains as a base, and then add specific ingredients for the individual horses or herds as needed.

Pasture management

Horse owners willing to make changes to pasture management need to research the organic grass farming publications (*Stockman Grass Farmer*) and local grass-based farmers (found at www.eatwild.com). Each part of the country has different soil types and needs. Also, as good organic farmers know, each field on an individual farm can have different needs. Grass-fed farms successfully raising livestock (cattle, sheep, and pigs) are increasing rapidly in many states. Much of what they are doing applies to pasture for horses, with a few exceptions. Managing grass for optimum health of the horse involves the rotation of pastures, improvements in soil health, and increased biodiversity in the plants.

One of the most important aspects of pasture management is rotation of pastures on a regular basis. Grass grows best when it is quickly grazed short, and then allowed to regrow. Animals eat grass best that is 2–9 inches tall; for grass height higher than that it becomes too tough. If grass is overgrazed and kept too short for too long, regrowth will be poor and weeds that indicate poor soil health will appear.

Horses that tend to be too fat can and should be kept in overgrazed paddocks. The weeds that do grow should be mowed. Be aware that the grass they are eating in overgrazed paddocks will be lower in quality. Horses do not graze as evenly as cattle and sheep, so mowing will have to be done on the grassy areas the horses refuse to eat, or graze other livestock (cattle, sheep, goats) with the horses.

Grass farmers looking for optimal performance of their livestock (growth, milk production, reproduction) want to keep the animals with the highest demand for energy on the richest and freshest pastures. These farmers will move the stock daily in many cases. Mature horses in light to moderate work generally do not need as rich a pasture as livestock to meet their energy requirements; however, they need healthy soil and diverse plant population. Rotation frequency will depend on the acreage, number of animals grazing, rainfall, and types of grasses. Small properties in areas with good rainfall can support several horses per acre during the grass growing season if pastures are small, rotated, and mowed regularly.

Electric fencing can be used to divide pasture spaces. Horses do well with electric fence as long as they can see it, so wide tapes work better than small wires. When space is limited, it may be best to use one small area in the winter, with the knowledge that the soil will become compacted and the grass left in poor condition.

Treatment of disease

Once the basic nutrition has been corrected, the alternative practitioner can then use herbs and homeopathy to treat specific diseases, as well as targeted nutrition to correct or support the tissue involved. Herbal medicine refers to the use of raw or processed herbs in their whole form. Homeopathy refers to the science of using very dilute substances to treat diseases that are similar to those that can be created in a healthy individual if that individual takes the substance in a concentrated form.

A detailed history and thorough physical exam are the most important parts of the diagnostic decision making in a holistic practice. All of the traditional veterinary diagnostics, such as blood tests and radiographs, are utilized but are often given a lower priority. Alternative medicine requires more detailed information than conventional medicine in order to tailor the treatment to the individual rather than the disease.

Homeopathy

Homeopathy is one of the most versatile modalities used in natural healing. The remedies are made according to international standards and their manufacture is regulated by the FDA. Education of the practitioner is vitally important to the success of the prescription.

The remedies can be used to treat many different conditions. Infections are readily treated with skillful use of the remedies, depending on the experience of the practitioner. These can range from a simple cut or cold to a sinus infection or osteomyelitis (bone infection). Many types of eye problems such as corneal ulcers and "moon blindness" and internal imbalances such as liver, kidney, and reproductive diseases respond well to homeopathic remedies. Colic and stomach ulcers can also be treated, though it must be remembered that a complete diagnosis is required to be sure there are no life threatening problems being overlooked. Respiratory diseases including allergic conditions can be treated. Musculoskeletal conditions such as laminitis, tendonitis, navicular, and bone spavin are frequently alleviated homeopathically.

Basic first-aid homeopathy is fairly straightforward. Required information includes appearance, amount of pain, colors of discharges, odors, and modalities (what conditions influence animal or affected body part for better or worse—cold, hot, pressure, touch, motion, weather) (Day, 1984). A quick response to treatment can be expected. Common traumatic injuries such as open wounds and bruises respond very well.

Treating chronic disease with homeopathy, often called constitutional treatment, requires a complete history. With a complex case this may take up to an hour, though often a limited history is all that is available. All body systems must be covered completely. The condition present needs to be described in as much detail as possible, especially how the condition responds to heat, cold, touch, motion, and weather. The response to the remedy will be much slower than when treating an acute condition. Results may not be seen for up to 2 weeks, so the horse owner must be patient.

Herbal medicine

Herbs have been used by all cultures for centuries; each area of the world uses herbs local to that area. Western herbs tend to work slowly to restore health and balance to the body, while Chinese herbology contains some fast acting herbs (antibacterials and antivirals). Chinese formulas can be much deeper acting and can cure problems faster; however, in general the practitioner needs to have knowledge of Chinese medicine to prescribe accurately. Chinese herbology has been used in animals for centuries. There are many animal studies published on Chinese herbs; however, the translations are not complete at this time. Clinical experience with Chinese herbal formulas used in the United States is growing.

Herbs are generally used together in a formula, so the effectiveness of a formula depends on the skill of the person putting it together. The efficacy and potency of a formula is affected by the quality of the raw ingredients. The best manufacturers test each batch for purity and strength but many companies cut corners by using inferior quality raw materials.

Herbal medicine can be used to treat arthritic conditions, immune system problems, diarrhea, colic, and other digestive upsets. Internal medical problems including liver, heart, stomach, lung, and kidney imbalances can be cured with many herbal formulas. Behavior can be altered with herbs by relaxing the muscles or toning down the nerves. Premade formulas for animals (Western and Chinese) are becoming more commonly available and are an excellent way to use herbs in practice.

Nutrition for the intestine

Since the intestinal tract is so frequently bombarded with antibiotics and nonsteroidal anti-inflammatories, many horses will need therapy directed at repairing the intestine. High quality probiotics should be used to help replace the intestinal flora. *Lactobacillus sporogenes* is one probiotic (healthy bacteria) that does not need refrigeration, and so is well adapted to use in the barn. Fermented probiotics with enzymes can help repair the gut wall, while the amino acid L-glutamine provides energy for the cells lining the intestinal tract. Certain herbs such as Slippery Elm can sooth the digestive tract and promote healing. The acidity of the stomach needs to be maintained for protein and mineral digestion, so the use of alkalinizing agents such as bicarbonates and antacid drugs should be discouraged. Homeopathic remedies can also be used to help heal the intestine provided they are carefully selected to fit the profile of the patient.

Conclusion

The role of the horse in agriculture is important. Equine health from a holistic perspective relates closely to soil and plant health. When treating horses using alternative medicine it is important to consider all aspects of health form, identifying subtle signs of ill health to treating the soil where the food is grown.

References

Clarke, L.L. 1990. Feeding and digestive problems in horses. *Vet. Clin. North Am. Equine Prac.* 6(2):433–450.

Day, C. 1984. *Homeopathic Treatment of Small Animals.* C.W. Daniel Co., Ltd. Saffron Walden, England.

DeMaar, T.W. 1993. Zoopharmacognosy: a science emerges from Navajo legends. *Ceres* 25(5):5–9.

Dodds, W.J. 1993. Vaccine safety and efficacy revisited: autoimmune and allergic diseases on the rise. *Vet. Forum* May:68–71.

Folino, M, A. McIntyre, and G.P. Young. 1995. Dietary fibers differ in their effects on large bowel epithelial proliferation and fecal fermentation-dependent events in rats. *J. Nutr.* 125(6):1521–1529.

Kimbrough, D.R., N. Martinez, and S. Stolfus. 1995. A laboratory experiment illustrating the properties and bioavailability of iron. *J. Chem. Educ.* 72(6):558–560.

Krimsky, S. 2000. *Hormonal Chaos.* Johns Hopkins University Press, Baltimore, MD.

Lipske, M. 1993. Animal, heal thyself. *Natl. Wildl.* 32(1):46–50.

McCaman, J.L. 1994. *Weeds and why They Grow.* Sand Lake, MI.

Ridzone, L. and C. Walters. 1994. *The Carbon Cycle.* Acres USA, Kansas City, KS.

Schmidt, M.A, L.H. Smith, and K.W Sehnert. 1993. *Beyond Antibiotics.* North Atlantic Books, Berkley, CA.

Walters, C. and C.J. Fenzau. 1996. *Eco-Farm.* Acres USA, Kansas City, KS.

White, N.A., M.K. Tinker, and P. Lessard. 1993. Equine colic risk assessment on horse farms: a prospective study. *Proc. Am. Assoc. Equine Pract.* 39:97.

Xie, H. 1994. *Traditional Chinese Veterinary Medicine.* Beijing Agricultural University Press, Beijing.

Section III
Concerns about Conventional Therapies

Chapter 11

The Ecology of Antimicrobial Resistance and Use of Alternatives to Antimicrobials in Food Animal Production in the United States

Stephen J. DeVincent

Introduction

The tale of Alexander Fleming's serendipitous discovery of penicillin in 1928 is legendary, in part because it appeals to our sense of possibility. Less widely known, however, is the fact that the growth-promoting effect of antibiotics was also discovered by accident. Scientists at Lederle Laboratories, where chlortetracycline was discovered in 1947, were searching for bacterial sources of the (Dewey et al., 1999) nutrient (later discovered to be vitamin B12) to add to chicken feed. One day they stumbled upon a vat of *Streptomyces* bacteria that had been used in the production of tetracycline. Administration of the bacteria in the feed produced dramatic results in growth that were eventually attributed to trace amounts of the drug (Levy, 2002). Since that time, it has been demonstrated that low levels of antimicrobials administered to food animals increase daily rates of weight gain and improve feed efficiency in livestock in addition to their ability to treat, prevent, and control disease. However, evidence also suggests that there are correlations between drug resistant bacteria and administration of levels of antimicrobials below therapeutic levels (Cohen and Tauxe, 1986).

Many antimicrobials used in food animal production are the same as, or closely related to, drugs used in human medicine. Tetracyclines, penicillins, and other antibiotics important in human and veterinary medicine now have been used to promote growth and enhance feed efficiency in food animal production for over 50 years. However, the exact mechanisms by which they confer growth promotion and enhance feed efficiency have not yet been determined. The increasing instances of multiple-drug-resistant infections in humans have led to greater attention to the use of antimicrobials in agriculture, and most intense in regard of antimicrobial growth promoters. However, it has been recognized by most medical experts that the greatest risk of antimicrobial resistance emanates from the inappropriate use of antimicrobials in human medicine (McNamara and Miller, 2002).

Calls for complete bans in the United States on the use of antimicrobials in animal feed have escalated, in part due to enacting of such policies in Europe. The majority of criticism emanates from public health officials, elected representatives, government agencies, and consumer and environmental groups. Other key stakeholders in the controversy are livestock producers, physicians, veterinarians, farm groups, ecologists, economists, scientists, and government agencies.

Arguments for a ban on the use of antimicrobials in animal feed generally include the following elements: 1) the long duration and low dosage use patterns typical of administration for growth promotion may exert a stronger selective pressure for resistance; 2) resistant bacteria within the gut flora of food animals may pose a particular threat to humans via resistant foodborne infections; and 3) the economic benefits of nontherapeutic use may not outweigh the costs it imposes on society. In response to these concerns, stakeholders such as agricultural producers, farm groups, the animal health pharmaceutical industry, and some scientists counter that the microbiological and epidemiological evidence is not conclusive to establish food animals as a source of infections caused by resistant pathogens from exposure of animals to antimicrobials.

However, there is increasing evidence that demonstrates use of antimicrobials in agriculture is resulting in increases in antimicrobial resistance in food animal bacteria, with the resultant transfer of resistant bacteria and genetic elements to humans, and infection of humans by these pathogens (National Research Council, 1999). There are studies in which scientists trace animal sources of antimicrobial-resistant pathogens in human infections (Luster et al., 1988; Holmberg et al., 1984; McDonald et al., 2001; Clark and Gyles, 1993). Overlap of resistant bacteria and opportunities for transfer are represented in Figure 11.1.

The debate on the use of antimicrobials in food animals has at its core a conflict between human health and economic concerns. Human health concerns include the impacts on public health as well as the economic costs of treating antimicrobial resistant infections. Economic concerns, however, are not limited to the health care sector. The safety of the food supply and public health is dependent on the production methods and costs that farmers invest in raising their herds and flocks. In the United States, the intensive stocking of food animals that has arisen to meet the increasing consumer

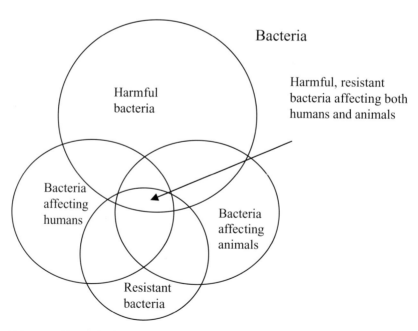

Fig. 11.1 Universe of bacteria (courtesy of Economic Research Service of the United States Department of Agriculture).

demand for inexpensive meat necessitates the nontherapeutic administration of antimicrobials. This is especially true for all phases of swine production. While stakeholders debate the issues of levels of transfer and percentage of resistance from animals to humans, and quantity of use in animals versus humans, there is overwhelming consensus for further development and implementation of alternatives to the use of antimicrobials in agriculture to decrease antimicrobials use in agriculture and the incidences of antimicrobial resistance. Examples of alternatives include competitive exclusion products, probiotics, novel therapeutics, vaccines, new rapid diagnostic methodologies, and targeted interventions to prevent the emergence and spread of resistant pathogens.

Ecology of antimicrobial resistance

The Report of the Joint Committee on the use of antibiotics in animal husbandry and veterinary medicine, issued in 1969, and referred to as the Swann report, is most often cited as the earliest report that theorized the potential that drug-resistant bacteria may be transferable to humans through the food chain (Swann, 1969). Since that time, commensurate with evidence of the rise in antimicrobial resistance in humans from foodborne pathogens, numerous other scientific analyses, reports and studies that focus on the debate concerning the risks of antimicrobial use in food animals on human health have been released (Institute of Medicine, 1980, 1989; CAST, 1981; Lederberg, 1992; ASM, 1995; World Health Organization, 1998a).

In 1999, the Alliance for the Prudent Use of Antibiotics (APUA) initiated a 2-year project entitled "Facts about Antimicrobials in Animals and the Impact on Resistance" (FAAIR). The purpose of FAAIR was to review and analyze scientific data on the subject of antimicrobial use in agriculture with an ecological perspective in order to better inform about public health policy. Figure 11.2 illustrates the multiple potential pathways by which antimicrobial use in food animal production could directly or indirectly affect the quality of the food supply.

As part of FAAIR, APUA convened a Scientific Advisory Panel of nationally recognized micro-biologists, physicians, statisticians, and veterinarians that developed the report, *The Need to Reduce Antimicrobial Use in Agriculture: Ecological and Human Health Consequences.* The APUA "FAAIR Report" considers the food animals and farms as part of a complex dynamic of selective pressures within the ecosystem that contribute to the development of resistant pathogens. However, factoring in the food animal and farm environment as potential methods of transfer also demonstrates that these farm reservoirs comprise a small portion of the total microbial ecosystem.

O'Brien (2002) explains that genes for resistance may be passed between bacterial communities. Therefore, levels of antimicrobial resistance in a given bacterial population in part reflect the total number of bacteria ever exposed to antimicrobials. Summers (2002) also recognizes that certain ecological dimensions of the resistance problem, such as the importance of commensal (non-disease-causing) bacteria and the linkage of resistance traits, have often been overlooked or underestimated by microbiologists.

Commensurate with most discussions regarding the relative percentages of contribution to resistance from antimicrobial use in humans and animals is the controversy over the total quantity and proportion of use in the two populations. Although few reliable data describing the extent and quantity of antimicrobial use in animals are publicly available in the United States, most food animals in the United States are exposed to antimicrobials in feed, water, or by injection at some point during their lives (McEwen and Fedorka-Cray, 2002). Estimates of U.S. populations of food animals are greater than 8 billion poultry, 100 million beef cattle, 160 million swine, 1 million dairy cattle,

ECOLOGICAL IMPACT OF THE USE OF ANTIBIOTICS IN
FOOD ANIMALS:
The Flow of Antibiotic-Resistant Bacteria
Antibiotic Use for Therapy, Prophylaxis or Growth Promotion
(selects for emergence of resistant bacteria)

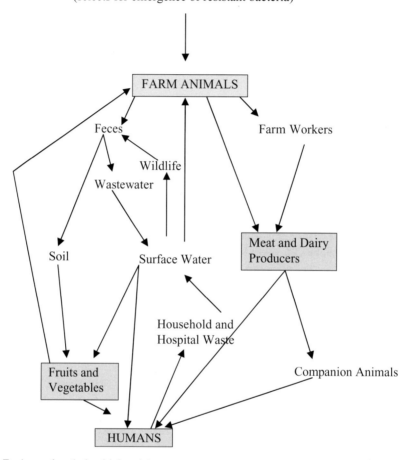

Fig. 11.2 Ecology of antimicrobial resistance.

and 10 million sheep (National Research Council, 1999). A report by Dewey et al. (1999) showed that in 1990, 88% of swine producers used antimicrobials in feed; they also reported that the most commonly used antimicrobials were tetracyclines, carbadox, and bacitracin and they were fed on a continual basis.

It is simultaneously argued that antibiotic use in livestock comprises the largest proportion of total antimicrobial use for both humans and animals, while others contend that use of antimicrobials in food animals, whether for therapy, prophylaxis, or growth promotion, is only a minor percentage in comparison to human use. Contributing to confusion in these discussions is the use of terms to describe the indications for use of antibiotics. In this document, as in the FAAIR Report, the term "therapeutic" refers to use of antimicrobials for the treatment of a symptom of disease. "Nontherapeutic" use includes use of antimicrobials for prophylaxis, growth promotion, and enhanced feed efficiency.

It is necessary in the determination of the effects of the use of antimicrobials in food animal production to include data on the extent of their use. However, the quantity of use in the United States remains unknown, and estimates must be used in risk assessment and public policy. Estimates from three studies on human and animal uses of antibiotics in the United States are most often cited to highlight the use of antimicrobials for growth promotion (Institute of Medicine, 1989). The most recent figures are from the Union of Concerned Scientists, a consumer advocacy group, which determined that 70% of antibiotic use in the United States is for nontherapeutic purposes (Mellon and Fondriest, 2001). In great contrast are the figures of a year earlier from the Animal Health Institute (AHI). Representing the animal health pharmaceutical industry, AHI released an estimate of 13% for nontherapeutic use (Animal Health Institute, 2000). The earliest and only objective estimate of the three is from the Institute of Medicine, in which a figure of 50% for nontherapeutic uses in animals of all use of antibiotics in humans and animals (Institute of Medicine, 1989) has been known.

There is epidemiological evidence for a linkage between the use of antibiotics in food animals and infections due to resistant strains of foodborne pathogens in humans. Several lines of direct and indirect evidence link antimicrobial use in food animal production to resistant foodborne infections in humans. Examples of direct evidence include a study that shows a clear chain of evidence between the illicit uses of chloramphenicol in farm animals and chloramphenicol-resistant *Salmonella* newport infection in humans (Centers for Disease Control and Prevention, 1999). Examples of indirect evidence include studies of fluoroquinolone resistance in *Campylobacter* in poultry and humans after the addition of fluoroquinolones to animal feed (World Health Organization, 1998b), vancomycin-resistant *enterococci* after the use of avoparcin in poultry (Institute of Medicine, 1989; National Research Council, 1999), and the emergence of resistance in vancomycin-resistant *enterococci* to streptogramin antibiotics used in poultry (Levy et al., 1976).

Utilization of risk assessment contributes to the evidence that the agricultural use of antibiotics imposes a burden on human health. Barza and Gorbach (2002) suggest that antimicrobial resistance may increase disease and adversely affect human health in a variety of ways. These include the following:

1. When antimicrobials are taken for any reason, they indiscriminately kill susceptible bacteria—bacteria that do not ordinarily cause disease (commensals) as well as pathogens. In this environment of reduced competition, any bacteria (even ordinarily harmless ones) that can withstand the effects of the antimicrobials may flourish, leading to additional (and resistant) infections.
2. In many organisms, including bacteria, certain gene combinations are commonly linked. Evidence suggests that, in bacteria, genes for resistance may be associated with genes for virulence, or the capacity of a pathogen to cause infection. Accordingly, resistance in pathogenic bacteria increases the number, severity, and duration of infections.
3. Infections caused by resistant pathogens may be more difficult to treat because several different drugs may have to be used before a drug (or combination of drugs) is found that is effective.
4. Antimicrobial resistance may increase the disease burden in food animals that may ultimately increase the number of infections passed to humans through the food supply.
5. Antimicrobial resistance may affect human health even when it develops in commensals, because these populations may serve as reservoirs of resistance genes that can be transferred to pathogens.

Barza and Travers (2002) examine the first mechanism above in detail, attempting to calculate the excess number of *Salmonella* and *Campylobacter* infections in patients taking antimicrobials for other reasons. This increase in human disease due to resistance is thought to occur because antimicrobials facilitate colonization by eliminating susceptible commensal bacteria. They determined that resistance accounts for 29,379 additional *Salmonella* infections per year in the United States, leading to 342 hospitalizations and 12 deaths. Similarly, resistance accounts for an additional 17,668 *Campylobacter jejuni* infections, resulting in 95 hospitalizations.

Travers and Barza (2002) also examined medical records of hospital patients with *Salmonella* and *Campylobacter* infections to test whether antimicrobial resistance led to longer and more severe infections. They estimated that resistance to fluoroquinolones, the drug of choice for severe food poisoning in humans, results in an estimated 400,000 more days of diarrhea per year in the United States.

Bailar and Travers (2002) reviewed evidence on increased virulence and delays in recovery due to initial choice of an antibiotic to which the pathogen is resistant. In a number of previously published studies, researchers have attempted to quantify the collective risk to human health from antimicrobial use in agriculture, but all have likely underestimated that risk. The most serious limitations in those studies include failure to adequately consider ecological aspects of the resistance problem, such as the cumulative nature of resistance and the transfer of resistance from environmental bacteria to pathogens.

Swedish and Danish models

In comparison to the United States, all antimicrobials used in human medicine have been banned from use in food animal feed by the European Union (EU). At present, in the EU, the four antimicrobials that remain approved for use in animal feed are flavophospholipol, salinomycin sodium, avilamycin, and monensin sodium (AFIA, 2002). However, effective in 2006, these four remaining antimicrobials will be also banned from use in animal feed. The 4-year time period allows for further development and implementation of alternatives to use of antimicrobials. The European Union invoked the precautionary principle in its ban of the use of antimicrobial growth promoters in animal feeds despite the lack of direct evidence linking such use to human infections.

Sweden banned antimicrobials for the purpose of growth promotion in 1996. In Denmark, after four classes of drugs were banned from use for growth promotion, it was concluded that it was possible to decrease the occurrence of antimicrobial resistance in a national population of food animals when use of the drugs was discontinued (Aarestrup et al., 2001). In Denmark, there were also initial increases in morbidity and mortality of flocks and herds associated with the ban, as well as increased therapeutic use of antimicrobials. These results were similar to those from Sweden, in which initially there was a 2-day increase to 30 kg body weight for pigs, and increases in incidences of necrotic enteritis (Wierup, 2001).

Increases in incidences of disease and rise of fecal shedding of pathogens, and production costs were also consequences of the ban. However, it was also concluded that the reductions in use were followed by reductions in antimicrobial resistance in food animal bacteria and a reduction of resistance in the food supply (Aarestrup et al., 2001).

In a very recent retrospective analysis of the discontinued use of antimicrobial growth promoters in Denmark, contrary to concerns that pathogen load would increase, investigators found a significant decrease in *Salmonella* in broilers and swine, and in pork and chicken meat, and no change in the prevalence of *Campylobacter* in broilers (Evans and Wegener, 2003). A complementary study exhibited results that the withdrawal of the growth promoters has taken place without significant effects on the productivity in broilers and swine (Shryock, 2000). While the conclusions reached by the respective study authors signify advances in strategies to limit the transfer of foodborne pathogens by banning the use of antimicrobials in animal feed, the magnitude of animal populations, and relative number and size of food animal production operations in the United States should not allow for analogous comparisons of the Scandinavian results with expectations of similar results. The disparity in food animal populations and the production management systems cannot be underestimated in any decisions on limiting the use of antimicrobials in food animals and economic losses that would result for American farmers.

It is also highly unlikely that a complete ban on the use of antimicrobials in animal feed, as in Europe, could be enacted in the United States. However, there are no recent estimates of the effects of banning only some antimicrobials for nontherapeutic use (Secchi and Babcock, 2002). The economic costs on the food animal industry in case of a partial (or complete) ban in the United States would have to be weighed against the benefits of reductions in antimicrobial resistance resulting from foodborne illnesses (Secchi and Babcock, 2002).

A case for alternatives

Significance of the results from both the Danish and Swedish bans on antimicrobials in animal feed is that the authors of the respective analyses concluded that the elimination of antimicrobial growth promoters could take place without significant adverse effects on food production provided that sufficient attention was given to the implementation of alternative intervention strategies to antimicrobials in food animal production. The Swedish Animal Health Service concluded that poultry, calves, and pigs could be raised without ongoing use of nontherapeutic doses of antimicrobial growth promoters with the implementation of superior hygiene practices (Wierup, 2001).

The authors of the Danish study concluded that the elimination of the growth promoters could be applied in both industrialized and developing countries without overwhelming economic losses with the adequate integration of the use of alternatives in livestock production (Statens Serum Institut, 2001). Similarly, in the multisite study in the United States mentioned above, the study authors concluded that the basis of success of the trials was the significant advantage of the utilization of strict hygiene practices that limited the spread of infectious agents and reduced the need for antimicrobials (Dritz et al., 2002).

In addition to strict controls on hygiene, other strategies to reduce the incidence of disease and reduce use of antimicrobials in food animals include disease eradication, population dynamics, feed quality, and environmental conditions to reduce stress, nutrition optimization and feeding regimens to boost natural immunity, breeding for genetically disease-resistant food animals, and substitutes for growth promotants.

As a result of the scrutiny focused on the use of antimicrobials in agriculture, there is an increasing number of articles, reports, and studies from high-profile institutions and organizations that include recommendations for research, and increased funding for the study of alternatives to the propalaytic use of antibiotics to fill current and projected gaps in methods to decrease antimicrobial use in agriculture and limit the foodborne transmission of resistant pathogens to humans (Barza and Gorbach, 2002; National Research Council, 1999; Torrence, 2001).

In the research on alternatives, goals must be attained that would have incorporated the development and implementation of appropriate and extensive risk management procedures to compensate for the loss of bacteriostatic and bacteriocidal aspects of antimicrobials. The alternatives must also be analyzed for their human and animal safety risk assessments before they are commercially used.

Their varied mechanisms of action and other potential beneficial or detrimental effects of their use, alone or in combination with other alternatives, must also be considered.

Research on the use of alternative strategies at multiple critical control points may potentially compensate for the prevention and control of disease and growth-promoting effects of antimicrobials. The potential benefits of intervention strategies involving multiple management and product alternatives that reduce the incidence of foodborne illness due to human food pathogens are both promising. However, such combinations of alternatives also increase the need for consideration of the ecology of antimicrobial resistance and measures that must be integrated into research and risk assessment.

Current examples of comprehensive and informative reviews of alternative methods to antimicrobials in livestock production include a report from Health Canada, (Advisory Committee on Animal Uses of Antimicrobials and Impact of Resistance and Human Health, 2002); a report from the United Nations FAO (Hughes and Heritage, 2002); a report by the Commonwealth Department of Agriculture, Fisheries and Forestry in Australia (Joint Expert Technical Advisory Committee on Antibiotic Resistance (JETACAR), 1999); National Research Council reports (NRC, 1980, 1999); and a report from Sweden (Wierup, 2001). Reviews specific to the swine industry include Doyle (2001); Goransson (1997); and Turner et al. (2001); and for poultry include Hooge (1999).

In this review, discussion is limited to major species of food animals for which increased performance and enhancement of feed efficiency are part of livestock production, which include beef, dairy cows, poultry (broilers), and swine. Alternatives to antimicrobials will be defined as products or practices that seek to replace antimicrobial use by treating, preventing, or controlling infectious disease or promoting animal growth. With a focus on antimicrobial-resistant pathogens, interest in growth promoters will be limited to products and practices likely to impact microbial ecology. While there is some overlap of these functions, nonantimicrobial growth promoters typically consist of feed supplements, while treatment, control, and prevention measures may involve feed additives, medications, or alterations in management practices. Table 11.1 summarizes key alternative interventions. More detailed examples of alternative interventions are shown after Table 11.1, and the interventions are categorized in these areas: breeding and genetics, environment and behavior, biosecurity, competitive exclusion, immune modulation, nutrition, probiotics, and target-specific antibacterials.

These examples of alternative interventions in farm management, technology, and products are not inclusive of all opportunities available or in research as strategies to decrease the use of antimicrobials and the incidence of disease. They the reflect author's review of current scientific literature on alternatives to the use of antimicrobials. Particularly lacking is more information on biotechnology, and more so the production of animals through biotechnology for research and commercial purposes. The research being conducted on new methods of selecting animals possessing desirable traits through the utilization of genetics and genomics and its ramifications is beyond the scope of this review.

Breeding and genetics

Control of response to infectious disease is influenced by genetics. The use of molecular biology enables the development of biological products to enhance the immunity of the individual and its offspring. Genetic selection can be applied to enhance selection for advantageous traits, including resistance to disease in livestock. However, breeding for resistance traits is difficult because resistance

Table 11.1   A summary of select examples of alternatives

Alternative interventions	Possible mechanism of action	Purpose
Probiotics and competitive exclusion products	Modify gut flora	Disease prevention and control
Organic acids	Help assimilation of nutrients by acidifying the gut environment	Growth promotion
Antibodies, cytokines, and spray-dried plasma	Enhance immune response	Disease prevention and control
Oligosaccharides (e.g. FOS and MOS)	Enhance nutrient absorption	Growth promotion
Trace elements in feed (e.g. vitamins, CLA, minerals, phospholipids, amino acids, carnitine, carbohydrates, spices, herbs, and homeopathics)	Various	Disease prevention and control growth promotion
Changes in the physical environment such as housing, hygiene, watering, and feeding	Help to reduce stress levels	Disease prevention and control growth promotion
Biotechnology innovations such as pathogen-free breeds	Increase resistance to pathogens	Disease prevention and control
Target-specific antibacterials such as bacteriocins, bacteriophages, antimicrobial peptides, and recombinant proteins	Eliminate targeted pathogens while minimizing cross-resistance	Therapy
Vaccines and autogenous biologics	Enhance immune response in individual animals	Disease prevention and control
Biosecurity measures	Prevent transmission of disease by farm workers	Disease prevention and control
All-in-all-out management	Prevent transmission of pathogens between populations	Disease prevention and control
Vaccines and autogenous biologics	Enhance immune response in individual animals	Disease prevention and control
Biosecurity measures	Prevent transmission of disease by farm workers	Disease prevention and control

is regulated by genes at numerous loci and is greatly influenced by environmental factors. For example, breeding programs for dairy cows have resulted in genetic increases in milk yield, but have led to higher incidences in mastitis (National Research Council, 1999).

Expected progeny differences

Scientists are currently developing expected progeny differences (EPD) as a breeding tool to select for efficient feed utilization. EPD are ratings for economically important traits in beef production that represent the estimated genetic potential of an animal as a parent. EPD is a broadly accepted tool in the beef industry and considered as the standard for genetic improvement. EPD ratings include birth weight, weaning weight, yearling weight, and milk production. Researchers offer the new EPD ratings as an alternative to improve efficiency of feed utilization without any major indirect effect on maturity size or maintenance requirements (Crews, 2003).

BISHOP BURTON COLLEGE
LIBRARY

Environment and behavior

Animals are more susceptible to disease during the period of environmental stress (Smith and Hogan, 1993). Therefore, introducing alternatives in management that limit environmental factors can lead to improved immunity and ability to withstand infectious disease in the animal. As a result, the need for use of antimicrobials is lessened.

Feed

Feed changes or feeding practices can disturb the normal flora of the intestine and promote transient colonization resulting in increased shedding of pathogens. Changes in feed have been associated with increased shedding of pathogens during lactation and weaning, as well as for cattle recently placed on feedlots (Sanchez et al., 2002).

Diets formulated for appropriate stages of growth and production may promote disease resistance; in a recent study it was demonstrated that beef steers grazed on dormant native tall grass prairie had a greater rate of gain when grain supplements were balanced for total degradable intake protein (Bodine and Purvis II, 2003).

Another recent study evaluated factors related to determining optimal feeding and management programs for increasing net returns from marketing cull sows. The results suggested that mating sows as they return to estrus post weaning and providing ad libitum access to a corn-soybean meal diet improved growth performance and feed efficiency (Shurson et al., 2003).

In addition, recent evidence from Europe demonstrates organic and free-range, and similar methods of food animal production, were found to increase the risk of infections in herds with microbial pathogens. Pigs with access to outdoor facilities had higher incidence of *Salmonella*, *Toxoplasma*, and helminths than indoor-bred pigs. Poultry from free-ranging operations had similar occurrences with *Campylobacter*.

Scientists at the USDA Agricultural Research Service (ARS) have discovered new formulas to determine the amount of energy required to maintain basal metabolism in farm animals. The researchers present data about factors other than weight, such as age, breeding, and nutritional history, that need to be considered when predicting basal metabolism. Their findings should lead to more efficient use of feed through the development of low-cost feeding strategies that should provide economic advantages to producers (Elstein, 2002).

Production systems and traditional and organic feed were compared for the occurrence of *Campylobacter* and *Salmonella* in broiler chickens. In the four treatment groups there were no instances of *Campylobacter* contamination and no significant effect of feed type on the occurrence of *Salmonella*. However, there was a pronounced farm effect; samples in which *Salmonella* was detected were limited to two of nine farms (Lund et al., 2003).

Fly control

The presence of flies and other ectoparasites can cause sufficient stress to adversely affect growth or milk production, and create greater likelihood of disease emergence (National Research Council, 1999). Therefore greater attention to fly control is a practical and effective management strategy that can be easily implemented or improved.

Housing

Researchers have found that small changes in the practice of housing sows in crates, such as allowing groups of sows more movement and social contact than in gestation stalls for long periods during pregnancies, result in greater weight gain for piglets born to group-housed sows (Freetly, 2003).

The results of a recent study supported the hypothesis that fence line contact between dams and calves at weaning results in decreased indices of stress compared with an abrupt separation of the cow and calf. The increased contact between dams and calves minimized losses in weight gain. This modification in management benefited the producer economically as well as improved the welfare of the animals (Shurson et al., 2003).

Manure and moisture

Moisture provides an immediate source for microbial proliferation and is the predominant environmental factor that predisposes animals to infection and re-infection (National Research Council, 1999). Disease-causing environmental pathogens in bedding and feces must be separated from the target animal by methods which include cleaning, use of a drainable or slatted floor, and dry and clean bedding materials. Inorganic materials such as crushed limestone or sand are preferable to finely chopped organic materials (such as sawdust and shavings) to reduce the bacterial load (Hogan et al., 1989; National Research Council, 1999). Proper bedding has demonstrated improved health in both piglets and poultry (Holmgren, 1994) and the addition of lime to sawdust bedding decreases bacterial populations and prevents udder infection in dairy cows (Hogan et al., 1989).

Transportation

Transport can trigger a subclinical infection or colonization of pathogens in healthy animals (Isaacson, 1997) as well as a negative impact on growth rates (Ekkel et al., 1995). Co-mingling of weaned pigs without regard to farm of origin when transported to grower facilities causes social stress that increases susceptibility to *Salmonella typhimurium* (Callaway et al., 2003a).

In pigs, farrow to finish (FTS) production provides an alternative to transportation of pigs required in multisite production. In the FTS system, the pigs are placed in the same pen from birth to the time they are slaughtered.

Research is continuing to determine if the products from yeast cell walls in conjunction with ascorbic acid might help alleviate physiological stress in dairy calves resulting from transportation (Freetly, 2003).

Ventilation and ambient temperature

Air quality and temperature control are very important for the animals to maintain their immune system and resistance to disease. Poor ventilation in broiler houses has resulted in necrotizing enteritis during episodes of high temperatures (Wierup, 1999). However, warmth prevents diarrhea in newborn piglets and is necessary for newly hatched chicks (Madelin and Wathes, 1989). Researchers at the USDA Agricultural Research Service (ARS) are developing objective means by which to measure stress in farm animals to improve existing, and invent new, practices that increase the efficiency of dairy, swine, and poultry production (Comis, 2001).

Biosecurity

General practices enlisted in biosecurity of herds include restricting access by nonfarm personnel, internal replacements of livestock, and animal quarantine, and/or isolation. Utilization of such measures prevents the introduction of infectious disease to farms and vertical transmission of diseases amongst the animals. Food animals that are segregated from other herds or flocks in a facility are less vulnerable to infectious agents and therefore need less feed for an increased rate of growth and days to market weight.

The geographic location, species, size of facility, weather conditions, and seasonality are all factors in the implementation of biosecurity measures on the farm. Individual producers must decide on the feasibility and prioritization of these and other measures to decrease the spread of potential pathogens.

Biosecurity measures that may prevent the dissemination of bacterial pathogens on farms may include isolation of new animals for a suitable period before introduction into a herd and isolation of all sick animals from healthy animals; changes of clothing and boots for visitors, bird and rodent control, footbaths containing active disinfectants inside and outside of houses, and limiting access to the site by visitors and trucks. Other examples include the following.

All-in, all-out systems

Where applicable for poultry, swine, and beef, all-in, all-out systems prevent the spread of pathogens and infections between consecutive groups of animals raised in the same unit. Generally it is a system of infection control more often used for swine, in which pigs weaned within a week are reared without mixing with other pigs. Investigators have demonstrated that it is possible to keep pigs free from, or reduce the level of, *Salmonella* when raised in a clean and disinfected environment (McEwen and Fedorka-Cray, 2002; Tielen et al., 1997).

Multisite locations

Use of multisite swine production methods decreases vertical transmission of pathogens from adults to growing pigs and lateral spread amongst groups of growing pigs. This reduces the pathogen load and results in less need for nontherapeutic use of antimicrobials (Ruen et al., 1992; Dritz et al., 2002). However, the transport of animals entailed in multisite production may not always be appropriate.

In multisite production of swine, "segregated early weaning" is a combined form of controlling infection by age segregated production and an all-in all-out system. The very young pigs are removed from sows early in production, as the sows are considered to be significant sources of pathogens (Pond et al., 1992).

Vector control

Transport vehicles should not be allowed into the farm unless they have been cleaned and disinfected before entry. Nonessential personnel should be excluded from the farm. Visitors, farmers, and farm workers should take showers and be provided clean clothing before entering the farm. Farm personnel also should not come in contact with animals outside the herd.

Competitive exclusion

Competitive exclusion (CE) implies the prevention of entry into a given site because that space is already occupied. CE products are unspecified mixtures of live bacteria (whereas probiotics are specified mixtures) isolated from the intestinal tract of animals and provided in feed to colonize the gastrointestinal tract prior to its colonization by potential pathogenic bacteria. The competing organism is better suited to establish and maintain itself in that environment or in producing a substance toxic to the pathogenic organisms. Because some of the claims for CE products are therapeutic, they are listed as drugs and are regulated by the Center for Veterinary Medicine (CVM, 1997).

In the early 1970s, Nurmi and Rantala demonstrated that *Salmonella* infections could be prevented by feeding chicks anaerobic cultures of normal intestinal adult fowl flora, which they referred to as "competitive exclusion" (Nurmi and Rantala, 1973; Rantala and Nurmi, 1973). Since that time the efficacy of the CE concept has been demonstrated in many laboratories (Barnes et al., 1980; Bailey, 1987) and in commercial field trials (Goren et al., 1988; Blankenship et al., 1993). A competitive exclusion mixture of *Escherichia coli* isolated from cattle feces has demonstrated reduced shedding with *E. coli* 0157:H7 (McEwen and Fedorka-Cray, 2002; Brashears, et al., 2003).

A new product, Mucosal Starter Culture (MSC), was compared with two other CE products to evaluate their ability to protect newly hatched chickens against colonization by a strain of *Salmonella kedougou*. The MSC treatment yielded the lowest mean level of cecal carriage and the smallest proportion of *Salmonella*-positive birds of the three products tested (Ferreira et al., 2003).

Generally, these healthy cultures of bacteria are administered to neonatal pigs to boost immune function, and to young poultry to prevent *Salmonella* and *Campylobacter* infections. USDA ARS is conducting field trial demonstrations at commercial swine operations at various geographical locations in the United States, testing defined, swine-derived CE products to prevent or reduce colibacillosis in nursery-age pigs (Harvey et al., 2002). For similar reasons to probiotics, CE products are also provided to animals to recolonize their gastrointestinal tracts with beneficial flora after having been administered antibiotics for therapeutic reasons.

Immune modulation

Immunologically active substances such as antibodies, cytokines, and spray-dried plasma added to animal feed may improve resistance to disease. These immune system modulators function by comparable means to which antimicrobials prevent low-grade infections or inhibit competitive intestinal bacteria.

Antibodies

Antibodies are molecules evoked by an antigenic stimulus in men or animals that react specifically with the antigen in a demonstrable way. One method by which antibodies have been produced in vitro is by immunizing hens that secrete antibodies against swine pathogens in egg yolks. The antibodies function by inhibiting the attachment of pathogenic bacteria to the intestine. Other examples are the use of egg yolks or freeze-dried eggs containing antibodies of calf diseases, which have been used with some success in calf milk replacers, and hyperimmunized spray dried egg protein has reduced mortality to piglet diarrhea and improved weight gain and growth conversion.

Colostrum

Adequate colostrum in the initial feeding will prevent failure of passive transfer in newborn calves. The recommended volume of colostrum is four quarts for the initial feeding to prevent failure of passive transfer in newborn calves (CEAH, 1993). However in a study by APHIS of the USDA, only 32% of calves received four quarts during their initial feeding, and 22% of deaths of dairy calves could be prevented by ensuring that calves receive the adequate intake of colostrum (NAHMS, 1993).

Chlorate

Not all species of animals are equipped with the physiological process through which the reduction of chlorate to chlorite kills select bacteria. Therefore, it has been suggested that ruminants be supplemented with chlorate prior to shipment to slaughter in order to reduce the incidence of foodborne illnesses. In a recent study, it was concluded that chlorate supplementation in ruminants immediately prior to slaughter is an effective method for the reduction of fecal concentrations of *E. coli* O157:H7 populations: in sheep (Callaway et al., 2003b) and in cattle (Callaway et al., 2002). Treatment of *E. coli* O157:H7-challenged pigs with chlorate also caused reductions in gut concentrations of the bacteria (Lowenthal et al., 1999; Anderson et al., 2001).

Preadaptation with sodium nitrate followed by experimental chlorate product supplementation immediately preharvest could be a potential strategy for the reduction of *S. typhimurium* in broilers (Jung et al., 2003).

Cytokines

These molecules are released from specific or generalized immune and nonimmune cells to function either locally or distantly from the site of origin (Babiuk et al., 1991). In dairy cows, prophylactic use of Interferon-γ (gamma) shortly before or after calving has reduced incidence of coliform mastitis.

Granulocyte and macrophage colony-stimulating factor (GMCSF) might be useful as an alternative to conventional dry-cow antimicrobial therapy. Interleukin-2 promotes resistance to invasive bacteria during the dry period (Nickerson et al., 1993).

Chicken interferon gamma has been shown to have potential therapeutic application as a growth promotant (Lowenthal et al., 1999).

Spray-dried plasma

The addition of spray-dried porcine plasma proteins to a corn-soy diet resulted in improved growth rates in swine (Chae et al., 1999; Coffey and Cromwell, 1995; Owusu-Asiedu et al., 2003) and provided a level of protection against experimental challenge with *E. coli* K99 similar to the antibiotic colistin (Torrallardona et al., 2003).

Dairy calves fed milk replacers containing 5% spray-dried bovine plasma or spray-dried porcine plasma reduced morbidity and mortality (Quigley et al., 2002; Quigley and Wolfe, 2003).

Vaccines

Vaccines control infection through the use of natural defense mechanisms. The control of viral and other infections can reduce the likelihood of secondary bacterial infections, thereby reducing the need for use of antimicrobials. The advantage of vaccines is that they specifically target pathogens while antimicrobials affect general populations of bacteria. Vaccines are available for bacterial and viral infections of our major livestock animals, including the following.

- Cattle. Vaccinations against bovine viral diarrhea (BVD) virus, infectious bovine rhinotracheitis (IBR) virus, *Leptospira*, and parainfluenza type 3 (PI3) are those most commonly practiced by producers (CEAH, 1993).

  Researchers in Canada have started efforts to advance developments in edible vaccine technology by genetically modifying alfalfa that they hope will protect against shipping fever by exposing the tonsils of beef cattle to *Mannheimia haemolytica albicans* (Shewen et al., 2003), as well as using transgenic white clover expressing *M. haemolytica* as an edible vaccine against bovine pneumonic *pateurellosis* (Lee et al., 2001). Another vaccine developed in Canada has shown a significant decline in the incidence of *E. coli* O157:H7 shedding in manure (AMI, 2003).

- Swine. In swine production, vaccinations used by most producers include protection against bacterial pneumonia, *E. coli*, erysipelas, *Haemophilus pleuropneumonia*, *Pasteurella pneumonia*, leptospirosis, and viral diarrhea. A vaccine designed to protect pigs against ileitis has recently been developed to decrease the amount of antibiotics used to protect the pigs from the disease (Cochrane, 2003).

- Poultry. Vaccines for poultry include protection against *Pasteurella* infection and Marek's disease. Research is underway to produce multispecies live vaccine to be used for the control of avian coccidiosis (Anonymous, 2002). An oil emulsion vaccine, considered more effective than current commercial vaccines of inactivated *Salmonella enteritidis*, is being developed to reduce the passage of the organism into chicken eggs (Durham, 2003).

Nutritional supplements

Deficiencies in proteins, vitamins, and trace elements and any imbalance in feed composition can result in outbreaks of disease and decreased efficiency of the immune system and feed conversion. Increases in select additives may also create suitable situations for improvements in immune function and other benefits without the use of antimicrobials.

Amino acids

Amino acids are organic acids that are nutritionally required by an organism and that must be supplied in its diet (essential) or may be synthesized by the organism and are therefore not required in the diet (nonessential). Supplementation of lysine, methionine, and threonine with barley, wheat, and soybean has improved growth performance of swine (Askbrant et al., 1994).

Carnitine (synthesized from lysine and methionine) has been utilized to increase performance on grazing calves and finishing lambs. The combination of L-carnitine and ascorbic acid may have positive effects on performance in broiler chicks under high temperature conditions (Celik and Ozturkcan, 2003). In broiler chicks, supplemental L-carnitine or L-carnitine and niacin could have positive effects on body weight gain and feed intake during the early stages of growth. However, supplemental L-carnitine or L-carnitine and niacin were not of benefit during the complete growth period (Celik et al., 2003). In other studies L-carnitine also had no effect. However, in one study in swine, providing L-carnitine to sows in feed during lactation had little effect on sow and litter performances (Musser et al., 1999); and in laying hens, in one study, dietary L-carnitine did not influence laying performance (egg production rate, mean egg weight, daily feed intake, daily egg mass, and feed conversion) or external egg quality (Rabie et al., 1997).

Conjugated linoleic acid

Conjugated linoleic acid is a group of polyunsaturated fatty acids found in beef, lamb, and dairy. Livestock feed supplemented with conjugated linoleic acid (CLA) have shown increased lean tissue and weight gain (Muller et al., 2000), decreased body fat in pigs (Ostrowska, et al., 2003), improved feed efficiency, decreased subcutaneous fat, and improved meat quality in stress-genotype pigs (Wiegand et al., 2001); and dairy cattle have had enhanced milk productivity (Mackle et al., 2003).

Distiller's dried grains with solubles

Distiller's dried grains with solubles (DDGS) is one of the three coproducts produced by the dry milling ethanol distillery industry. The process decreases digestibility of protein while increasing the value of the protein. DDGS is a source of vitamins, low in fiber and high in fat, yielding a product with much greater digestible energy than corn. In dairy cattle, substituting the DDGS for corn has been shown to increase milk yields, reduce acidosis, and improve rumination in high-producing cows. In swine, light colored (high quality) DDGS improves gut health, decreases mortality, and improves growth performance. In research with poultry, DDGS was found to serve as an effective partial replacement for corn and soybean meal. Light colored 5% DDGS resulted in 17–32% improvement gain and 3% in diets increased egg numbers and hatch in turkey breeder hens (Buchheit, 2002).

Enzymes

Gastrointestinal enzymes added to feed catalyze the breaking down of certain components of the feed, e.g., phytates and proteins, thereby increasing their digestibility. Enzymes have been shown to enhance the digestive efficiency in swine and poultry as well as beneficially alter the microbial micro flora of the gastrointestinal tract. In young swine it is thought that supplementing the amounts of enzymes may increase the animal's own enzyme activity or in adult swine enable the utilization of the energy in complex carbohydrates that normally pass through the GI tract undigested (Hughes and Heritage, 2002). Research efforts are underway to both improve the quality of enzymes currently in use and broaden the range of feed components for which enzymes may improve digestion and feed conversion.

Phytase decreases the effects of phytate that binds a large proportion of phosphorus in vegetable matter. It has also been found to increase weight gain and decrease feed conversion ratios in swine fed select diets, including barley-corn, soybean-corn, and low phosphate pearl millet-soy (Doyle, 2001).

A combination of enzymes extracted from *Trichoderma viride* improved average daily growth and feed conversion in swine fed hulless barley (Doyle, 2001). Other enzymes used as feed additives are alpha-amylase (*Bacillus subtilis*), aminopeptidase, and cellulase.

Fatty acids

Omega-3 fatty acids, of which fish such as salmon and tuna have high concentrations, have been evaluated in young weaned pigs as a means of improving the development of their immune systems.

Studies have demonstrated that fish oil diets improved the immune systems of the pigs and should serve as alternatives to antimicrobials in swine feed (Gaines et al., 2003). Oilseeds supplemented to fattening cows reduced rumen fluid protozoa counts and carcasses tended to be leaner with the fat supplements, but daily gains were similar to those for control groups (Sutter et al., 2000).

Fermentation

Fermentation is a potentially less expensive and equally effective means of acidification of diets. Fermented liquid by-products of food industries, containing sugars and starch (wheat, cheese whey, potato steam peel), have increased weight gain and improve feed conversion ratios (Scholten et al., 1999).

Genistein

Genistein is an isoflavone found in soybeans and soy feed products (e.g., soybean meal). It is considered a promising natural product for preventing and treating disease, as well as for promoting growth (Bingham et al., 2003). Low concentrations of genistein have been reported to elicit natural killer cell activity. The objective of a recent study was to quantify the effects of dietary genistein on pig growth and immune response during a viral challenge. Effects of the dietary genistein on daily pig gain and feed intake were dependent upon its concentration and stage of viremia. The data indicated that dietary soy genistein at 200–400 ppm is an orally active immune modulator that enhances systemic serum virus elimination and body growth in virally challenged pigs (Greiner et al., 2001).

Minerals and salts

Research suggests that the definition of specific micronutrient (e.g. trace mineral and antioxidant) requirements for the proper health status of food animals may be important factors in defining the relationship between nutrition and antimicrobial resistance (Tengerdy, 1990a, 1990b). Some mineral oxides and salts have antimicrobial activity and have demonstrated growth promotion. Use of zinc oxide in Denmark improved performance of piglets and reduced severity and duration of diarrhea (Holm, 1996).

Zinc oxide (3,000 ppm) and copper sulfate (250 ppm) minerals have been added to diets containing antimicrobials and have increased weight gain, feed intake, and feed efficiency in animals. However, the use of zinc and copper has been criticized and curtailed due to their accumulation in the environment and adverse effects on plants and in humans.

Chromium has been used in animal feed as an immune system stimulant in agricultural production. Administration to stressed feedlot cattle has been associated with lower morbidity and improved weight gain, feed efficiency and immune responsiveness, and increased milk yield (Kegley et al., 1997).

Oligosaccharides derived from cell walls of yeast provide decoy attachment sites for certain pathogens, thereby preventing or inhibiting their attachment to bacteria and subsequent colonization in the gastrointestinal tract.

Mannanoligosaccharides (MOS) is the most widely used oligosaccharide in both poultry and swine. One study on swine indicated that highest gains were reported for swine that were fed both MOS and an antimicrobial, suggesting that there was an additive or synergistic effect on growth in weanling pigs. However, it was concluded that there was no benefit to the use of MOS in finishing pigs (Turner et al., 2001).

Polysaccharides have been shown to improve the performance of pigs. Treatment of barley and maize with polysaccharides (Medel et al., 1999) and the addition of polysaccharides to Jerusalem artichoke meal (Farnworth and Chambers, 1996) have resulted in weight gain and improved feed efficiency in piglets.

Organic acid ions that act by controlling bacterial populations in the upper gastrointestinal tract are responsible for the beneficial antimicrobial effects of these acidifiers (Roth, 1998). Organic acids administered to weaned piglets have improved growth performance: fumaric acid, formates, and citric acid were more effective in young pigs (Roth et al., 1996; Overland et al., 2000), and formic acid was more effective in weight gain in fattening pigs (Overland et al., 2000).

Organic acids, malate, fumarate, and aspartate potentially provide an alternative to ionophores by stimulating rather than inhibiting specific ruminal microbial populations (Martin, 2003). Current evidence indicates no direct or environmentally mediated risk to human health through the use of ionophores and coccidiostats. Ionophores have been used to minimize lactate accumulation within the rumen and maintain production efficiency. The accumulation of lactate in the rumen decreases ruminal pH, from which the increasing acidity lessens the appetite of the animal. Organic acids, primarily malate, acted similarly to ionophores (decreased lactate, increased pH) that significantly improved performance of cattle, after having been fed a high-grain diet, in two of three feedlot studies (Martin, 2003).

Slow release forms of organic acids that consist of acids mixed with fatty acids and mono- and diglycerides to form microgranules have resulted in greater feed intake and growth in comparison to free acids (Cerchian, 2000).

Vitamins

Vitamin A and its precursor, beta carotene, have stimulated immunity and reduced incidence of mastitis and mammary infection in early dry periods. Vitamin E has facilitated improved immune response to bacterial challenge in mastitis. It has also been found to reduce weanling diarrhea (Lamberts, 1997).

Yeast

Two experiments were conducted to evaluate the effects of live yeast supplementation on nursery pig performance, nutrient digestibility, and fecal microflora and to determine whether live yeast could replace antibiotics and growth-promoting concentrations of zinc and copper in nursery pigs. Results indicated that live yeast supplementation had a positive effect on the nursery pig performance when diets contained antimicrobial growth promoters. Overall, however, the responses were variable (van Heugten et al., 2003).

Probiotics

Probiotics consist of live culture of bacteria that are used to control and promote the proper environmental conditions for establishing an ideal microbial population in the digestive tracts of animals. Similar to competitive exclusion products, probiotics promote digestive balance by supplementing intestinal microflora with beneficial bacteria, thus creating unfavorable conditions for pathogen growth. Probiotics have also been demonstrated to increase average daily gain, feed consumption, and feed efficiency (Abe et al., 1995; Hofacre et al., 1998).

The FDA requires manufacturers of probiotics to use the term "direct-fed microbial" (DFM) instead of the term "probiotics." They are regulated by the CVM, and the microorganisms administered to animals in DFM (probiotics) are defined and specified. The Association of American Feed Control Officials lists the organisms in these products.

The addition of the probiotic bacteria to the gut flora is believed to perform several beneficial functions: (1) heighten the level of immunity, thereby stimulating circulation of white blood cells that limit colonization by potential pathogens; (2) bolstering the physiological activities within the intestinal tract to enhance production of bacteriocins, organic acids and other substances that are bacteriocidal to other bacteria; (3) adherence to intestinal mucosa thereby preventing attachment by pathogens; and (4) competition with pathogens for nutrients. Examples of probiotics used in food animals include *Lactobacillus* spp., *Bifidobacteria, Streptococcus* spp., and *Bacillus* spp. Overall the results for the effectiveness of probiotics are varied. In a 1998 study, results from a study supported the use of probiotics as an effective alternative to antimicrobials that can reduce the severity of *Clostridium perfringens*-associated necrotic enteritis in broiler chickens (Hofacre et al., 1998).

Research at the USDA Agricultural Research Service indicates that bacterial microvesicles may act as a delivery system for bacterial-derived bactericidal compounds and contribute to the beneficial effects of competitive exclusion cultures (Anonymous, 2003a). However, overall results are varied and most successes with probiotics have been with in vitro studies. In addition, a report in Australia from the Scientific Committee for Animal Nutrition concerning the safety of a probiotic product determined that the two principal strains contained in the product, *Pediococcus acidilactici* and *Lactobacillus plantarum*, were resistant to tetracyclines. The Committee concluded that the use of the product in food animals posed a risk of dissemination of tetracycline resistance genes into the microbial ecosystem (Hughes and Heritage, 2002). The combination of the lack of evidence of the exact mechanisms of action of probiotics and the potential that some strains are harmful demonstrates the need for additional studies to determine the impact on animal health and welfare.

Target-specific antibacterials

Bacteriocins

Bacteriocins are proteins produced by certain bacteria possessing genetic elements that can exert a lethal effect on closely related bacteria. Generally, they have a narrower range of activity and are more potent than antimicrobials (Anonymous, 1995). A recent study of the potential use of *Streptococcus bovis* HC5 by the Agricultural Research Service of the USDA has demonstrated the effectiveness of bacteriocins of ruminal bacteria as an alternative to antimicrobials (Russell and Mantovani, 2002).

Lactobacillus lactis subsp. *lactis* A164 and *L. lactis* BH5 were demonstrated to have the strongest antibacterial activity against *Helicobacter pylori* species strains of seven bacteriocins produced by lactic acid bacteria (Kim et al., 2003).

Bacteriophages

Bacteriophages are viruses with specific affinity for bacteria by which they can invade and kill them, thereby facilitating prevention of disease and limitation of foodborne pathogens. Scientists at the USDA Agricultural Research Service discovered a usage that protects broiler chickens from respiratory infection through the use of a bacteriophage mixed with a particular strain of *E. coli* that causes disease in poultry (Huff et al., 2002).

Bacteriophages inoculated with *E. coli* O157:H7 have been found to reduce the shedding of 0157:H7 (Sanchez et al., 2002).

Phage-based interventions for *Salmonella enterica* serotype typhimurium DT104 are being explored for potential applicability at several stages of animal production and processing (Whichard et al., 2003).

Recombinant proteins

These are altered proteins resulting from insertion into the proteins by elements not originally part of the protein by biological, chemical, or enzymatic means. Scientists have recently filed a patent application on a cloned gene that produces a protein to treat or prevent bacterial infections that cause mastitis in dairy cows. The recombinant protein, CD14, binds to and neutralizes toxins made by the mastitis-causing bacteria (Anonymous, 2003b).

Animal product regulation

(Information included in this section is principally derived from the animal feed portion of the Center for Veterinary Medicine, http://www.fda.gov/cvm/index/animalfeed)

The use of animal food products is governed by the provisions of the Federal Food, Drug, and Cosmetic Act (FFDCA), and the regulations issued under its authority. These regulations are published in the Code of Federal Regulations (CFR). Any product for which the intention is to use as an animal feed ingredient, to become part of an ingredient or feed, or to add to an animal's drinking water is considered a "food" and thus, is subject to regulation. The Center for Veterinary Medicine (CVM) monitors and approves safe food (feed) additives and manages the FDA's medicated feed program through its Division of Animal Feeds.

Association of American Feed Control Officials

Association of American Feed Control Officials (AAFCO) is composed of state, federal, and international regulatory officials who are responsible for the enforcement of state laws regulating the safe production and labeling of animal feed, including pet food. FDA cooperates with AAFCO and the States for the implementation of uniform policies for regulating the use of animal feed products. This includes the establishment of uniform feed ingredient definitions and proper labeling to assure the safe use of feeds.

Biotechnology

Biotechnology products are a growing proportion of the feed components regulated by the Center for Veterinary Medicine (CVM). CVM anticipates that "new" biotechnology will become an even greater source of products in the future.

Federal Food, Drug, and Cosmetic Act

The FFDCA does not require premarket approval of "food." Foods that animals consume, e.g., grains, hays, etc., are considered safe. Most mineral and vitamins are "generally recognized as safe" (GRAS) as sources of nutrients; however, some ingredients added to an animal feed must be used in accordance with a food additive regulation. The basis for a food additive regulation is an approved "food additive petition" (FAP). A list of approved food additives for use in animal feed and a partial list of GRAS substances for use in animal feed are found in the CFR.

Products marketed as dietary supplements or "feed supplements" for animals fall under the FFDCA, and they are considered "foods," "food additives," or "new animal drugs" depending on the intended use. The regulatory status of a product is determined by CVM on a case-by-case basis. FDA carries out its responsibility for the regulation of animal feed in cooperation with state and local partners through a variety of mechanisms: cooperative agreements, contracts, grants, memoranda of understanding, and partnerships.

Feed ingredients

A feed ingredient is a component or constituent or any combination/mixture added to and comprising the feed. Feed ingredients might include grains, milling by-products, added vitamins, minerals, fats/oils, and other nutritional and energy sources. Animal feeds provide a practical outlet for plant and animal by-products not suitable for human consumption. The Official Publication of the Association of American Feed Control Officials (AAFCO) contains a list of feed ingredients with their definitions. Many of these ingredients are not approved food additives and may not meet the criteria needed to be recognized as GRAS (21 CFR 570.30). Nevertheless, FDA has not objected to the listing of certain ingredients (e.g., those used as sources of nutrients, aroma, or taste) in the AAFCO Official Publication or their marketing in interstate commerce, provided there were no apparent safety concerns about the use or composition of the ingredient.

Food additive petition

The basis for a food additive regulation is an approved food additive petition. Use of a food ingredient that is neither GRAS nor an approved food additive can cause a "food" to be adulterated, which cannot be legally marketed in the United States.

Under the FFDCA the FDA is not to approve a food additive petition if a fair evaluation of the data fails to establish that the proposed use of the food additive, under the conditions of use to be specified in the regulation, will be safe. Only if the petitioner meets this criterion can the food additive be approved. Regulations, which apply specifically to food additives in feeds, are published in Title 21, Part 570 of the CFR. Part 571 prescribes the kinds of data that should be submitted by the petitioner and the required format for the petition itself.

While the actual content may vary from petition to petition, depending primarily on the composition of the food additive and its intended use, each of the following subject areas should be addressed: (a) human food safety; (b) target animal safety; (c) environmental impact; (d) utility (intended physical, nutritional, or other technical effect); (e) manufacturing chemistry; (f) labeling (cautions, warnings, shelf life, directions for use); and (g) proposed regulation. A list of approved food additives for use in animal feed is found in Part 573 and a partial list of GRAS substances for use in animal feed is found in section 582 of Title 21 of the CFR. Substances affirmed as GRAS for use in animal feeds are listed under 21 CFR 584.

Labeling and claims

Products that are advertised with expressed or implied claims that establish the intended use to cure, treat, prevent, or mitigate disease, or affect the structure/function of the body in a manner other than food (nutrition, aroma, or taste), identify the intent to offer the product as a "drug" under the FFDCA. Unless the "drug" product has been shown to be safe and effective for its intended use via approval of a New Animal Drug Application (NADA), it could be subject to regulatory action as an adulterated drug. It is noted that, on a case-by-case basis, CVM has allowed references to "nutritional support" for specific organs or body functions.

New animal drug application

As mandated by the Federal Food, Drug and Cosmetic Act, a new animal drug may not be sold in interstate commerce unless it is the subject of a new animal drug application (NADA). The veterinary drug approval process consists of a series of consultative procedures and reviews. An approved application demonstrates that the product is safe and effective for its intended use and that the methods, facilities, and controls used for the manufacturing, processing, and packaging of the drug are adequate to preserve its identity, strength, quality, and purity.

Veterinary feed directive

The Food and Drug Administration (FDA) has amended the new animal drug regulations to implement the veterinary feed directive (VFD) drugs. A VFD drug is intended for use in animal feeds, and such use of the VFD drug is permitted only under the professional supervision of a licensed veterinarian.

Next steps

There are promising results from research showing that the identification and implementation of optimal alternative farm practices and products will reduce use of antimicrobials in food animals and the transfer of resistance from animals to humans. There are trade-offs and counterbalances amongst advocates of animal health, consumers, producers, and public health that comprise the intense debate on the use of antimicrobials in agriculture that must be considered in the limitations on growth promotants and their substitution by alternatives.

Research is needed so that agreement on risks can be obtained. It is on the farm that alternative changes will facilitate, and could serve as the basis for, a transformation of the long-held belief that these drugs are necessary at all stages of production to ensure healthy animals, safe products into the food chain, and agricultural economic sustainability. However, agreement will remain elusive until there is evidence to convince farmers that the costs attributable to utilization of a wide range of alternatives to antimicrobials outweigh the incremental benefits of nontherapeutic use of antimicrobials for growth promotion by farmers. Since the removal of antimicrobial growth promotants in European countries, there has been a decrease in the incidence of resistance in bacteria isolated from food animals. However, no data have yet shown a concomitant decrease in resistance in human infections although such a decrease in resistance may become apparent over time (DANMAP, 2000). Therefore, the economic effects of decreases in use of antimicrobials for nontherapeutic purposes on farmers remains of paramount importance.

There have been numerous studies of the economic impacts of various partial and complete bans on the use of antimicrobials in animal feeds; however the studies did not address the effects of such bans on human health (Wade and Barkley, 1992; National Research Council, 1999). The results varied amongst the studies, but overall they demonstrated higher costs to producers and price increases to consumers. On an industry level, assuming 93 million pigs annually, a decline of $0.79 per hog represents a decline in profits of approximately $73.5 million annually (McNamara and Miller, 2002). As a result, it seems apparent that the issues within the ongoing debate will be more effectively addressed through economic models and social welfare analyses.

There exist economic models of the optimal use of antimicrobials in humans and animals and the interplay with social welfare. McNamara and Miller (2002) recently put forth a timely discussion on the problem being faced in the development of social welfare analyses of agricultural use of antimicrobials. They emphasize the point that without strong agreement amongst the scientists about the risks posed by antimicrobial use in agriculture, conclusions from social welfare analysis will reflect the lack of scientific consensus on the issue.

While there are data in agricultural economic research for costs attributable to complete bans on antimicrobials as growth promotants, there is a need for estimates of the effects of a ban on some of the antimicrobials used in feed. However it is presumed that the costs would be substantially lower than the costs of the total ban, provided suitable alternatives to antimicrobials exist (Secchi and Babcock, 2002). It should be anticipated that a partial ban on these drugs will take place in the United States, affecting all species, and therefore future economic models need to include the impact of alternative management and practices that are substitutes for the banned antimicrobials.

Conclusion

A compelling need exists to begin using alternatives to antimicrobials in food animal production. Alternative therapies offer viable solutions to decrease the use of antimicrobials in livestock, which would limit the transfer and spread of antimicrobial resistance in the food chain and in the environment. Practical improvements in farm management, which include improved hygiene and biosecurity, should serve as the mainstay of intervention strategies on the farm. With the use of non-antimicrobial alternatives in animal feed, there is a much reduced risk of developing antimicrobial resistance to drugs used for human infections, and a much reduced risk of residues in meat or meat products.

The greatest scrutiny of use of antimicrobials in agriculture is on growth promotants. Therefore, the focus on alternatives needs to be on replacing nontherapeutic use of antimicrobials. However, due to the importance of certain infectious diseases in livestock production, and the unpredictability of the outcome on bans on nontherapeutic use, initial research should target the growth promoting effects of alternatives and the prevention of liver abscesses in feedlot cattle. In addition, the use of non-antimicrobial regimens for the prevention of "shipping fever" in feedlot cattle and the control of such infections as postweaning diarrhea in swine and necrotic enteritis in poultry should also be specific targets for initial substitutes for antimicrobials.

Widescale implementation of alternatives to antimicrobials that could provide comparable benefit of higher priced antimicrobials could lessen the profits of the pharmaceutical companies that produce, market, and sell antimicrobials as growth promotants. However, the cost of research and development limits the introduction of a potentially greater number of new alternative products. In addition, animal feed companies are probably also hesitant to support research that will not result in a proprietary product. Therefore, consideration should be given to awarding tax breaks to pharmaceutical and feed companies that invest and market suitable novel alternative therapeutics, and similarly new technologies. Commensurate consideration, and implementation, must be given to compensation to farmers as a result of expected initial rises in morbidity and mortality with the introduction of alternatives and with the removal of antimicrobials from their production system.

Although the development and promotion of alternative products and methods was designated as a "Top Priority Action Item" by the Interagency Task Force on Antimicrobial Resistance in 2001, no government agency is responsible for coordinating related activities and no mechanism currently exists to integrate and assimilate available knowledge regarding alternatives. With the exception of the Agricultural Research Service of the USDA, too little government effort has gone into evaluating the effectiveness of the various alternatives in reducing antimicrobial resistance and protecting the food supply. In addition, there are little or no extension materials or prepared curricula to make the information on alternatives accessible to food animal producers, veterinarians, and other stakeholders responsible for ensuring food safety.

The lack of definitive data on the extent of transfer of antimicrobial resistance from animals to humans is also an impediment to increased action on alternatives. Without substantial agreement amongst scientists concerning the risks involved in antimicrobial use in food animals, decisions on substitute strategies and novel therapeutics rendered from analyses of economic, food safety, and public health policy will reflect the lack of scientific consensus on the issue and adversely affect funding for research. However, sufficient evidence exists that the potential benefits of alternatives are worthy of investment. The option is to wait until limitations on antimicrobial use force the use of inadequately tested alternatives that pose significant risks to animals, consumers, and environment, or act preemptively in a substantial effort to demonstrate their safety and effectiveness through adequate field studies and as evidence to avoid the need for limitations on therapeutic use.

Alternatives to the use of antimicrobials in agriculture should become an integral part of disease prevention methods used in food animal production in the United States. Stakeholder groups that are vehemently opposed on other issues relating to the use of antimicrobials in food animals are in agreement of the need for additional research and funding, and long-term benefits to human, animal, and environmental health. The rare consensus on this issue signifies a tremendous opportunity to influence economic and social welfare. Improved collaboration and coordination are essential to maximize the opportunities presented by the use of alternative interventions. We need to move forward with alternatives because our unwillingness to do so is disingenuous with our commitments to improve human and animal health, agricultural sustainability, and the safety of our food supply.

References

Aarestrup, F.M., et al. 2001. Effect of abolishment of the use of antimicrobial agents for growth promotion on occurrence of antimicrobial resistance in fecal enterococci from food animals in Denmark. *Antimicrob. Agents Chemother.* 45(7):2054–2059.

Abe, F., N. Ishibashi, and S. Shimamura. 1995. Effect of administration of bifidobacteria and lactic acid bacteria to newborn calves and piglets. *J. Dairy Sci.* 78:2838–2846.

Advisory Committee on Animal Uses of Antimicrobials and Impact of Resistance and Human Health. 2002. *Uses of Antimicrobials in Food Animals in Canada: Impact on Resistance and Human Health*, Chapter 12, pp. 145–164. Vet. Drugs Directorate, Health, Canada.

American Feed Industry Association (AFIA). 2002. EU plans to phase out antibiotics in feed. American Feed Association Feedgram Newsletter, April 2.

AMI. 2003. New research highlights progress towards *E. coli* O157:H7 vaccine for live cattle, Am. Meat Inst. Media Release.

Anderson, R.C., T.R. Callaway, et al. 2001. Effect of oral sodium chlorate administration on *Escherichia coli* O157:H7 in the gut of experimentally infected pigs. *Int. J. Food Microbiol.* 71(2–3):125–130.

Animal Health Institute. 2000. The antibiotics debate: antibiotics and safe food, at http://www.ahi.org/antibioticsDebate/antibioticsandsafefood.asp. Accessed Dec. 29, 2004.

Anonymous. 1995. *Stedman's Medical Dictionary*. Williams and Wilkins, Baltimore, MD.

Anonymous. 2002. Production of vaccine strains suitable for incorporation in a live vaccine for avian coccidiosis. USDA Ag. Res. Serv. Available at: http://www.ars.usda.gov/research/projects/projects.htm?accn_no=405195. Accessed Dec 29, 2004.

Anonymous. 2003a. Probiotics and their use in food animal production: a novel explanation for antibacterial properties. USDA Ag. Res. Serv., Available at: http://www.ars.usda.gov/research/publications/publications.htm?SEQ_NO_115=132182. Accessed Dec 29, 2004.

Anonymous. 2003b. Researchers develop effective mastitis treatments. USDA Ag. Res. Serv. Vol. 15, July.

Askbrant S, H.J. Andersson K. Svensson, and C. Malmof. 1994. A short note on the effects of low-protein diets supplemented with biosynthetic amino acids on growing-finishing pig performance. *Swed. J. Agr. Res.* 24(3):115–118.

ASM. 1995. *Report of the ASM Task Force on Antibiotic Resistance*. Am. Soc. for Microbiology, Washington, DC.

Babiuk, L.A., et al. 1991. Application of interferons in the control of infectious diseases of cattle. *J. Dairy Sci.* 74(12):4385–4398.

Bailar, J.C. and K. Travers. 2002. Review of assessments of the human health risk associated with the use of antimicrobial agents in agriculture. *Clin. Infect. Dis.* 34(Suppl. 3):S135–S144.

Bailey, J.S. 1987. Factors affecting microbial competitive exclusion in poultry. *Food Technol.* 47:88–92.

Barnes, E.M., C.S. Impey, and D.M. Cooper. 1980. Competitive exclusion of *Salmonellas* from the newly hatched chick. *Vet. Rec.* 106:61.

Barza, M. and S.L. Gorbach. 2002. The need to improve antimicrobial use in agriculture: ecological and human health consequences. *Clin. Infect. Dis.*: 34(Suppl. 3):S71–144. Available at: http://www.journals.uchicago.edu/CID/journal/contents/v34nS3.html. Accessed Dec 29, 2004.

Barza, M. and K. Travers. 2002. Excess infections due to antimicrobial resistance: the attributable fraction. *Clin. Infect. Dis.* 34(Suppl. 3):126.

Bingham, A.K., et al. 2003. Potential for dietary protection against the effects of aflatoxins in animals. *J. Am. Vet. Med. Assoc.* 222(5):591–596.

Blankenship, L.C., J.S. Bailey, N.A. Cox, N.J. Stern, R. Brewer, and O. Williams. 1993. Two-step mucosal competitive exclusion flora treatment to diminish *Salmonellae* in commercial broiler chickens. *Poul. Sci.* 72:1667–1672.

Bodine, T. and H. Purvis II. 2003. Effects of supplemental energy and/or degradable intake protein on performance, grazing behavior, intake, digestibility, and fecal and blood indices by beef steers grazed on dormant native tallgrass prairie. *J. Anim. Sci.* 81:304–317.

Brashears, M., et al. 2003. Isolation, selection, and characterization of lactic acid bacteria for a competitive exclusion product to reduce shedding of *Escherichia coli* O157:H7 in cattle. *J. Food Prot.* 66(3):355–363.

Buchheit, J. 2002. Alternative agriculture: distiller's dried grains with solubles, *Rural Enterprise and Alternative Ag. Dev. Initiative Rep.* No. 11, 1–4.

Callaway, T.R., et al. 2002. Sodium chlorate supplementation reduces *E. coli* O157:H7 populations in cattle. *J. Anim. Sci.* 80(6):1683–1689.

Callaway, T., et al. 2003a. *Escherichia coli* O157:H7 populations in sheep can be reduced by chlorate supplementation. *J. Food Prot.* 66(2):194–199.

Callaway T.M., J.L. Morrow, T.S. Edrington, K.J. Genovese, R.O. Elder, J.W. Dailey, R.C. Anderson, and D.J. Nisbet. 2003b. Effect of co-mingling stress on fecal shedding of *Salmonella typhimurium* by early weaned piglets. *J. Anim. Sci.* 80(Suppl. 1)/*J. Dairy Sci.* 85(Suppl. 1): 157.

CAST. 1981. *Antibiotics in Animal Feed.* Counc. Ag. Sci. Tech., Ames, Iowa.

CEAH (1993). *Transfer of Maternal Immunity to Calves.* National Dairy Heifer Project. Centers for Epidemiology and Animal Health, Fort Collins, CO.

Celik, L. and O. Ozturkcan. 2003. Effects of dietary supplemental L-carnitine and ascorbic acid on performance, carcass composition and plasma L-carnitine concentration of broiler chicks reared under different temperature. *Arch. Tierernahr.* 57(1):27–38.

Celik, L., et al. 2003. Effects of L-carnitine and niacin supplied by drinking water on fattening performance, carcass quality and plasma L-carnitine concentration of broiler chicks. *Arch. Tierernahr.* 57(2):127–136.

Centers for Disease Control and Prevention. 1999. FoodNet—foodborne diseases active surveillance network. *CDC's Emerging Infections Program—1999 Surveillance Results*, Atlanta, GA.

Cerchian, E. 2000. Active matrix technology making more of acids. *Pig Progr.* 16(4):34–35.

Chae, B.J., J.H. Kim, C.J. Yang, J.D. Hancock, I.H. Kim, and D.A. Anderson. 1999. Effects of dietary protein sources on ileal digestibility and growth performance for early-weaned pigs. *Livestock Prod. Sci.* 58(1):45–54.

Clark, R.C. and C.L. Gyles. 1993. *Salmonella. Pathogenesis of Bacterial Infection in Animals*, 2nd edn. (ed. C.L. Gyles and C.O. Thoen), pp. 133–153. Iowa State University Press, Ames, IA.

Cochrane, B. 2003. *New Ileitis Vaccine Reduces Producer Reliance on Antimicrobials.* World Pork, Farmscape, June.

Coffey, R.D. and G.L. Cromwell. 1995. The impact of environment and antimicrobial agents on the growth response of early-weaned pigs to spray-dried porcine plasma. *J. Anim. Sci.* 73(9):2532–2539.

Cohen, M. and R. Tauxe. 1986. Drug resistant *Salmonella* in the United States: an epidemiological perspective. *Science* 234:964–969.

Comis, D. 2001. High-tech spying-on livestock. USDA Ag. Res. Serv., 4–7, June.

Crews, D.H., Jr. 2003. New breeding tool developed to increase feed efficiency in beef cattle, Lethridge Res. Centre, Lethridge, Alberta, Canada.

CVM. 1997. *New Animal Drug Determination.* Cent. Vet. Medicine, Washington, DC.

DANMAP. 2000. *Consumption of Antimicrobial Agents and Occurrence of Antimicrobial Resistance in Bacteria from Food Animals and Human Beings in Denmark.* Danish Integrated Antimicrobial Resistance Monitoring and Research Programme. Danish Vet. Lab., Copenhagen.

Dewey, C.E., et al. 1999. Use of antimicrobials in swine feeds in the United States. *Swine Health Prod.* 7(1):19–25.

Doyle, M.E. 2001. FRI briefing: alternatives to antibiotic use for growth promotion in animal husbandry http://www.wisc.edu/fri/briefs/antibiot.pdf. Accessed Dec. 29, 2004.

Dritz, S.S. et al. 2002. Effects of administration of antimicrobials in feed on growth rate and feed efficiency of pigs in multisite production systems. *J. Am. Vet. Med. Assoc.* 220(11):1690–1695.

Durham, S. 2003. A possible new vaccine to ko salmonella in chicken eggs. USDA Agric. Res. Serv., 7 May.

Ekkel, E.D., et al. 1995. The specific-stress-free housing system has positive effects on productivity, health, and welfare of pigs. *J. Anim. Sci.* 73(6):1544–1551.

Elstein, D. 2002. Estimating farm animals' feed efficiency, USDA Agric. Res. Serv., News and Information. Dec. 24, 2002.

Evans, M.C. and H.C. Wegener. 2003. Antimicrobial growth promoters and *Salmonella* spp., *Campylobacter* spp. in poultry and swine, Denmark. Emerg Infect Dis [serial online] April. Available from: URL: http://www.cdc.gov/ncidod/EID/vol9no4/02-0325.htm. Accessed Dec. 29, 2004.

Farnworth, E.R. and M.H. Chambers, Jr. 1996. Technical aspects related to the incorporation of bifidobacteria and bifidogenic factors in feed materials. *Bull. Int. Dairy-Fed* 313:52–58.

Ferreira, A., et al. 2003. Research note comparison of three commercial competitive exclusion products for controlling *Salmonella* colonization of broilers in Brazil. *J. Food Prot.* 66(3):490–492.

Freetly, H.C. 2003. Researchers seek methods to control farm animal stress, USDA Agric. Res. Serv., Newsletter, March 14, 2003.

Gaines, A.M., et al. 2003. Effect of menhaden fish oil supplementation and lipopolysaccharide exposure on nursery pigs. II. Effects on the immune axis when fed simple or complex diets containing no spray-dried plasma. *Domest. Anim. Endocrinol.* 24(4):353–65.

Goransson, L. 1997. Alternatives to antibiotics—the influence of new feeding strategies for pigs on biology and performance. In *Recent Advances in Animal Nutrition* (ed. P.C. Garnsworthy and J. Wiseman), pp. 45–56. Nottingham University Press, Nottingham, UK.

Goren, E., W.A. DeJong, P. Doornenbal, N.M. Bolder, R.W.A. Mulder, and A. Jansen. 1988. Reduction of *Salmonella* infection of broilers by spray application of intestinal microflora: a longitudinal study. *Vet. Q.* 10:249–255.

Greiner, L.L., T.S. Stahly, et al. 2001. The effect of dietary soy genistein on pig growth and viral replication during a viral challenge. *J. Anim. Sci.* 79(5):1272–1279.

Harvey, R.B., et al. 2002. In vitro inhibition of *Salmonella enterica serovars choleraesuis* and *typhimurium*, *Escherichia coli* F-18, and *Escherichia coli* O157:H7 by a porcine continuous-flow competitive exclusion culture. *Curr. Microbiol.* 45(3):226–229.

Hofacre, C.L., et al. 1998. Use of Aviguard and other intestinal bioproducts in experimental *Clostridium perfringens*-associated necrotizing enteritis in broiler chickens. *Avian Dis.* 42(3):579–584.

Hogan, J.S., et al. 1989. Bacterial counts in bedding materials used on nine commercial dairies. *J. Dairy Sci.* 72(1):250–258.

Holm, A. 1996. Zinc oxide in treating *E. coli* diarrhea in pigs after weaning. *Compend. Contin. Educ. Pract. Vet.* 18(1 Suppl. S):S 26.

Holmberg, S., et al. 1984. Drug-resistant *Salmonella* from animals fed antimicrobials. *New Engl. J. Med.* 311:617–622.

Holmgren, N. 1994. The therapeutic need of meidicates feed in Swedish piglet producing herd (Swedish). *Svensk Veterinartidning* 45:57–64.

Hooge, D.M. 1999. Antibiotics and their alternatives for poultry examined. Feedstuffs, 17 May 1999, p. 59.

Huff, W.E., G.R. Huff, N.C. Rath, J.M. Balog, H. Xie, P.A. Moore, Jr., and A.M. Donoghue. 2002. Prevention of *Escherichia coli* respiratory infection in broiler chickens with bacteriophage (SPR02). *Poult. Sci.* 81:437–441.

Hughes, P. and J. Heritage. 2002. Antibiotic growth-promoters in food animals, AGRIPPA, FAO.

Institute of Medicine. 1980. *The Effects on Human Health Of Antimicrobials in Animal Feeds*. Nat. Acad. Press, Washington, DC.

Institute of Medicine. 1989. *Human Health Risks with the Subtherapeutic Use of Penicillin or Tetracyclines*. Nat. Acad. Press, Washington, DC.

Isaacson, R.E., et al. 1997. The effect of transportation stress and feed withdrawal on the shedding of *Salmonella typhimurium* by swine. In *Proc. of the Second International Symposium on Epidemiology and Control of Salmonella in Pork*, Copenhagen, Denmark.

Joint Expert Technical Advisory Committee on Antibiotic Resistance (JETACAR). 1999. The use of antibiotics in food-producing animals: antibiotic-resistant bacteria in animals and humans. Dept. of Health and Aging, Gov. of Australia. Available at: http://www.health.gov.au/internet/wcms/Publishing.nsf/Content/health-pubs-jetacar.htm. Accessed Dec. 29, 2004.

Jung, Y.S., R. Anderson, J. Byrd, T. Edrington, R. Moore, T. Callaway, J. McReynolds, and D. Nisbet. 2003. Reduction of *Salmonella typhimurium* in experimentally challenged broilers by nitrate adaptation and chlorate supplementation in drinking water. Available at: http://www.ars.usda.gov/research/publications/publications.htm?SEQ_NO_115=137274. Accessed Dec. 29, 2004.

Kegley, E.B., et al. 1997. Effect of shipping and chromium supplementation on performance, immune response, and disease resistance of steers. *J. Anim. Sci.* 75(7):1956–1964.

Kim, T., et al. 2003. Antagonism of *Helicobacter pylori* by bacteriocins of lactic acid bacteria. *J. Food Prot.* 66(1):3–12.

Lamberts, F. 1997. Vitamin E as a potential agent to control diseases on pig farms—a field trial. *Tijdschrift Voor Diergeneeskunde* 122(7):190–192.

Lederberg, J. 1992. The interface of science and medicine. *Mt. Sinai J. Med.* 59(5):380–383.

Lee, R.W., et al. 2001. Towards development of an edible vaccine against bovine pneumonic pasteurellosis using transgenic white clover expressing a Mannheimia haemolytica A1 leukotoxin 50 fusion protein. *Infect. Immun.* 69(9):5786–5793.

Levy, S. 2002. *The Antibiotic Paradox: How the Misuse of Antibiotics Destroys Their Curative Powers*, 2nd edn. Perseus Publishing, Cambridge, MA.

Levy, S.B., G.B. Fitzgerald, and A.B. Macone. 1976. Spread of antibiotic-resistant plasmids from chicken to chicken and from chicken to man. *Nature* 260:40–42.

Lowenthal, J.W., et al. 1999. Cytokine therapy: a natural alternative for disease control. *Vet. Immunol. Immunopathol.* 72(1–2):183–188.

Lund, M., T.K. Welch, K.N. Griswold, J.B. Endres, and B.N. Shepherd. 2003. Occurrence of *Campylobacter* and *Salmonella* in broiler chickens raised in different production systems and fed organic and traditional feed. *Food Prot. Trends* 23(3):252–256.

Luster, A.D., et al. 1988. Molecular and biochemical characterization of a novel gamma-interferon-inducible protein. *J. Biol. Chem.* 263(24):12036–12043.

Mackle, T.R., et al. 2003. Effects of abomasal infusion of conjugated linoleic acid on milk fat concentration and yield from pasture-fed dairy cows. *J. Dairy Sci.* 86(2):644–652.

Madelin, T.M. and C.M. Wathes. 1989. Air hygiene in a broiler house: comparison of deep litter with raised netting floors. *Br. Poult. Sci.* 30(1):23–37.

Martin, A. 2003. Alternatives to antibiotics. The Scientist. Feb. 10, 2003.

McDonald, L.C., et al. 2001. Quinupristin-Dalfopristin–resistant *Enterococcus faecium* on chicken and in human stool specimens. *New Engl. J. Med.* 345:1155–1160.

McEwen, S.A. and P.J. Fedorka-Cray. 2002. Antimicrobial use and resistance in animals. *Clin. Infect. Dis.* 34(Suppl. 3):S93–S106.

McNamara, P.E. and G.Y. Miller. 2002. Pigs, people, and pathogens: a social welfare framework for the analysis of animal antibiotic use policy. *Am. J. Agric. Econ.* 84:1293–1300.

Medel P, S.S. de Blas, and J.C. Mateos. 1999. Processed cereals in diets of early weaned piglets. *Anim. Feed Sci. Technol.* 82(3–4):145–156.

Mellon M. and S. Fondriest. 2001. Union of concerned scientists. Hogging it: estimates of animal abuse in livestock. *Nucleus* 23:1–3. Also available at: http://www.ucsusa.org, by choosing "antibiotic resistance" and choosing report from the right-hand menu. Accessed Dec 29, 2004.

Muller, H.L., M. Kirchgessner, F.X. Roth, and G.I. Stang. 2000. Effect of conjugated linoleic acid on energy metabolism in growing-finishing pigs. *J. Anim. Physiol. Anim. Nutr.* 83(2):85–94.

Musser, R.E., et al. 1999. Effects of L-carnitine fed during lactation on sow and litter performance. *J. Anim. Sci.* 77(12):3296–3303.

NAHMS. 1993. *Dairy Herd Management Practices Focusing on Preweaned Heifers*, April 1991–July 1992. National Animal Health Monitoring System (USDA), Fort Collins, CO, p. 8.

National Research Council. 1999. Approaches to minimizing antibiotic use in food-animal production. *The Use of Drugs in Food Animals: Benefits and Risks*, pp. 188–209. National Academy Press, Washington, DC.

National Research Council. 1999. The use of drugs in food animals, benefits and risks. Natl. Res. Counc., National Academy of Press, Washington, DC.

Nickerson, S.C., et al. 1993. Effects of interleukin-1 and interleukin-2 on mammary gland leukocyte populations and histology during the early nonlactating period. *Zentralbl Veterinarmed* B 40(9–10):621–633.

NRC. 1980. *The Effects on Human Health of Subtherapeutic Use of Antimicrobials in Animal Feeds.* Natl. Res. Counc., Washington, DC.

Nurmi, E. and M. Rantala. 1973. New aspects of *Salmonella* infection in broiler production. *Nature* 241:210–211.

O'Brien, T.F. 2002. Emergence, spread, and environmental effect of antimicrobial resistance: how use of an antimicrobial anywhere can increase resistance to any antimicrobial anywhere else. *Clin. Infect. Dis.* 34 (Suppl. 3):S78–84.

Ostrowska, E., et al. 2003. Conjugated linoleic acid decreases fat accretion in pigs: evaluation by dual-energy X-ray absorptiometry. *Br. J. Nutr.* 89(2):219–229.

Overland, M., et al. 2000. Effect of dietary formates on growth performance, carcass traits, sensory quality, intestinal microflora, and stomach alterations in growing-finishing pigs. *J. Anim. Sci.* 78(7):1875–1884.

Owusu-Asiedu, A., et al. 2003. Response of early-weaned pigs to an enterotoxigenic *Escherichia coli* (K88) challenge when fed diets containing spray-dried porcine plasma or pea protein isolate plus egg yolk antibody, zinc oxide, fumaric acid, or antibiotic. *J. Anim. Sci.* 81(7):1790–1798.

Pond, W.G., et al. 1992. Effect of dietary fat and cholesterol level on growing pigs selected for three generations for high or low serum cholesterol at age 56 days. *J. Anim. Sci.* 70(8): 2462–2470.

Quigley III, J. and T. Wolfe. 2003. Effects of spray-dried animal plasma in calf milk replacer on health and growth of dairy calves. *J. Dairy Sci.* 86:586–592.

Quigley, J.D., III, et al. 2002. Effects of spray-dried animal plasma in milk replacers or additives containing serum and oligosaccharides on growth and health of calves. *J. Dairy Sci.* 85(2):413–421.

Rabie, M.H., et al. 1997. Effects of dietary L-carnitine on the performance and egg quality of laying hens from 65–73 weeks of age. *Br. J. Nutr.* 78(4):615–623.

Rantala, M. and E. Nurmi. 1973. Prevention of the growth of *Salmonella infantis* in chicks by the flora of the alimentary tract of chickens. *Br. Poult. Sci.* 14:627–630.

Roth, K.M. 1998. Organic acids as feed additives for young pigs—nutritional and gastrointestinal effects. *J. Anim. Feed Sci.* 7(Suppl. 1):25–33.

Roth, F., et al. 1996. Nutritive use of feed additives based on diformats in the rearing and fattening of pigs and their effects on performance. *Agribiol Res Zeitschr Agrarbiol Agrikulturchemie Okologie* 49(4):307–317.

Ruen, P.D., et al. 1992. Breeding and gestation facilities for swine. Matching biology to facility design. *Vet. Clin. North Am. Food Anim. Pract.* 8(3):475–502.

Russell, J.B. and H.C. Mantovani 2002. The bacteriocins of ruminal bacteria and their potential as an alternative to antibiotics. *J. Mol. Microbiol. Biotechnol.* 4(4):347–355.

Sanchez, S., et al. 2002. Animal issues associated with *Escherichia coli* 0157:H7. *J. Am. Vet. Med. Assoc.* 221(8):1122–1126.

Scholten, R.H.J., et al. 1999. Fermented co-products and fermented compound diets for pigs: a review. *Anim. Feed Sci. Technol.* 82(1–2):1–19.

Secchi, S. and B.A. Babcock. 2002. Pearls before Swine? Potential trade-offs between the human and animal use of antibiotics. *Am. J. Agricul. Econ.* 84(5):1279–1286.

Shewen, P.E., et al. 2003. Efficacy of recombinant sialoglycoprotease in protection of cattle against pneumonic challenge with *Mannheimia* (Pasteurella) *haemolytica* A1. *Vaccine* 21(17–18):1901–1906.

Shryock, T.J. 2000. Growth promotion and feed antibiotics. In *Antimicrobial Therapy in Veterinary Medicine*, 3rd edn (ed. J.F. Prescott, J.D. Baggot, and R.D. Walker). Iowa State University Press, Ames, IA.

Shurson, G., et al. 2003. Impact of energy intake and pregnancy status on rate and efficiency of gain and backfat changes of sows postweaning. *J. Anim. Sci.* 81:209–216.

Smith, K.L. and J.S. Hogan. 1993. Environmental mastitis. *Vet. Clin. North Am. Food Anim. Pract.* 9(3):489–498.

Statens Serum Institut (2001). DANMAP 2000. *Consumption of Antimicrobial Agents and Occurrence of Antimicrobial Resistance in Bacteria from Food Animals, Foods, and Humans in Denmark.* Danish Medicines Agency, Danish Vet. Lab., Danish Veterinary and Food Administration, Copenhagen, Denmark.

Summers, W.C. 2002. A historical introduction. In *Bacterial Resistance to Antimicrobials: Mechanisms, Genetics, Medical Practice, and Public Health* (ed. K. Lewis, A.A. Salyers, H.W. Taber, and R.G. Wax.). Marcel Dekker, New York, NY.

Sutter, F., et al. 2000. Comparative evaluation of rumen-protected fat, coconut oil and various oilseeds supplemented to fattening bulls. 1. Effects on growth, carcass and meat quality. *Arch. Tierernahr.* 53(1):1–23.

Swann, M.M. 1969. *Report of Joint Committee on the Use of Antibiotics in Animal Husbandry and Veterinary Medicine.* Cmnd. 4190. Her Majesty's Stationary Office, London.

Tengerdy, R.P. 1990a. Immunity and disease resistance in farm animals fed vitamin E supplement. *Adv. Exp. Med. Biol.* 262:103–110.

Tengerdy, R.P. 1990b. The role of vitamin E in immune response and disease resistance. *Ann. N.Y. Acad. Sci.* 587:24–33.

Tielen, M.J.M., F.W. van Schie, P.J. van der Wolf, A.R.W. Elbers, J.M. Koppens, and W.B. Wolbers. 1997. Risk factors and control measures for subclinical salmonella infection in pig herds. In *Proc. Second Inter. Sym. Epidemiology and Control of Salmonella in Pork*, Copenhagen, Denmark, Aug. 20–22. Federation of Danish Pig Producers and Slaughterhouses, Copenhagen, Denmark.

Torrallardona, D., et al. 2003. Effect of fishmeal replacement with spray-dried animal plasma and colistin on intestinal structure, intestinal microbiology, and performance of weanling pigs challenged with *Escherichia coli* K99. *J. Anim. Sci.* 81(5):1220–1226.

Torrence, M. 2001. Activities to address antimicrobial resistance in the United States. *Prev. Vet. Med.* 51:37–49.

Travers K. and M. Barza. 2002. Morbidity of infections caused by antimicrobial-resistant bacteria. *Clin. Infect. Dis.* 34 (Suppl. 3):S131–S134.

Turner, J.O., S. Dritz, and J.E. Minton. 2001. Review: alternatives to conventional antimicrobials in swine diets. *Prof. Anim. Sci.* 17:217–226.

van Heugten, E., D.W. Funderburke, and K.L. Dorton. 2003. Growth performance, nutrient digestibility, and fecal microflora in weanling pigs fed live yeast. *J. Anim. Sci.* 81:1004–1012.

Wade, M. and A. Barkley. 1992. The economic impacts of a ban on subtherapeutic antibiotics in swine production. *Agribusiness* 8(2):93–107.

Whichard, J., et al. 2003. Suppression of *Salmonella* growth by wild-type and large-plaque variants of bacteriophage Felix O1 in liquid culture and on chicken frankfurters. *J. Food Prot.* 66(2):220–225.

Wiegand, B.R., et al. 2001. Conjugated linoleic acid improves feed efficiency, decreases subcutaneous fat, and improves certain aspects of meat quality in stress-genotype pigs. *J. Anim. Sci.* 79(8):2187–2195.

Wierup, M. 1999. The Swedish experience of limiting antimicrobial use. Available at: http://www. gov.on.ca/OMAFRA/english/livestock/animalcare/amr/facts/wierup.htm. Accessed Dec. 29, 2004.

Wierup, M. 2001. The Swedish experience of the 1986 year ban of antimicrobial growth promoters, with special reference to animal health, disease prevention, productivity, and usage of antimicrobials. *Microb. Drug Resist.* 7:183–190.

World Health Organization. 1998a. *The Medical Impact of the Use of Antimicrobials in Food Animals.* Report of a WHO Meeting, Berlin, Germany, Oct 13–17, 1997. Available at http://www. who.int/emc/diseases/zoo/zoo97_4.html on Dec. 29, 2004. Accessed Dec. 29, 2004.

World Health Organization. 1998b. *Use of Quinolones in Food Animals and Potential Impact on Human Health.* Report of a WHO meeting held in Geneva, Switzerland, June 2–5, 1998. World Health Organization publication, WHO/EMC/ZDI/98.10.

Chapter 12
Use of rbST and Implications for Cow Health in the Dairy Industry

Alan H. Fredeen

Introduction

Recombinantly derived bovine Somatotrophin (rbST) significantly increases milk yield of dairy cows. However, rbST use is also associated with higher risk of a number of health disorders that reduce animal welfare and increase culling rate. Product precautions draw attention to these risks, which include higher incidence of mastitis, reproductive failure, and feet and leg problems. Studies and analyses conducted after rbST was approved for use in the United States in 1993 supported a precautionary approach to its use. Clear risks to cows had been identified and there was a lack of scientific data on the impact of the drug relative to these risks. Society regularly approves drugs and practices that have unknown associated risks, often with warning clearly issued. The precautionary approach can be applied by society to prevent product use until sufficient data from research, designed to rigorously assess impact, are available. In the case of rbST, risks to cow health are issued, but the adjoiner that type and degree of risk are influenced by the goals of farmers and their husbandry skills mutes the warning. Farmers with excellent husbandry skills may wrongly conclude from this that their cows will not experience adverse effects from rbST use.

In 1994, after perhaps the largest expenditure on efficacy testing of an animal drug in history, rbST (Posilac7, Monsanto) was approved for use in the United States to increase milk production in dairy cows (Bauman et al., 1999). Production was obviously the focus of the testing. Acceptance in the industry, by large herds particularly, has been widespread, and use of rbST in the United States has been increasing. Selected herds in 21 states were tracked between 1996 and 2002 (APHIS, 2002). Over 15% of herds and 22.3% of cows in the study received the hormone in 2002; use was more prevalent with increasing herd size. There was a 5.8% increase in herds using rbST between 1996 and 2002. Before the turn of the century, rbST had been approved in 40 countries (Bauman et al., 1999). Its popularity is related to the obvious link between milk yield and revenue for dairy farmers in unrestricted markets.

Related animal health and welfare consequences have received little attention despite Monsanto's own warnings of lower pregnancy rate, and increases in number of days open, occurrence of cystic ovaries, disorders of the uterus, retained placenta at subsequent calvings, clinical and subclinical mastitis, elevated milk somatic cell count, indigestion, off-feed, bloat, and diarrhea, increased number of enlarged hocks and lesions of the knee (carpal region) and disorders of the foot region. Unlike those evaluating efficacy, studies designed to examine health impacts of rbST are lacking in the scientific literature. In the majority of the efficacy studies, animal health and welfare costs were not adequately measured, nor were they designed to measure such effects in the first place. Consequently it is not possible to draw reliable conclusions on the effect of rbST on herd health from the literature without further statistical manipulation.

In an industry that seems to be ignoring the dawning of the postindustrial age, higher and higher yield is still sought as a means of increasing revenue. Even with an export avenue for dairy products, the industrial model of converting fossil fuel to milk makes less and less sense. Oddly, focus on higher yield is accompanied by less interest in, or knowledge of the nonfinancial costs involved. In the dairy industry, it seems the end, in this case higher milk production per cow, justifies the means. Effects of management aimed at increasing yield on animal health and welfare are largely hidden and, therefore, are seemingly accepted by the industry as necessary costs of doing business. To keep pace with society's evolving ethic and the need to control all costs, production practices in the dairy industry must be continually reevaluated, particularly as they affect animal health. Societal concerns have changed greatly within the span of a single generation of agricultural scientists and farmers demand simply for more, cheaper food to one that is multidimensional. Dairy researchers have been caught by surprise when research and technology focused only on production is not universally accepted because of implications for environment and welfare (Rollin, 2004).

In March 1993, before rbST was approved, a US Food and Drug Administration (FDA) advisory committee concluded that the use of rbST might increase risk of mastitis. In its first year of use, however, 14 million doses were sold to 13,000 commercial dairy farms (11% of dairy farmers in the United States). The FDA and some veterinarians seemed unconcerned about possible negative effects of rbST on cow health. Bauman (1999) subsequently contrasted dairy herd improvement records from herds that did or did not use rbST. The 4-year study examined more than 2,000 lactations from 340 commercial herds, 164 of which used rbST on at least 50% of cows in the herd. Supporting their hypothesis that rbST was safe, the authors reported no observed effects of the drug on vet costs, somatic cell count (SCC), or herd life. As specific indicators of cow health and welfare, however, these variables are limited.

Part of the obvious impact on cows is higher yield. The mammary gland of cows is an extremely demanding organ that often tests the limits of a cow's ability to provide substrates for milk synthesis. Naturally secreted somatotrophin (ST) is the enabler that plays a major role in coordinating the supply of metabolites for lactation. The use of rbST (additional ST) adds to the stress of lactation by increasing the demand for metabolites, which have to be consumed, absorbed, processed, and either secreted or excreted. More walking to acquire feed and water and the consumption of a more nutrient dense diet may be part of this stress. The hormone is not normally injected until after peak yield and initial rebreeding (60–90 days); however, the period of stress due to high yield is extended by rbST, and length of dry periods is probably reduced. Steady selection pressure in the dairy industry has increased the yield potential of cows, and along with it, adaptation to the associated metabolic stress. Considering the genetic potential of modern cows, it is usually argued that high yield in itself is not a stress. However, higher milk yield may amplify a variety of environmental stresses (lack of comfort, improper nutrition, etc.).

Evaluation of the separate effects of rbST and higher yield on cow health is only possible through comparison of paired animals in double blind experiments, one receiving rbST and the other a placebo, both producing equivalent milk yields. Such research has not been conducted. Consequently, distinction of effects must be based on observations in the literature where treated cows were compared with control cows producing similar quantities of milk pretreatment only. In these experiments, cows receiving rbST would have been influenced by differential treatment. Based on an analysis of these studies, however, Dohoo et al. (2003a) suggested that the effects of rbST and high yield on cow health may be different. Higher yield may, therefore, explain part of the effect of rbST on cow health.

Despite the large volume of literature on its yield enhancing effects, up to 2001 there had not been a single study of the effects of rbST on cow health under commercial conditions (Collier et al., 2001). Those that had attempted to evaluate the effects of rbST on cow health are few. Furthermore, the number of cows used in these experiments and length of trial were usually inadequate to detect differences in key health parameters.

A full-lactation study of the health effects of rbST was conducted postapproval (Collier et al., 2001). It involved a total of 1,128 cows on 28 commercial farms in four regions of the United States. This postapproval monitoring program (PAMP) showed that rbST increased the percentage of primiparous and multiparous cows with mastitis from 14.71 to 18.48 and from 22.51 to 28.71 representing increases of 25.6 and 27.7%, respectively. This effect resulted in more cow-days of medication in rbST treated cows and more days with discarded milk. A 27% increase in use of nonmastitis therapies was attributed to a greater incidence of musculoskeletal (MS) disorders in cows given rbST. The 48.9% increase in MS disorders of primiparous cows was not statistically significant, while the 88.9% increase in MS disorders in multiparous cows was. The study concluded that "label directions were compatible with safe use," although it identified that the increase in incidence of foot and hock lesions was associated with rbST use.

Unlike the United States, the effect on cow health was more central to Canada's decision regarding licensing the drug. A study was conducted for Health of Canada on the overall health impact of rbST use on cows. The government's decision not to approve rbST was based, in part, on its findings. This study based its evaluation on existing data from research conducted largely in the research dairy herds at universities across North America. Most of this research was conducted in association with the efficacy testing of rbST, or from studies conducted in-house by Monsanto itself (Dohoo et al., 2003a, b). Over 1,700 papers (mostly refereed), published between 1981 and 1989, were obtained using main literature search engines. This represented at least 60% of all publications on all biological effects of somatotropin in existence at that time (Bauman et al., 1999). Publications were screened for data that could be used to calculate statistics on cow health. After combining data, Dohoo et al. (2003a, b), assessed the overall impact of rbST on health using meta analysis, a statistical technique used to pool data and identify trends across studies (Dohoo et al., 2003b). This overarching evaluation (Dohoo et al., 2003a, b) permitted an evaluation of the effects of rbST on health, with each study weighted for number of animals it used. Significance of the effect of parity (multiparous or primiparous) and source of data (Monsanto study or study published in the dairy database) were also examined. Only controlled studies (i.e., where treated cows were compared with paired herd-mates receiving none) were included. In these studies allocation of cows to treatment (control or rbST) was random and groups were balanced pretreatment, with respect to key production variables. Only studies where a subcutaneous dose of rbST similar in amount to that approved (35.7 mg/d) was administered were used.

Obvious limitations in these studies were their short-term nature, primary focus on productivity, and that they were not conducted in double blind fashion. Observation and reporting of health problems in research facilities is usually meticulous, but efficacy studies are generally not designed to provide a rigorous evaluation of animal health. Since it can be assumed that husbandry in the research facilities that generated the data was superior, observed effects on health, though not definitive, may provide a "best case scenario" of the effect of rbST on cow health.

Neither Bauman et al. (1999) nor Dohoo (2003a) observed effects of rbST on SCC, an indicator of subclinical mastitis. Without data on incidence and cause of clinical mastitis, however, SCC alone is an inadequate indicator of the overall effect of rbST on mastitis. For example, in the same database

Table 12.1 Effects of rbST use on indices of mammary health (Dohoo et al., 2003a)

Aspect	Unit of evaluation	Effect
Clinical mastitis	Incidence rate[a]	1.24
	Incidence risk ratio[b]	1.27
Subclinical mastitis	SCC[c]	NS[d]

[a] Cases/cow days at risk
[b] Incidence in treated cows/incidence in controls
[c] SCC = somatic cell count (log10)
[d] NS = not significant

that showed no effect on SCC, Dohoo et al. (2003a) observed effects on the risk of clinical mastitis. Based on 18 groups of cows from 9 studies, and 29 groups of cows from 20 studies, both risk and rate of clinical mastitis respectively were significantly increased by rbST (Table 12.1). In each case, rbST use resulted in risk and incidence both 20% higher than those for controls.

Limited data existed to assess the impact of rbST on gestational parameters including retained placenta, gestation length, and abortion rate (Dohoo et al., 2003a). This is in part because efficacy studies typically end at or before the end of lactation, missing a relevant period following the subsequent calving. Despite some evidence of higher risks of retained placenta and abortion, there were insufficient data to draw a firm conclusion on rbST effects.

Despite variation among studies regarding how it was defined, clinical lameness was consistently increased by the use of rbST (Dohoo et al., 2003a). Of particular interest is the fact that even short-term application of rbST appears to increase lameness. A 50% increase in rate of lameness was observed when all reported types of lameness were combined (Table 12.2).

Injection site reactions occur in some cases. Dohoo et al. (2003a) found insufficient data to adequately assess the frequency or severity of these reactions. Genetic predisposition may be important.

Bauman et al. (1999) concluded from an evaluation of more than 2,000 dairy herd improvement records over 4 years that rbST, through its association with extended lactations, may decrease the risk of disease associated with calving. Huber et al. (1990) reported significantly less ketosis and parturient paresis in the carryover period succeeding rbST use. Similarly, Lean et. (1991) observed a tendency for less clinical ketosis. Dohoo et al. (2003a) concluded that use of rbST might reduce the risk of metabolic disease during the subsequent calving period, potentially through body condition reduction/appetite stimulation.

Digestive effects of rbST are likely related to the feeding management of higher yielding cows, and consequently would be similar in treated and untreated herds at similar levels of production and under similar management.

Table 12.2 Effect of rbST on incidence of other health disorders (Dohoo et al., 2003a)

Aspect	Unit of evaluation	Effect
Lameness (all types)	Incidence risk ratio[a]	1.55

[a] Incidence in treated cows/incidence in controls

Table 12.3 Effects of rbST use on indices of reproductive health[a] (Dohoo et al., 2003a)

Aspect	Unit of evaluation	Effect
Days open	Days	5.1
Nonpregnancy	Incidence risk ratio[b]	1.42
Services to conception	Services	NS[c]
Incidence of cystic ovaries	Incidence rate[d]	NS
Incidence of twinning	Incidence rate	NS

[a] Based only on cows that eventually conceive
[b] Incidence in treated cows/incidence in controls
[c] NS = not significant, $P < 0.05$
[d] Cases/cow days at risk

Parameters related to breeding that were evaluated by Dohoo et al. (2003a) included incidence of cystic ovaries, services to conception (STC), days open (DO), incidence of twinning, and nonpregnancy risk (Table 12.3). Effects on both STC and DO were computed only for cows that conceived. Overall, rbST marginally increased the risk of cystic ovaries by approximately 25% ($P = 0.11$). Based on six studies, no effect of rbST on STC was observed, while DO (i.e. the number of days between calving and conception) was significantly increased in treated cows. Based on 18 groups the mean increase in DO was 5 days. However, effects on both STC and DO could be underestimated because they were calculated only for cows that conceived and rbST could have an impact on conception rate, which was not evaluated. Treatment with rbST appeared to increase the risk of cystic ovaries by approximately 25%, although this increase was marginally significant ($P = 0.11$). Incidence of twinning was evaluated in cows for the parturition following the lactation in which rbST was given. Consequently, the evaluation was based on the few studies that reported data on this period (five groups of cows from three studies, with a total of 791 observations). Collier (1996) provided most of the data, wherein risk for primiparous cows tended to be lower, while that for multiparous cows tended to be higher. Dohoo et al. (2003a) noted that to detect a doubling in the risk of twinning (from 2.5% to 5%), 2,000 cows (1,000 cows in each treatment group) would be required (Table 12.3).

Effect of rbST on culling rate is difficult to interpret. Where it is related to a failure to reproduce, mastitis or lameness rbST may increase premature culling. Conversely, culling rate may be reduced because animals with minor health problems, those of genetically inferior type or production, and cows that don't conceive could be kept in herds longer through use of rbST. The difficulty in evaluating overall effect of rbST on culling rate is that, even if culling rate is reported, culling criteria vary among studies. Collier (1996) reported a statistically significant increased risk of culling in multiparous, but not primiparous cows (risk ratio = 1.38). This interaction may reflect health problems and extended lactations, both a result of rbST use. Based on results from a small data set (eight groups of cows in five herds), Dohoo et al. (2003a) observed a similar and significant ($P = 0.01$) risk ratio of culling associated with the use of rbST (1.36) in multiparous cows (Table 12.4). Again, the increase was not significant for primiparous cows. Ruegg et al. (1998) and Bauman et al. (1999) reported that

Table 12.4 Effect of rbST on culling rate (Dohoo et al., 2003a)

Aspect	Unit of evaluation	Effect
Culling rate (multiparous cows)	Incidence risk ratio[a]	1.36

[a] Incidence in treated cows/incidence in controls

rbST use did not affect survivability of dairy cattle. Data from these studies were not included in the evaluation by Dohoo et al. (2003a) because they were not randomized clinical trials and were, therefore, prone to bias.

Conclusion

The extensive database existing on rbST focuses on its impact on production, not health. These efficacy studies were either too small or collected insufficient data for statistically rigorous conclusions on health. Health-related research generally requires more cows.

When studies were combined to generate sufficient data for analysis, use of rbST was associated with substantially increased risks of mastitis, lameness, and reproductive failure. These effects concur with the few other studies that reported most directly on cow health issues, and with label precautions. Overall, these effects lead to increased rate of culling of multiparous cows.

Since control cows were managed under similar conditions to those of rbST treated cows in the efficacy trials used, environment can be ruled out as a significant factor affecting response to rbST in this analysis. A heavier mammary gland may result in part of the observed impact of rbST on cow health. Changes this incurs in cow behavior, locomotion, ability to lay comfortably, position in a stall, or stand with good posture may explain part of the effects. These effects on cows treated with rbST would be compounded in cows that likely make more trips to the milking parlor, feed bunk, and water source.

Because rbST use is more common in large herds, the management system treatment is less likely to include pasture and activity away from concrete surfaces. However, effects were shown in research where influence of animal management was well controlled. Despite this rbST cows would have consumed more dry matter and thus more nonstructural carbohydrate to support the higher yield. Where diets result in suboptimal rumen function, health issues arise.

Somatotropin (growth hormone) is released naturally from the anterior pituitary within a complex, well-regulated system. It receives positive feedback from a low level of somatotropin relative to set points established by physiological state of the animal. The signal involved is received from growth hormone releasing factor (GRF). Somatostatin (SS) is released in response to high ST levels. Injecting rbST overrides this loop (Burton et al., 1994). Secretions of IGF-1 and its binding proteins from liver are stimulated by endogenous and exogenous ST. Associated with this, among other effects, is the stimulation of growth of somatic tissue. A 2–10 fold elevation in blood IGF-1 level accompanies use of rbST (Burton et al., 1994). Receptors for ST and IGF-1 are found in many cell types including chondrocytes and osteoblasts, which are upregulated by rbST. Thus, rbST would be expected to affect animal structure as well as function.

Cells of the immune system are among those stimulated by rbST with potentially positive effects on the health of stressed cows. Overall, however, based on published data rbST has a detrimental effect on many aspects of cow health. Effects of rbST are well recognized by both the manufacturer and the scientific community. Its use, therefore, is based on a decision to accept the costs to cow health in pursuit of higher revenue.

References

APHIS, 2002. Bovine somatotropin. Info Sheet, December.

Bauman, D. 1999. Bovine somatotropin and lactation: from basic science to commercial application. *Domest. Anim. Endocrinol.* 17:101–116.

Bauman, D.E., R.W. Everett, W.H. Weiland, amd R.J. Collier. 1999. Production responses to bovine somatotropin in northeastern dairy herds. *J. Dairy Sci.* 82:2564–2573.

Burton, J.L., B.W. McBride, E. Block, D.R. Glimm, and J.J. Kennelly. 1994. A review of bovine growth hormone. *Can. J. Anim. Sci.* 74:167–201.

Collier, R.J. 1996. Post-approval evaluation of Posilac7 bovine somatotropin in commercial dairy herds (#93–051). Monsanto Study Report. St. Louis, MO.

Collier, R.J., C. Byatt, S.C. Denham, P.J. Eppard, A.C. Fabellar, R.L. Hintz, M.P. McGrath, C.L. McLaughlin, K. Shearer, J.J. Veenhuizen, and J.L. Vicini. 2001. Effects of sustained release bovine somatotrophin on animal health in commercial dairy herds. *J. Dairy Sci.* 84:1098–1108.

Dohoo, I.R., L. DesCoteaux, K. Leslie, A. Fredeen, W. Shewfelt, A. Preston, and P. Dowling. 2003a. A meta-analysis review of the effects of recombinant bovine somatotropin 2. Effects on animal health, reproductive performance, and culling. *Can. J. Vet.Res.* 67:252–264.

Dohoo, I.R., K. Leslie, L. DesCoteaux, A. Fredeen, P. Dowling, A. Preston, and W. Shewfelt. 2003b. A meta-analysis review of the effects of recombinant bovine somatotropin 1. Methodology and effects on production. *Can. J. Vet. Res.* 67:241–251.

Huber, J.T., D.E. Bauman, W.A. Samuels, R.C. Lamb, and D.L. Hard. 1990. Long term evaluation of zinc methionyl bovine somatotropin treatment in a prolonged release system for lactating multiparous cows at four U.S. clinical trial sites (85-039, 85-038, 85-021, 85-003). Monsanto Study Report, St. Louis, MO.

Lean, U., M.L. Bruss, H.F. Troutt, et al. 1991. Bovine ketosis and somatotrophin: risk factors for ketosis and effects of ketosis on health and production. Bovine somatotropin (bST) and the dairy industry. *Res. Vet. Sci.* 57(2):200–209.

Rollin, B.E. 2004. Animal agriculture and emerging social ethics for animals. *J. Anim. Sci.* 82:955–964.

Ruegg, P.L., A. Fabellar, and R.L Hintz. 1998. Effect of the use of bovine somatotropin on culling practices in thirty-two dairy herds in Indiana, Michigan, and Ohio. *J. Dairy Sci.* 81(5):1262–1266.

Section IV
Ideas to Promote Alternative Methods

Chapter 13
Funding for Testing Alternative Livestock Methods:
Developing and Performing Grants to Help Fund Sustainable Livestock Production

Randy Kidd

Section I: An Introduction to Grant Writing

Introduction

Grants are a legitimate way to fund a wide spectrum of farm-related projects. For our purposes in this chapter, the more common of these types of projects include producer projects, research and education projects, and professional development projects. There are, from a number of sources, millions of dollars of grant monies available for partial or full funding of a great variety of projects. While there is considerable money available specifically for farm-related projects, one only needs to extend his/her thinking slightly outside the traditional farm circle to include many other sources for grant funding that would apply quite nicely to the farm or rural family.

However, even though grant money is readily available from numerous sources, the process of obtaining a grant can be tedious work, and the results of the grant writer's efforts are never guaranteed, no matter how well the grant is written. In fact, one professional grant writer has said that writing a grant is a lot like making a visit to the race track or the craps table in a casino in the following ways:

- You know you will never win them all
- The "house" holds all the cards
- You will never get a straight flush unless you are in the game
- The trick is finding the grant (the bet) that holds the best odds

The difference between this analogy of gambling and the actual practice of grant writing is this: while you may think of grant money as "free" or "gambling-generated" money, you will absolutely work for any grant money you receive, and chances are, you will work hard for it.

This chapter is directed toward helping put you in a position of making the best "bet" to increase your "odds" of winning a grant.

Opening strategies for obtaining grants

Find a need

When gambling, you may be able to win some money with the luck of the draw, and there are almost unlimited places where one can gamble to one's heart's content, trying for that one big win. When we're dealing with grant money, on the other hand, the money is only put on the table when a grant provider determines there is a need. You can, therefore, only win the game if you find the "table" where grant money is being offered, and it is the "dealer" (the grant provider) who decides when and where to put up the money. Those are the rules of the game, and you will only waste your time if you try to play with different rules.

This is not to say that it is hopeless to try to find available grants for a project you want to do. Even given the limitations of the rules of the game, whether you are a producer, a farm-based educator, or a researcher with a bent toward working with farm-related research, you still have a good shot at obtaining grant funds for a project you feel needs to be funded.

You can increase your odds of finding available grants if you approach the process from the following perspectives:

1. Grant money is most often offered to someone who wants to learn something so that someone else can benefit from the findings.
2. Ask yourself the basic question: "What needs to be done?" Is there something in your day-to-day operations that you think could be made to work more efficiently, function better, generate a higher yield on the money expended, be more sustainable, provide better health for your livestock, create a more cost-efficient product, or make your family time more rewarding? If you can see a "need" in your sphere of operation, it is likely someone else will also have seen a need to answer that same question.
3. Ask another basic question: "What are the barriers I encounter and how could I overcome them?"
4. Realize that your questions, or ones very similar, are likely being asked by other producers or educators. When enough people have the same or similar needs and questions as yours, or when enough folks become fed up with the barriers they face daily and are ready to find an easier way to overcome them, then the grant money will become available. The key is to find that specific grant provider whose concerns correspond to yours.

Love what you are doing

Grant writing is a chore that can be quite difficult and lengthy, and at times extremely perplexing. In addition, performing the actual trials and actions stipulated in the grant will take time and effort. It's been estimated that more than 80% of the time requirement should be allocated to performance, to actually doing the work; the process of grant writing itself should only consume 20% of the total time you have available to fulfill the objectives of the grant.

And remember that grant monies are typically dispersed with the objective in mind of obtaining some form of information that will ultimately be helpful to future producers, educators, and/or professional development, or to the public in general. This, of course, almost always requires that the person(s) performing the grant requirements will need to keep some form of accurate, accessible, and easy-to-comprehend documentation of their results. In other words, you will need good written records. Further, grant funding agencies usually require recipients to provide some form of understandable summary so others will benefit from their efforts.

All this means extra work, and it is not always work that fits into a farmer/livestock producer's daily routine, nor is it the type of work he/she particularly enjoys or is necessarily good at. In short, in order to carry you through all that is necessary for writing and acquiring a successful grant, you will need to find a way to enjoy, if not love, the actual work involved.

Read, read, read

There are literally thousands of sources of grant money available from local, regional, and national sources. An example of a federal source of grant money is the USDA Sustainable Agriculture Research and Education program (SARE), and this chapter will focus primarily on SARE grants. However, grant seekers greatly increase their odds for writing a "winning" grant if they avidly read about as many of the available grants as they can, from whatever sources they have available. Professional grant writers spend a portion of each day simply reading the ever-changing information on the wide spectrum of grants currently available.

The appendix at the end of this chapter gives several potential grant-funding sources, and other sources for information pertaining to the specific areas of sustainable agriculture and the broader areas that might apply to agriculture in general. Note that most of these sources are available via the Internet, and many have contact phone or fax numbers along with postal mail addresses. In addition, many of these sources have the contact person details that you can use for further information.

You can often download information about the qualifications for grants from the specific provider; written copies of the requests for grants; archives of successful proposals in the past; and proposal application forms. If you don't have in-house access to Internet service, most libraries do. Many libraries will, for a fee, allow you to download the grant information from the Internet for later appraisal at home.

The point is that the more time you spend reading about the various grants available, the better are your chances to find the one grant that fits the need or question you feel needs answered.

Review other grants

For a better understanding of the grant writing process, read other successful grants. Most grant providers have archives of past grants on file. Read several of these grant projects, and as you read, get a general feel for how a successful grant is written. Observe the general flow of the grant: the outline, format, manner and order of presentation, and style of writing. Take a close look at what type of projects were funded in the past, who obtained the grants and who carried them out (producers, educators, or researchers), the dollar amount of the budget, where they were located, and what conclusions or solutions to problems were generated from the grant. Finally, if possible, try to get a feel for a possible trend or direction this grant-funding agency seems to be taking.

As you continue your review, notice how the grants were formulated so as to create the "best odds for success."

Determine the "best odds"

Following is a quick checklist to be used for evaluating a grant proposal to see if it is appropriate for your project.

- Determine eligibility. Each grant will specifically say who is and who isn't eligible to apply. You are either eligible, or you are not. If there are questions of eligibility, contact the granting agency.

- Identify geographic restrictions. Some grants are offered nationally, some regionally, and some will only be offered in a certain state or possibly in one small local area.
- Determine competitiveness. As a general rule, the more money available, the more muscle you will need to get the grant. Smaller grants can also be competitive, but a smaller operation has a better chance to obtain one of these. If you are a one-man-farm operation, it probably does not make much sense to apply for a nationally funded, several-million dollar grant, at least not without involving other area and regional agencies.
- Recognize deadlines. Know the date for the "call for proposals." This is when upcoming grants are announced, and this is the time when you will begin to formulate your final plan for making an application. It is also important that you know the final date when grant applications can be submitted. Determine the deadline date for submission of the applications, and be sure you can meet the deadline. It probably does no good to begin work on an application that is due next week; it is better to wait for next year's proposals. Also check the due date for the completion of the project, and be certain you can fulfill the requirements by then.
- Review selection criteria. Do you (and the people you will be working with) fit the criteria, and if you do, how and when can you present this information to the grant reviewers?

Establish ongoing relations with grant writers and grant officers

If you are really serious about obtaining grants, both short-term and in the future, it is extremely beneficial to establish ongoing relationships with other grant writers and grant officers. Grant writers are an excellent source for information about techniques, successful grants they have written, and grants that are available from areas outside your own explorations. And, like any other type of personal networking, an ongoing relationship with grant officers assures that your grant will at the very least have a "familiar face" when it is being reviewed.

Collaborate and get help

Most grant funding agencies are more apt to fund projects that involve several people with a variety of abilities and backgrounds. In addition, when you are developing a grant, two or more heads are better than one—by collaborating with a number of people with different skills and training, you enhance your chances of writing a successful grant. Further, it often makes good sense to divide the performance workload between several interested participants.

SARE feels it is especially important to obtain help and/or collaboration for all phases of your project. In many regions SARE sponsors workshops that assist grant writers in the writing of their grants. They also strongly recommend getting assistance in the design of your project, urging grant seekers to find someone at their county extension office or land-grant university with experience in setting up and conducting research on farms to work with you as a collaborator.

If you cannot find an experienced helper, SARE has a list of guidebooks and farmer research networks that can walk you through the process of designing a valid research project. Check their Web site www.sare.org and read the handbook *How to Conduct Research on Your Farm or Ranch*. This handbook contains a list of available publications.

Finally, SARE is partial to grants that include a wide spectrum of people and/or institutions that are working together in collaboration on all phases of the grant, from conception, to performance, to analysis and dissemination of the results, and on to outreach to others in the community.

Grant writers can also get help from several sources outside the general farming community. Many institutions and private entrepreneurs offer grant writing workshops. Check with your local library and university for sources.

One of the better-known sources for grantsmanship training is The Grantsmanship Center (www.TGCI.com). This Center offers week-long training courses in grantsmanship, and their membership services include free access to federal and foundation grants databases, a quarterly informational magazine, and access to job and consulting opportunities. While the Grantsmanship Center's focus is more directed toward the arts and humanities, education, and health services, they could be an excellent training source for the would-be serious grant writer.

The grant review process

Characteristics of the grant review process

There are several general characteristics of the grant review process that pertain to most, if not all, funding organizations.

- Subjectivity. Even the most standardized grant reviews contain subjectivity and allow for reviewer subjectivity.
- Reviewers often look for the negative. Don't give them a chance to find any negatives. Read and reread the criteria for the grant, and conform to *these* criteria precisely.
- Effective proposals "flow" from the evaluation criteria and make it easy for the reviewer to follow and understand.
- One negative reviewer can influence an entire panel.

Understanding reviewers

People who review grants come from a diverse background, and their background will depend on the granting agency. The serious grant writer will want to know the general background of the reviewers for each funding agency he/she applies to. It is important to know if the reviewers are all academically oriented, for example, or do they come from a rural or urban background? Do they know and understand farming or do they all have Ph.D.s in nonfarming specialties?

The people who review SARE grant proposals are folks who have a rural background—either farmers, producers, or people associated with agricultural academic programs or agricultural production in general. SARE reviewers are strictly volunteers, and by SARE bylaws, they cannot submit a grant proposal during the time they serve as a reviewer.

Section II: Grant Writing

Final hints from SARE before you begin

Before you actually put pen to paper, there are some further tips to help you create the winning proposal. SARE has prepared a one-page summary, and it is included here:

How To Write A Winning Proposal:

1. Make sure SARE is the right granting program for your project. Take a few moments to review the proposal guidelines, focal areas, and evaluation criteria in the Call for Proposals for your region. Every year, we receive a number of well-written, well-designed proposals that don't clearly address SARE's unique goals and criteria.
2. Involve farmers early and in meaningful ways. The strongest proposals clearly demonstrate that the project will be relevant to producers, providing practical answers to their questions. The best way to accomplish this goal is to involve farmers and growers in the planning, design, and implementation of the project.
3. Collaborate. SARE encourages projects that examine multiple issues simultaneously. To be successful, such projects must involve a variety of disciplines.
4. Look beyond state lines, both in terms of direct project participants and your eventual outreach audience. SARE is a regional program. Your project stands a better chance if it addresses issues in a way that's relevant to several states and builds on the expertise and knowledge available regionally.
5. Keep the writing simple. Proposals with clear objectives and methods are generally the most successful.
6. Help reviewers understand the importance of your project. Don't assume reviewers are intimately familiar with the issues your proposal addresses. SARE's technical review panels are composed of farmers and experts in a variety of disciplines.
7. Avoid jargon. Also be sure to spell out the full names of any acronyms.
8. Make sure the methods and team are appropriate to accomplish your goals. If the project involves experimentation, are plot sizes, replications, and controls adequate to provide meaningful information? Be sure to consult with a statistician in developing your experimental design. Also, make sure the proposal shows that your team has both the background and expertise to carry out the project.
9. Have someone proofread your proposal. A fresh set of eyes can help you identify sections that are unclear and catch typographical errors.
10. Follow directions. Every year, proposals are disqualified because the writer failed to follow general format directions regarding the number of pages, appendices, fonts, spacing, etc. Reviewers rank proposals lower when writers fail to follow instructions regarding what content goes in which section of the proposal.

Key elements found in almost all grants

Most grants have similar key elements:

*   Mission Statements
*   Abstract
*   Needs Statement
*   Plan of Operation
*   Evaluation
*   Budget
*   Organization and Adequacy of resources
*   Collaboration/Dissemination of Results

Mission statements

Each proposal should have a mission statement that differentiates it from the rest. The best mission statements are short, often no more than one simple phrase or sentence. Effective mission statements are also what some writers have referred to as "bomb safe." That is, they are so inspiring and easy to remember, they could be recited during a bomb raid. The following are characteristics of a well-written mission statement:

- Short. Brief and simple statements are easy to understand and remember.
- Flexible. Flexible statements last a long time.
- Distinctive. Your statement differentiates your proposal from other applicants who might have proposals with a similar mission.
- Positive. Use positive terms and develop a mission statement that expects and anticipates positive results.
- Mission statements should motivate, excite, and inspire.

Abstract

An abstract is defined as a statement that summarizes the important points of a given text. In terms of a grant proposal, the abstract should specifically and precisely tell what it is you plan to do and very briefly tell how you plan to do it. The abstract, when done properly, should give anyone who reads it an understanding of what you are trying to accomplish and the manner in which you will be working to accomplish your goals.

Writing a precise abstract often helps the grant writers formulate exactly what it is they are proposing, and it gives them *time* to consider the best and most precise way to explain their objectives to others.

Finally, a well-written abstract should project an air of confidence, and it should demonstrate that the grant writers really believe in their project, in its usefulness, and in the likelihood of its successful completion.

Following are key elements to a well-written abstract:

- Provides a clear and concise summary of your proposal
- Should be no *longer* than one page, and most abstracts are only one or two paragraphs in length.
- Should *include* major goals and expected outcomes of the proposal
- Establishes a "perception of success"

Needs statement

The needs or problems statement describes the situation that caused you to prepare this proposal. The needs statement zeroes in on the specific problem or problems that you want to solve through your proposed program. In the needs section, you are given the opportunity to express what you see as a problem, and if you know of evidence to support it, you can address the problem on a larger, regional or national, scale.

Do not assume that everyone knows the problem exists. You are the "problem expert," and you are drawing on your personal experience to describe what you see as a problem that needs solving.

Make sure you make the case for a need to solve your problem on an individual or regional level; don't think the needs statement must apply on a national level. At the same time, don't assume you are the only one who has the problem you feel needs to be solved. If it is your problem, it is likely that someone else has the same or similar problem. And, if you are aware of a problem on a regional or national scale, be sure to indicate the extent of these needs as well.

Following are characteristics of a well-written needs statement

- Is very specific
- Avoids sensationalism
- Uses charts and tables sparingly
- Uses short sentences and paragraphs
- Avoids professional jargon
- Spells out any acronyms used
- Utilizes national, state, and local data if available

Plan of operation—methods

The plan of operation is your plan of action, the specific methods you will use to answer the needs or problems you have identified. A well-written plan of operation includes the following components:

- Develops goals, objectives, and activities that represent a solution to the problem
- Thinks specific and is narrow in focus and broad in terms of replication. That is, your plan of action is how you specifically will handle the problem; your plan of action should be easy for others to follow
- Establishes a clear plan to achieve the stated goals
- Identifies resources and strategies that will contribute to the project

Results and interpretations/evaluations

The data gleaned from the project, when summarized, give us an accurate picture of the overall results of the project. Results will always include a written summary, and they may also include charts or some type of graphic display. The idea is to make the (often cumbersome) data easier to interpret. The project leaders then take those results and give further meaning to them by offering their written interpretations and evaluations.

Some tips for writing results and interpretations are:

- The initial design of the project is the key to producing valid results. Get help as you are developing the project's design.
- Results should flow naturally from the needs statement and the objectives of the project.
- Results include hard data (weights and measurements) and personal observational data. The trained eyes of the farmer/rancher are often the best tools for data that may not fit exactly into the experimental design. Be sure to use these tools, record your observations, and share them with other producers. What you see may be as valuable for other producers as *are* the raw data that derive from the project.
- Look for unexpected results. Often these unexpected findings are more valuable than those you were seeking.

- Outside evaluators are often a plus. Have an ag-savy friend assist in collecting data and especially in helping to interpret the data.
- If possible include feedback from the target groups—other farmers/ranchers, educators, or community members.

Budget

The reason you have written the grant is to obtain funding for a project you feel will fulfill a need or solve a problem you have identified, and the budget is how you propose to be reimbursed for the work you will do to fulfill the activities for the grant. The best way to formulate a budget is to develop it as you write the proposal.

As you consider each activity and the personal time and effort it will require; as you think about what materials and supplies you will need, farm-related and project-related, such as printing and paper; as you are considering the barn, pen, and field space you will need for your project; as you add up the numbers of livestock that will be required; as you contemplate the outside man-hours that will be necessary to accomplish your goals including both manual labor and consultant time; and as you contemplate other possible expenses such as travel costs, attending seminars, or workshops, and the like, these are the times to put a sharp pencil to the costs you will be assuming.

If you will be doing your project as a collaborative effort with an outside institution such as a university, they will most likely have an indirect, administrative fee, and this fee is usually a percentage of the total cost of the project. This fee can seem to be considerable (some may be as high as 40–50% of the total budget), so you need to be sure your budget planning includes it from the beginning. Check with the collaborating institution for the format they use for determining the fee.

Writing a budget that is acceptable to the granting agency and that will make it beneficial for you to carry out the activities of the project can be a most daunting task, and it is likely one area where expert help can almost always be utilized. Professional grant writers can be a tremendous help here, if nothing more than to proof read the project and make suggestions where you should include a request for more funds just to cover expenses. Most people in the academic world are fairly well versed in writing grant (obtaining and performing grants are typically an integral part of their job description), and they too can be invaluable aids for helping to develop a valid budget—one that supports the costs you will incur and one that matches the type of budget the granting agency will provide.

Some key points to writing the budget portion of your proposal include:

- Develop the budget as you write the proposal.
- Justify each line-item and expenditure.
- The budget should reflect the nature and scope of the project.
- Avoid miscellaneous expenditures, that is, specify most, if not all of the expenses in a line-item request. Grant providers generally hate to see miscellaneous expenses in a budget.
- Write the budget to be user friendly.

Personal and group strengths and abilities to perform the objectives

This section of the grant proposal is your chance to shine, your opportunity to tout the specific skills and abilities of all those who will perform the objectives. Take the time to give a fair and accurate assessment of all the human resource skills that will be brought to the project. This is, of course, not the time to overstate your abilities, credentials, or past history; but it is the time and place to be very positive about all your abilities, capabilities, and past successes. Include the following:

- Describe the strengths of the personnel who will be involved in any of the activities of the project.
- Outline resources that are available for the project.
- Describe the things that make you, your farm, and your organization better than others.
- Include a brief history of success. Include your relevant farming successes as well as any other grants you have obtained and successfully completed in the past.

Outreach

Outreach is an important component of many grants, but it is especially important for SARE grants. Grant funding institutions want to see the fruits of their investment being put to good use, and the way to insure this is to make certain the information gleaned from the project gets to as many people as possible.

The grant proposal should show specifically how the project will benefit others as well as how the information from the performance of the project will be distributed to others. Following are some tips for demonstrating your ability to produce and disseminate outreach information:

- Describe how the project will benefit other individuals, farms, institutions, and/or the general public.
- Identify other individuals, farms, and/or agencies that will support the project and receive services.
- Describe the coordination that will exist within the community and the region.
- Describe how you will help others address similar needs.

If at first you don't succeed

If you don't succeed with your first grant proposal, don't give up. Use the process as a learning experience, and set about making the next grant proposal. Here are some tips for helping you move on to the next grant writing adventure, and for helping you make the next one a successful one.

- Always request the reviewer's comments in an effort to improve your application the next time.
- Read, read, read. Read other agency proposals, funded proposals, and nonfunded proposals. Pay special attention to those proposals that were funded instead of yours.
- Resubmit the same project/idea to a different funding source.
- Volunteer to review grants for agencies in an effort to gain a better understanding of what reviewers look for in successful applications.
- Try, try again.

Section III: Sustainable Agriculture Research and Education (SARE)

SARE (Sustainable Agriculture Research and Education) is a USDA federal competitive grants program. It was first authorized by the 1985 farm bill and first funded in 1988. Each year Congress allocates funds that are distributed among four regions and the central office in Washington, DC. SARE provides funds for projects led by researchers, educators, producers, nonprofit organizations, and others exploring environmentally sound, economically viable, socially responsible agriculture.

SARE's mission statement is: "We strive to create and manage a system designed to encourage the involvement of farm and nonfarm citizens in the process of discovery and learning that leads to achieving a more sustainable, environmentally benign agriculture."

Goals include to foster site-specific, integrated farming systems; satisfy human food and fiber needs; enhance environmental quality, natural resource conservation, and the integration of on-farm and biological resources; enhance the quality of rural life and support owner-operated farms; protect human health and safety; and promote crop, livestock, and enterprise diversity and the well-being of animals.

SARE is divided into four regions. Each has its own specific goals, and its regional administrative council comprising a variety of agriculture shareholders.

SARE grants are awarded in three major programs: Research and Education Grants, the Professional Development Program, and Producer Grants.

Research and Education Grants are awarded to teams of researchers, educators, nonprofits, producers, and others. These competitive grants are provided to examine sustainable agriculture and are generally in the range of $10,000–$100,000.

The Professional Development Program supports competitive training grants and state-specific planning that help agriculture educators assist producers in maintaining viable operations. Grants are awarded to teams developing sustainable ag education programs and educators learning about sustainable ag; grants generally range from $10,000 to $100,000.

The Producer Grant Program is designed with the recognition that there is a huge base of farmer ingenuity and know-how that can help alleviate many troublesome issues. Farmers and ranchers throughout each SARE region are awarded grants to explore profitable, environmentally sound alternatives on-farm that enrich their lives and their communities. The Producer Grant Program examines sustainable agriculture on-site. Grants may run from $500 to $15,000, but generally are capped at $5,000 for individuals; groups of three or more producers can usually apply for more money. As a rule, producer grant projects last 1 year, although no-cost extensions have been granted.

Each of the SARE programs has its specific dates for: "call for proposals"; "proposals due"; and "funds available"—visit www.sare.org to download calls for proposals, check deadlines, and learn about grant requirements. SARE also provides an annual report for each region, and they maintain an extensive archive of past grants awarded.

Section IV: Requirements for Farm-Based Research Projects

This brief section is provided to give potential researchers some idea for the commitment of time, space, and effort they will likely need when conducting a research project. It should be recognized that implementing any farm-based project requires the willingness to put some of your time and land "at risk" for experimentation, and the idea of this section is to help you understand how much "risk" might be involved. The rewards are that you will likely help solve a problem you have personally identified, and the information you gain may be extremely helpful to other farmers.

Available free from SARE is a 12-page bulletin, "How to Conduct Research on Your Farm or Ranch" that is a much more extensive resource for the actual process of conducting research. The bulletin contains an additional list of resources: free or low-cost on-farm research bulletins and reports; market research resources; and, farmer/researcher networks.

Farm-based research is limited only by your imagination. The type of project—be it crops, livestock, or marketing—will dictate project design. Assistance with designing your project is key. SARE recommends that you find someone at your county extension office or land-grant university with experience in setting up and conducting research on farms who wants to work with you as a collaborator. If you cannot find an experienced helper locally, additional resources are available from SARE. A mistake at the planning stage can render your data unusable, or worse, misleading.

When doing on-farm research with crops, the best way to have faith in your results is by designing research plots that you can compare against each other again and again. This means replicating your treatments, which will allow you to distinguish between random variation in the system and the real effects of treatments. Analyzing data in a valid statistical manner is virtually impossible without replicated treatments. Most scientists would advise at least three replications.

Crop researchers, especially at first, should keep it simple. As an example: use three replication plots of one or two treatment applications tested against plots with no treatment application. Individual plots will need to be harvested and the harvest analyzed separately. Even this simplified experimental design requires planting, monitoring, and analyzing 6–8 plots of ground.

Likewise, livestock research projects require replications of treatments, and this means several side-by-side pens for comparisons. Materials needed then include good reliable scales, several pens or paddocks of the same size for side-by-side, pen-to-pen comparisons, and separate feed storage bins if you are using different diets for feeding trials.

In all cases, whether the project includes livestock or crops, accurate measurements will be required and consistent monitoring will be necessary throughout the entire length of the project. Accurate records must be maintained, and with livestock, this may require day-to-day feed and activity records with periodic weighings.

A necessary part of most projects will be data analysis and interpretation, and this will involve the use of statistics. Don't let the specter of statistics scare you; many computer spreadsheet programs conduct statistical tests. Seek assistance when designing your project and again for data analysis.

Remember that the data you collect while performing a farm-based project can be invaluable for you and for others, both locally and nationally. Farm-based research is the vital cog in the wheel of sustainable agriculture.

Acknowledgments

I thank Bonnie Houk, Grant Manager for Greenbush Education Service Center, personal communications for her generous assistance in helping me formulate an outline and plan of action for seeking grants.

Resources

Note: Some of these listings were found at: www.sare.org.ncrsare/orgs.htm; others were obtained from various other sources.

Alternative Farming Systems Information Center
National Agricultural Library
Agricultural Research Service
U.S. Department of Agriculture
10301 Beltsville, MD 20705-2351
301-504-6559
www.nal.usda.afsic

American Farmland Trust
1920 N Street N.W. Suite 400
Washington, DC 20036
202-659-5170
202-659-8339 (fax)
info@farmland.org
www.farmland.org/

Appropriate Technology Transfer for Rural Areas (ATTRA)
P.O. Box 3657
Fayetteville, AR 72702
1-800-346-9140
askattra@ncatark.uark.edu
www.attra.org

Center for Holistic Management
1010 Tijeras NW
Albuquerque, NM 87102
505-842-5252
505-843-7900 (fax)
chrm@igc.apc.org

Center for Rural Affairs
P.O. Box 406
Walthill, NE 68067
402-846-5428
402-846-5420 (fax)
info@cfra.org
www.cfra.org

Consortium for Sustainable Agriculture Research and Education
University of Wisconsin
1450 Linden Drive, Room 146
Madison, WI 53706
608-265-6483
eabird@facstaff.wisc.edu
www.csare.org

FoodRoutes Network
P.O. Box 443
Millheim, PA 16854
814-349-6000
814-349-2280 (fax)
www.foodroutes.org

Henry A. Wallace Institute for Alternative Agriculture
9200 Edmonston Road, Suite 117
Greenbelt, MD 20770-551
301-441-8777
301-220-0164 (fax)
hawiaa@access.digex.net
www.hawaiaa.org/index.html

Institute for Agriculture and Trade Policy
1313 5th St., S.E. Suite 303
Minneapolis, MN 55404
612-870-0453
612-870-4846 (fax)
iatp@iatp.org
www.iatp.org/

The Kerr Center for Sustainable Agriculture
P.O. Box 588
Poteau, OK 74953
918-647-9123
918-647-8712 (fax)
mailbox@kerrcenter.com
www.kerrcenter.com/home.htm

The Land Institute
2440 E. Water Well Road
Salina, KS 67401
785-823-5376
theland@midkan.com

Land Stewardship Project
2200 Fourth St.
White Bear Lake, MN 55110
612-653-0589 (ph/fax)
www.misa.umn.edu/lshp.html

Michael Fields Agricultural Institute
W 2493 Co. Road ES
East Troy, WI 53120
414-642-2202
414-642-4028 (fax)

Midwest Organic Alliance
400 Selby Ave., Suite T
St. Paul, MN 55102
www.organic.org

Midwest Sustainable Agriculture Working Group
Dave Butcher
R.R. 3, Box 168
Perquot Lakes, MN 56472
218-568-8624
davidb@uslink.net
or
Kris Thorp
Center for Rural Affairs
P.O. Box 406
Walthill, NE 68067
402-846-5428
402-846-5420 (fax)
krist@cfra.org
www.cfra.org

National Audubon Society
700 Broadway
New York, NY 10003
212-979-3000
www.audubon.org

National Campaign for Sustainable Agriculture
P.O. Box 396
Pine Bush, NY 12566
845-744-8448
845-744-8477 (fax)
campaign@sustainableagriculture.net
www.sustainableagriculture.net

National Organic Standards Program
USDA/AMS/TMD
Room 2510 – South
P.O. Box 96456
Washington, DC 20090-6456
202-205-7810 (ph/fax)
www.ams.usda.gov/nop/

Native American Farmers' Association
P.O. Box 170
Tesuque, NM 87574
505-983-2172

The Nature Conservancy
1815 North Lynn St.
Arlington, VA 22209
703-841-5300
www.tnc.org

Northwest Area Foundation
E 1201 1st Bank Bldg.
332 Minnesota St.
St. Paul, MN 55101-1373
612-224-9635
612-225-3881 (fax)

National Wildlife Federation
8925 Leesburg Pike
Vienna, VA 22184
704-790-4000
www.nwf.org/nwf/index.html

OrganicAgInfo
www.organicaginfo.org

Organic Crop Improvement Association
1001 Y St., Suite B
Lincoln, NE 68508-1172
402-477-2323
402-477-4325 (fax)
info@ocia.org
www.ocia.org

Organic Farming Research Foundation
P.O. Box 440
Santa Cruz, CA 95061
818-426-6606
research@ofrf.org

Rodale Institute
611 Siegfriedale Road
Kutztown, PA 19530
610-683-1487
610-683-9175 (fax)
rhartmn@rodaleinst.org

Seed Savers Exchange
Kent Whealy
3076 N. Winn Road
Decorah, IA 52101

Sierra Club
85 Second St.
Second Floor
San Francisco, CA 94105-3441
415-977-5500
415-977-5799 (fax)
www.sierraclub.org

Small Farms Program
USDA/CSREES
Stop 2220
868 Aerospace Center
901 D St. S.W.
Washington, DC 20250-2220
800-583-3071
202-401-5179 (fax)
smallfarm@reeusda.gov
www.reeusda.gov/agsys/smallfarm

Soil and Water Conservation Society
7515 N.E. Ankeny Road
Ankeny, IA 50021-9764
800-843-7645
515-289-1227 (fax)
swc@swcs.org
www.swcs.org

Sustainable Agriculture Coalition
Ferd Hoefner
110 Maryland Ave., NE Box 28
Washington, DC 20002
202-547-5754
202-547-1837 (fax)
fhoefner@msawg.org

Sustainable Agriculture Network
Andy Clark
10300 Baltimore Ave.
Bldg. 046 BARC-WEST
Beltsville, MD 20705-2350
301-504-6425
301-504-5207 (fax)
san@sare.org
www.sare.org

Sustainable Farming Connection
Craig Cramer
1769 Ellis Hollow Road
Ithaca, NY 14850
610-791-9683
cdcramer@clarityconnect.com
metalab.unc.edu/farming-connection

World Wildlife Fund
1250 Twenty-Fourth St. N.W.
Washington, DC 20037
202-293-4800
www.wwf.org/index.html

Additional Resources
Agribusiness Center
A project of the Institute for Agriculture and Trade Policy (www.iatp.org)
www.agribusinesscenter.org

American Farmland Trust
1200 18th Street NW #800
Washington, DC 20036
202-331-7300
202-659-8339 (fax)
www.farmland.org
Kansas Rural Center
www.kansasruralcenter.org

Leopold Center for Sustainable Agriculture
209 Curtiss Hall
Iowa State University
Ames, Ia 50011-1050
515-294-3711
515-294-9696 (fax)
www.leopold.iastate.edu

Missouri Alternatives Center
http://agebb.missouri.edu/mac/

Missouri Institute for Sustainable Agriculture
www.misa.umn.edu/main.html
National Institutes of Health
www.nih.gov

Nebraska Center for Applied Rural Innovation
www.unl.edu/ianr/csas/

Nebraska Sustainable Agriculture Society
www.nebsuag.org
New York State Integrated Pest Management Program
www.nysipm.cornell.edu

North Central Initiative for Small Farm Profitability
www.farmprofitability.org

Allan Savory Center for Holistic Management
www.holisticmanagement.org

Sustainable Agriculture Resources for Teachers K-12
(A 21-page list of resources compiled by Mary Gold of the Alternative Farming Systems
Information Center)
www.nal.usda.gov/afsic/AFSIC_pubs/k-12.htm

Sustainability Institute
www.sustainer.org

Practical Farmers of Iowa
www.practicalfarmers.org

The New Farm Web site
www.newfarm.org

University of California Sustainable ag Web site
www.sarep.ucdavis.edu

USDA
Cooperative State Research, Education, and Extension Service (CSREES)
Small Farm Program
Stop 2215
Washington, DC 20250-2215
Small farm phone : 800-583-3071
www.reeusda.gov/smallfarm/

USDA
Alternative Farming Systems Information Center
National Agriculture Library, Rm 132
10301 Baltimore Ave.
Beltsville, MD 20705-2351
301-504-6559
301-504-6927 (fax)
www.nal.usda.gov/afsic

USDA Funding Opportunities
USDAGRANTS-L@Linux08.UNM.edu

Chapter 14
Economics of Niche Marketing in Alternative Livestock Farming

Gary L. Valen

Value-added marketing

Value-added is a term often used by agricultural advisors to help farmers realize a higher income for their products. The term usually refers to actions the farmer can perform such as processing or packaging meat products that can command a higher price from the consumer.

This chapter deals with an emerging value-added strategy that improves farmer income by the adoption of production techniques or an adherence to specific practices that are valued by the consumer, for example, the use of labels such as pasture-raised or free-range appeals to food buyers who oppose intensive confinement livestock and poultry systems. These consumers will often pay higher prices for food purchases and only buy from certain producers due to their convictions and their preferences for specific agricultural practices. The growing consumer support for organic foods also offers farmers an opportunity to improve their incomes by adopting production strategies that appeal to a market niche.

While we can apply the value-added strategy to any food marketing effort, the focus of this chapter is on livestock production although the concept also works for dairy, poultry, and vegetable farmers. Meat production in the United States is a valued and lucrative business. Consumers demonstrate daily preferences for meat dishes and the export market for livestock products is a significant component in U.S. trade policies. In recent years the federal government has provided ever increasing subsidy payments to support livestock producers. The problem is that most of the income for meat production goes to only 8% of the total farmers who raise livestock (Kellogg, 2002).

The small and midsize farmers do not share the major economic benefits of livestock production and are therefore in danger of disappearing for viable businesses. Niche marketing based on consumer preferences is a way for these producers to sustain themselves without having to compete directly with the large livestock industries that are less flexible in changing their fundamental farming practices.

An alternative livestock farm operation requires creative marketing strategies and often a specific set of production methods. The place to start is the market. Why would consumers be willing to make special efforts and perhaps pay more to purchase products from alternative livestock farmers? The answer is that these farmers add value to their products by using alternative production methods or utilizing marketing techniques that meet the expectations of their customers. What are the values that will attract the special interests of consumers?

Marketing strategies

Local and regional food systems

One of the most important marketing strategies is to link farmers and consumers in the same community or region. A local food movement is sweeping the country as restaurants, school cafeterias, grocery stores, and individuals choose food products that come from farmers in the same locale. Consumers enjoy fresh food that has not endured the rigors of long distance travel. The money spent on food remains close to home and contributes to the economic vitality of the local region including the community based small and midsize farmers. When consumers know exactly where their food comes from, they can choose to patronize farmers they know are sensitive both to the environment and the humane treatment of farm animals.

Environmental sensitivity

Environmental sensitivity is a significant marketing strategy for some livestock producers. The use of rotational grazing practices maintains healthy pastures that prevent soil erosion and maintain air quality. Organic farmers avoid the use of synthetic fertilizers and herbicides that are potentially damaging to wildlife as well as streams and lakes. Setting aside areas for wildlife contributes to the overall health and vitality of a bioregion. Pasture raised livestock do not require waste lagoons that can leak and cause major environmental disasters. Rather than just relying on government regulations and enforcement to sustain the environmental integrity of a community, many consumers realize they can protect the environment by purchasing food from farmers who use production methods that are in harmony with the natural systems of their region.

Humane treatment of farm animals

The humane treatment of farm animals is another hot button issue for some food buyers. Media in recent years has documented negative conditions experienced by livestock and poultry housed in intensive confinement production systems. While advocates of animal confinement agriculture claim these systems are humane, the fact remains that a significant number of consumers prefer animals that have access to the outdoors, are not kept in small cages or pens, and are able to experience a positive social existence with other animals. A market opportunity exists for the farmer who meets the expectations of consumers who are concerned about farm animal welfare.

Health

A corollary that farmers can use to attract certain customers is the marketing of meat products that are free of grown hormones, antibiotics, and other veterinary medicines. Once again, recent media attention is focused on the growing human resistance to antibiotics that may be caused by consuming meat from animals that are routinely given drugs as growth stimulants or to keep the animal alive in confinement systems. Some consumers fear that hormones may cause unusual growth patterns in young people. Meat products marketed as hormone or drug free appeal to health conscious food buyers.

A national alarm is growing out of media reports about the high rate of human obesity and food related illness such as diabetes. While these concerns do not fall entirely on farmers, they do offer marketing opportunities for producers who promote pasture-raised or grass-fed livestock products as leaner sources of meat.

Parents and school officials are expressing concern about the diets of students, especially as food service operators often give in to student demand for fast food. While government purchasing policies often limit farmer access to school food services, there are growing demands to offer locally produced foods to students because the meals will have a nutritional balance of fresh food including healthy meat choices. We also see more healthy food choices in restaurants and grocery stores. Small and midsize meat producers can take advantage of the growing public awareness of the food related health issues by marketing special meat options.

Community based family farmers

Finally, there is a marketing strategy that appeals to food buyers who want to identify with community based farm families. Perhaps it is a sense of nostalgia connected with memories of how things "used to be" or possibly consumers feel they can trust the food produced by farmers who acknowledge that they care about the earth, their communities, and their families. An extension of this marketing strategy is a farmer owned cooperative or other organization that consists of producers the consumers deliberately choose to support. In the modern world, many of these farmers have Web sites with as many photos of their farms and family members as the products they have for sale.

Examples

The Internet is rapidly becoming a strong marketing tool for alternative agriculture producers. Farmers and their supporters use Web sites to convince potential consumers why they should buy food products produced in a special way. Text and photos are designed to appeal to buyers who will apply their values to food purchases. Special interest groups also use their Web sites to urge their members to support specific market products.

The following examples reveal different marketing strategies that are being employed across the country. They are used here as representative samples and reflect only a small number of farmers who are using niche marketing strategies.

Farmer network

A growing marketing strategy for alternative livestock producers is to join an alliance, cooperative, or for-profit company to gain maximum benefits from national advertising and brand recognition. The brand reflects certain values that apply to the production practices of all the member farmers. The California Company Niman Ranch is a good example.

Niman Ranch

Niman Ranch is one of best known marketing success stories for alternative livestock production in the country. The business started almost 20 years ago as an alternative to mass production of meats. Today it offers beef, pork, and lamb to a select group of retailers and restaurants and through an online store. The marketing strategy is an appeal to consumers who want great tasting meat products that are achieved by treating animals humanely, feeding them all-natural feeds, and allowing them to mature naturally (Niman Web site, 2004).

Niman Ranch uses networks of small family farmers to produce meat according to their established protocol. One of the more surprising outcomes of this niche marketing is that restaurants across the country feature Niman Ranch meat products by name on their menus. The Atlanta Opera recently offered its patrons a special dinner and opera package that featured Niman Ranch pork loins that it claimed would have been a favorite of Figaro.

Several years ago the Niman Ranch Company added pork to their line of beef and lamb products. The pork was raised largely in Iowa on family farms that used open pastures and the deep bedded pens, often referred to as hoop barns. Niman promotes its pork products by touting the taste and adding the fact the hogs were not housed in a confinement system and/or raised with the use of hormones.

The marketing of Niman Ranch pork has strong support from animal welfare groups. The Animal Welfare Institute (AWI) endorses Niman Pork and other pork producers who follow strict criteria that include access to pastures, freedom of movement, the ability to fulfill the natural instinct to build nests when they are about to give birth, and natural socializing behaviors. AWI goes further to offer a certification program that is only available to independent family farmers who own the animals, depend on the farm for a livelihood, and are involved in the day to day labor of managing the pigs (Halverson, 1999).

Hoop barns

A marketing strategy that draws attention from consumers with special interests is the promotion of value-added production practices by local and national organizations. Such an example is the growing use of hoop barns as an alternative to intensive confinement hog systems.

The Humane Society of the United States

Hoop barns are also endorsed by the Humane Society of the United States (HSUS) as "a humane and environmentally friendly methods of housing pigs" (HSUS, 2001). This is a strong example of how alternative livestock farmers receive marketing assistance at no cost from national organizations that promote animal welfare, environmental sensitivity, and public health.

The thrust of the HSUS position is that consumers can support a wide range of values when they purchase pork products that come from hoop barn systems. These include the protection of the environment because the bedded manure from hoop barns can be easily composted to avoid the odors and potential spillage from confinement system manure lagoons. Hogs enjoy more normal swine behaviors because they have more freedom to move than in conventional confinement systems. Since hogs raised in hoop barns enjoy a healthier environment, the HSUS notes that these systems do not require heavy use of antibiotics that can threaten public health by developing antibiotic-resistant strains of bacteria. The HSUS also endorses hoop barns because they are more affordable to small and midsize farmers and appeal to consumers who support animal welfare, the environment, and small family-based farmers.

The Leopold Center for Sustainable Agriculture

The promotion of hoop barns is also benefiting from some pioneering research done at The Leopold Center in Ames, Iowa that shows a growing niche pork market of consumers who prefer environmental-friendly and pig-friendly systems (Leopold Center News Release, 2002). In the

BISHOP BURTON COLLEGE
LIBRARY

spring of 2002, Pork Niche Working Group was formed in Iowa with the support of the Leopold Center that is made up of pork producers, distributors, retailers, agency representatives, and Iowa State University faculty.

The working group set three goals to help small and midsize Iowa farmers, promote environmentally sensitive approaches to pork production, and help revitalize rural communities. Specifically, the working group focuses on markets for hogs raised with "humane animal husbandry practices with no animal by-products, artificial growth promotants or antibiotics" (Leopold Center Newsletter, 2001). The marketing effort by the Iowa Pork Niche Working Group is a good example of how alternative farmers can partner with organizations and individuals to develop niche markets based on specific values.

Pastured livestock

Farmers and marketing organizations promote pastured beef as more sensitive to the environment and human health than beef raised in confinement systems or feedlots. Considerable attention is paid to the health benefits of grass-fed beef products. Three examples of this marketing effort are Eat Wild, Meadow Raised Meats, and The American Homestead Foods Family Farm Certification Program.

Eat Wild

Eat Wild is a Web site established and maintained by Washington State author Jo Robinson. Farmers who meet the criteria established by Eat Wild are listed on the Web site for an annual $25 fee. The unique marketing aspect of Eat Wild is that consumers are drawn to the site for health and environmental concerns. A well-documented case is made for the advantages of pastured beef products complete with references, health charts, and news items related to livestock production.

The health advantages of pastured beef are listed as lower fat content, reduced LDL cholesterol levels, and more health benefiting omega-3 fatty acids. Further documentation of health benefits include higher levels of conjugated linoleic acid that may reduce the risk of cancer in humans and four times more vitamin E than found in feedlot cattle. Pastured beef is also promoted as free of antibiotics, artificial hormones, and pesticides (Eat Wild, 2002).

The Eat Wild Web site offers information about research that finds raising beef on pastures is better for the environment than confinement or feedlot production systems. A strong benefit is the management of waste that is spread over a pasture as opposed to manure lagoons that can potentially damage the environment with an excessive release of nitrogen and phosphorus. Pastured beef naturally improve soil fertility and contribute to the biodiversity of plant life, both beneficial to the environment. Another environmental benefit is the reduction of greenhouse gases by pastures through carbon sequestration.

While Eat Wild does not market beef, it is a site where farmers can gain access to public who will purchase food products because of health and environmental issues. As alternative livestock farmers seek new markets, Web sites are a gateway to discriminating consumers.

Meadow Raised Meats

Meadow Raised Meats is a New York State cooperative made up of ten farmers who raise their animals on grass-based diets. The cooperative clearly states it was formed to fill a niche market of consumers who want meat products free of antibiotics and hormones. They are experiencing an increase in their market share because health-conscious consumers are concerned about dietary fats and obesity. Another marketing message is that the farmers in the cooperative use a way of farming that "harmonizes with their land and family life" (Smith-Heavenrich, 2002).

One of the cooperative farmers, Amy Kenyon of Skate Creek Farm states that her products are natural raised meat that is a healthy option for consumers and healthier for the environment. She markets her products to restaurants and uses the Meadow Raised Meat Web site to reach online shoppers.

American Homestead Foods Family Farm Certification Program

The American Homestead Foods Family Farm Certification Program is operated as a way for alternative livestock producers who raise pastured beef to gain access to consumers. The program uses a Web site hosted by American Pasturage, Inc., a for-profit company that retails pastured beef, veal, and lamb. Certified farmers pay a one time fee of $30 to market their products through the Internet retail outlet. American Homestead describes its producers as "a farm whose principle operator is a resident of the farm and from which a portion of the farm incomes is derived from sales directly to consumers" (American Pasturage, 2002).

The health benefits of the pastured livestock are promoted as being free of chemicals and pharmaceuticals. Animals that required medication for a health reason are removed from the herd. The Web site also promotes the environmental advantages of pastured livestock and the fact that family farmers are good stewards of the land.

A strong marketing message of American Homestead Foods is an appeal to consumers to support family farms in their region. The reasons given are that industrial agriculture depends completely on petroleum resources for production and distribution while regional food systems are less dependent on fossil energy. In addition consumers should seek local supplies of food as a way to preserve rural America and to ensure the future of safe food. The promotion of local and regional food systems offers exciting marketing opportunities for alternative livestock producers.

Local and regional markets

Sustainable Agriculture Network (SAN), an outreach program of the Sustainable Agriculture Research and Education (SARE) program, promotes alternative livestock systems by helping farmers emphasize the welfare benefits and environmentally friendly characteristics of their production methods. The Network adds to these marketing benefits the advantages of selling products locally. SAN profiles several operations on its Web site including Greg Gunthorp of LaGrange, Indiana.

Gunthorp discovered that he can market 1,000 hogs at ten times what he could get on the commodities market. His secret is regional marketing. He found a ready market in some of Chicago's restaurants once he personally delivered cuts of meat to the chefs. He also developed a catering business for wedding receptions, company picnics, and family barbecues (SARE Bulletin). Gunthorp's value-added niche is his personal relationship with customers he knows in a regional market.

Another example of local marketing is Barbara Wiand of Mifflinburg, Pennsylvania. She and her husband, Glenn, moved from a more conventional contract production system to a value-added local market system as a way to improve the farm income. While she uses an outside certified processing facility, she markets her products under her own label, Stonehouse Farm. She has a retail store and she sells hogs to local customers. Wiand may extend her operation to include beef and lamb. She found good markets in her own community and is able to sustain the family farm in the process (SAN Bulletin, 2002).

The newly formed New England Livestock Alliance (NELA) has also found a strong marketing niche in its region. Ridgeway Shinn admits that his regional market strategy has a great advantage because it includes New York City. NELA is a nonprofit steering group that helps for-profit grassland farmers and processing facilities in the Northeast region.

The Alliance is especially helpful to small and midsize farmers who are not able to compete with high-volume, commodity-priced beef producers. Instead NELA found customers who are willing to pay higher prices for value-added beef that meet specific guidelines. NELA lists its market advantages as: (1) locally produced; (2) no antibiotics or hormones in the beef; (3) humanely raised animals; (4) support of family farmers; (5) environmental protection; (6) support for the rural economy, and (7) food that is source-verified (Nation, 2002). NELA hopes to add grass dairy and pastured swine to its system in the future.

The growth of farmers' markets and Community Support Agriculture (CSA) programs over the last decade is a phenomenal testimony to the strength of local and regional marketing. These marketing systems usually support small producers who can spend the time selling at a market or in the preparation for a CSA distribution. Local and regional marketing strategies are becoming more important for midsize farmers who are presently trying to compete in the same markets as large intensive confinement systems.

Maryland Extension Livestock Specialist Scott M. Barao concluded in a recent editorial that alternative marketing is a way to stem the loss of farms and farm families in his state. He suggests that a "Maryland Grown" type of marketing structure is an obvious support for producers who are located in areas where consumers are willing to support farmers in their region. On the other hand he notes that producers are often not good marketers, so he calls for leadership to connect consumers and farmers in his region (Barao, 2002).

Corporate agricultural businesses know who their customers are and how they can be reached. Using the value-added approach, alternative livestock producers can do the same with niche markets, especially in a regional food system where they actually know their customers.

Marketing the farm family

A key advantage that alternative livestock producers have is that they are usually located on a specific farm with a family unit that cares about the land, animals, and their community or region. Farm families and their farms can be used to reach consumers who want to know where their food comes from and who produced it. A theme of all of the examples in this chapter is the ability of family farmers to use methods that will win consumer approval and support. The Practical Farmers of Iowa provides much information about marketing of local products to consumers. Their advice for marketing grass-fed products is shown in Table 14.1 (Ennis and Huber, 2003).

Four Winds Farm in Gardiner, New York has a Web site that markets pork, lamb, and beef that are "sustainably and humanely raised without antibiotics and hormones" (Four Winds, 2002). The Web site presents a production strategy that uses rotational grazing and discusses how the animals are processed in a small family-owned and USDA inspected abattoir. There is considerable information about the health and environmental attributes of pasture raised livestock.

One of the intriguing features of the Four Winds Farm Web site is the photos of animals in pastures or the barnyard and family members doing chores. A customer can see exactly where the food comes from and what production methods are used. Large food corporations often portray themselves in

Table 14.1 Marketing advice to livestock producers from Midwest focus group research

1. Promote direct benefits such as health and good taste
2. Advertise benefits such as hormone-free or animal well-being
3. Overcome perceptions that grass-fed meat products are tough by describing aging process
4. Explain price differences by showing how product is superior
5. Be clear about food safety strategies
6. Make products convenient for consumers to buy

television commercials or with slogans on their delivery trucks as family farms. Family farmers can do the same thing and have the photos, family members, and the farm to prove it. Ultimately, niche marketing will become mainline marketing as consumers become more selective about what they choose to eat.

A vision for the future

The loss of farmland, the decline of rural communities and the gradual disappearance of family farmers do not have to be our future. The reverse to these present conditions depends on forging new partnerships between people who produce food and people who eat food. The suggestion of this chapter is that marketing strategies can be used to make the farmer-consumer linkage a reality in the coming years. What it takes is for farmers to adopt value-added approaches to their production methods that will appeal to consumers.

Niche marketing requires commitment to a strategy, integrity to alternative production methods, and a solid business plan. One thing is for certain, the more consumers learn about their food, the more they will want to support alternative producers.

The vision of the future is that consumers will use their foodbuying dollars to support family farms, protect the environment, and sustain the more humane treatment of farm animals. In return these consumers will enjoy healthy and great tasting meals.

References

American Homestead Foods Family Farm Certification Program. 2002. American Pasturage Web site, www.homesteadfoods.com/aboutus.htm, pp. 1–2. Accessed Dec. 29, 2004.

Barao, S.M. 2002. Animal Agriculture Update. Maryland Coop. Ext. Newsletter, Fall, pp. 1–2.

Eat Wild. 2002. Pastured Products and Your Health. Eat Wild Web site, http://www.eatwild.com/health.html. Accessed Dec. 29, 2004.

Ennis, J. and G. Huber. 2003. Consumer messages for grass-based foods: exploring what works. Practical Farmers of Iowa Web site: http://www.practicalfarmers.org/resource/PFIResource_77.ppt#1. Accessed Dec. 29, 2004.

Four Winds Farm. 2002. Pastured Meat. Four Winds Farm Web site, http://users.bestweb.net/~fourwind/. Accessed Dec. 29, 2004.

Halverson, D. 1999. Niman Ranch: AWI Approved. *AWI Q.* 38(3):1–2.

Humane Society of the United States (HSUS). 2001. Why Hoop Barns? Halt Hog Factories. HSUS Web site, http://65.61.158.165/web-files/PDF/2003_HHF_brochure.pdf. Accessed Dec. 29, 2004.

Kellogg, R.L. 2002. Profile of Farms with Livestock in the United States: A Statistical Summary. Analysis Publication. USDA, Natural Resources Conservation Service, Feb. 4, 2002, p. 2.

Leopold Center for Sustainable Agriculture. 2001. Hoop Structure Changes Iowa Landscape. Leopold News Release, July 3, 2001, p. 1.

Leopold Center for Sustainable Agriculture. 2002. Hoops Gain Support, Group Revise Plans for more Work. Leopold Newsletter, Spring, pp. 1–2.

Nation, A. 2002. Small volume high margin market is profitable for Northeastern Grassfed Alliance. *Stockman Grassfarmer* 59(11):1.

Niman Ranch. 2004. Our Story. Niman Ranch Web site, http://www.nimanranch.com/is-bin/ INTERSHOP.enfinity/WFS/NimanRanch-NimanRanchStore-Site. Accessed Dec. 29, 2004.

Smith-Heavenrich, S. 2002. Meadow Raised Meats Cooperative Finds its Niche. Grassroots: The Voice of New York Farm Bureau. NY Farm Bureau Web site, http://www.nyfb.org/Grassroots/ grassroots.htm. Accessed Dec. 2004.

Sustainable Agriculture Network (SAN). 2002. Profitable Pork: Strategies for Hog Production. SAN Web site, http://www.sare.org/publications/hogs.htm. Accessed Dec. 29, 2004.

Index